Epidemiology of Pediatric and Adolescent Diabetes

Epidemiology of Pediatric and Adolescent Diabetes

Edited by

Dana Dabelea
University of Colorado HSC
Denver, Colorado, USA

Georgeanna J. Klingensmith
University of Colorado
Aurora, Colorado, USA

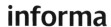

informa
healthcare

New York London

Informa Healthcare USA, Inc.
52 Vanderbilt Avenue
New York, NY 10017

© 2008 by Informa Healthcare USA, Inc.
Informa Healthcare is an Informa business

No claim to original U.S. Government works

Printed and bound by CPI Group (UK) Ltd, Croydon, CR0 4YY

Transferred to Digital Print 2012

International Standard Book Number-10: 1-4200-4797-3 (Hardcover)
International Standard Book Number-13: 978-1-4200-4797-4 (Hardcover)

Library of Congress Cataloging-in-Publication Data

Epidemiology of Pediatric and Adolescent Diabetes / edited by Dana Dabelea, Georgeanna J. Klingensmith.
   p. ; cm.
  Includes bibliographical references and index.
  ISBN-13: 978-1-4200-4797-4 (hardcover : alk. paper)
  ISBN-10: 1-4200-4797-3 (hardcover : alk. paper)
  1. Diabetes in adolescence—Epidemiology. 2. Diabetes in children—Epidemiology. I. Dabelea, Dana. II. Klingensmith, Georgeanna J.
  [DNLM: 1. Diabetes Mellitus, Type 1. 2. Adolescent. 3. Child. 4. Diabetes Mellitus, Type 1—epidemiology. 5. Diabetes Mellitus, Type 2—epidemiology. 6. Diabetes Mellitus, Type 2. 7. Risk Factors. WK 810 E642 2008]
  RJ420.D5E65 2008
  618.92'462—dc22

                               2007039134

For Corporate Sales and Reprint Permissions call 212-520-2700 or write to: Sales Department, 52 Vanderbilt Avenue, 16th floor, New York, NY 10017.

**Visit the Informa Web site at
www.informa.com**

**and the Informa Healthcare Web site at
www.informahealthcare.com**

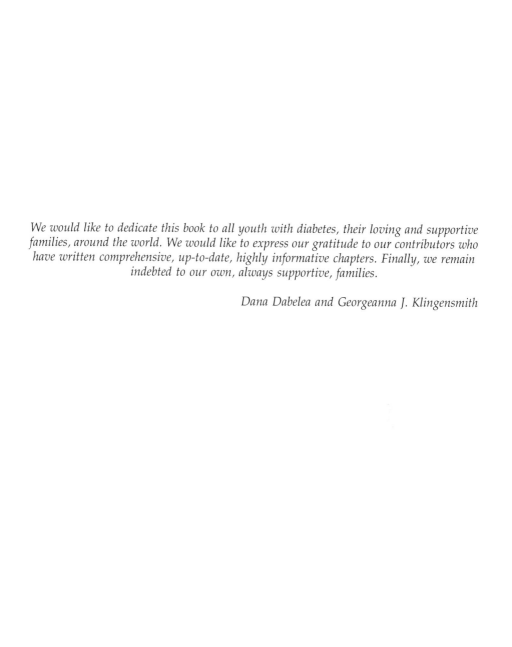

We would like to dedicate this book to all youth with diabetes, their loving and supportive families, around the world. We would like to express our gratitude to our contributors who have written comprehensive, up-to-date, highly informative chapters. Finally, we remain indebted to our own, always supportive, families.

Dana Dabelea and Georgeanna J. Klingensmith

Preface

Diabetes mellitus is the third most prevalent severe chronic disease of childhood. Despite this, there are currently no comprehensive books dedicated to the epidemiology of childhood diabetes. In addition, the epidemiology of diabetes in youth is changing. Until recently, diabetes diagnosed in children and adolescents was almost entirely considered to be type 1 (insulin dependent) diabetes, formerly known as "juvenile diabetes" or "IDDM." Now, as youth are becoming increasingly overweight, we are seeing more obese children with a clinical phenotype of type 2, or "adult onset" diabetes. Childhood diabetes, similar to adult diabetes, is now acknowledged to be a complex and heterogeneous disorder. Some patients not only exhibit the clinical features of type 2 diabetes but also have positive diabetes autoantibodies. This finding demonstrates the limits of the current diabetes classification scheme in youth and the need to better understand the natural history and long-term evolution of diabetes in youth, especially those with features of both type 1 and type 2 diabetes.

There is also a worldwide increase in childhood type 1 diabetes, and the reasons for this increase are still not known. New interesting data on the potential role of infant diet are emerging from longitudinal studies following youth from birth until the development of autoimmunity and type 1 diabetes. Genetic studies explore the heterogeneity of classical type 1 diabetes, as well as the genetic basis for monogenic forms of diabetes, including recently identified mutations responsible for neonatal forms. Challenging hypotheses that require careful testing are advanced, linking the worldwide obesity epidemic to the increasing incidence and earlier age at onset of both type 1 and type 2 diabetes. In both type 1 and type 2 diabetes, research is focusing on identifying early life, perinatal, and intrauterine exposures and new concepts such as "fetal programming" are increasingly being used in conjunction with diabetes risk. The development of elevated levels of cardiovascular risk factors and preclinical cardiovascular disease among youth with diabetes and the potential future impact on morbidity and mortality poses special challenges.

Our increasing understanding of the multifactorial etiology of childhood diabetes and its complications will hopefully translate into improved quality of life for youth with diabetes, and will ultimately lead to the successful prevention of diabetes.

The goal of this book is to review the epidemiology of diabetes from a worldwide perspective and to provide an overview of where this exciting field stands today. In its broadest perspective, diabetes epidemiology provides a framework for understanding the etiology, risk factors, acute and chronic complications, and the natural history of the disease, providing insight into population and clinical patterns of onset and course, and suggesting avenues for further basic science research. This book also includes a discussion of current technologies that provide promise for prevention or cure in the future.

At the beginning of the 21st century, we have now experienced several decades of increased risk for both type 1 and type 2 diabetes in youth and adults throughout the world. Projections indicate that these trends will worsen if the causes of diabetes are not rapidly identified and preventive strategies begun. Such strategies will require both individual clinically-based approaches and a much broader population initiative, targeting social and environmental factors that operate to alter energy balance, and lead to increases in viral or toxic exposures. The challenges are large for science and public health but the cost of not proceeding urgently will be truly immense. We hope that this book will provide a benchmark for our current understanding and suggest promising paths toward diabetes prevention and cure.

Dana Dabelea, MD, PhD
Georgeanna J. Klingensmith, MD

Contents

Contributors

Theresa A. Aly   Barbara Davis Center for Childhood Diabetes and Human Medical Genetics Program, University of Colorado at Denver and Health Sciences Center, Aurora, Colorado, U.S.A.

Barbara J. Anderson   Department of Pediatrics, Baylor College of Medicine, Houston, Texas, U.S.A.

Silva Arslanian   Division of Weight Management and Wellness, Children's Hospital of Pittsburgh, Pittsburgh, Pennsylvania, U.S.A.

Fida Bacha   Division of Pediatric Endocrinology, Metabolism and Diabetes Mellitus, and Division of Weight Management and Wellness, Children's Hospital of Pittsburgh, Pittsburgh, Pennsylvania, U.S.A.

Jennifer M. Barker   Barbara Davis Center for Childhood Diabetes, Aurora, Colorado, U.S.A.

Franziska K. Bishop   Barbara Davis Center for Childhood Diabetes, University of Colorado at Denver and Health Sciences Center, Aurora, Colorado, U.S.A.

Sonia Caprio   Department of Pediatrics and the Children's General Clinical Research Center, Yale University School of Medicine, New Haven, Connecticut, U.S.A.

Harvey K. Chiu   Division of Endocrinology, Children's Hospital and Regional Medical Center, University of Washington, Seattle, Washington, U.S.A.

Nancy A. Crimmins   Department of Pediatrics, Cincinnati Children's Hospital Medical Center and University of Cincinnati School of Medicine, Cincinnati, Ohio, U.S.A.

Dana Dabelea   Department of Preventive Medicine and Biometrics, University of Colorado at Denver, Denver, Colorado, U.S.A.

Stephen R. Daniels   Department of Pediatrics, The Children's Hospital, University of Colorado School of Medicine, Denver, Colorado, U.S.A.

Lawrence M. Dolan   Department of Pediatrics, Cincinnati Children's Hospital Medical Center and University of Cincinnati School of Medicine, Cincinnati, Ohio, U.S.A.

Kim C. Donaghue   Institute of Endocrinology and Diabetes, The Children's Hospital at Westmead, University of Sydney, Westmead, Australia

George S. Eisenbarth   Barbara Davis Center for Childhood Diabetes and Human Medical Genetics Program, University of Colorado at Denver and Health Sciences Center, Aurora, Colorado, U.S.A.

Philippe Froguel   Section of Genomic Medicine, Imperial College London, London, U.K.

Anders Green   Department of Epidemiology, Institute of Public Health, University of Southern Denmark and Department of Applied Research and Health Technology Assessment, Odense University Hospital, Odense, Denmark

Heikki Hyöty   Department of Virology, University of Tampere, and Department of Clinical Microbiology, Center for Laboratory Medicine, Tampere University Hospital, Tampere, Finland

Giuseppina Imperatore   Division of Diabetes Translation, Centers for Disease Control and Prevention, Atlanta, Georgia, U.S.A.

Lois Jovanovic   Department of Clinical Research, Sansum Diabetes Research Institute, Santa Barbara, California, U.S.A.

Georgeanna J. Klingensmith   Department of Pediatrics, University of Colorado at Denver and Health Sciences Center, Barbara Davis Center for Childhood Diabetes, Aurora, Colorado, U.S.A.

Mikael Knip   Hospital for Children and Adolescents, University of Helsinki, Helsinki, and Department of Pediatrics, Tampere University Hospital, Tampere, Finland

Elizabeth J. Mayer-Davis   Department of Epidemiology and Biostatistics and Center for Research in Nutrition and Health Disparities, Arnold School of Public Health, University of South Carolina, Columbia, South Carolina, U.S.A.

Fauzia Mohsin   Department of Pediatrics, BIRDEM and Ibrahim Medical College, Dhaka, Bangladesh

Kristen Nadeau   Department of Pediatrics, University of Colorado at Denver and The Children's Hospital, Denver, Colorado, U.S.A.

K.M. Venkat Narayan   Hubert Department of Global Health, The Rollins School of Public Health, Atlanta, Georgia, U.S.A.

Jill M. Norris   Department of Preventive Medicine and Biometrics, University of Colorado at Denver and Health Sciences Center, Denver, Colorado, U.S.A.

Reena Oza-Frank   Nutrition and Health Sciences Program, Hubert Department of Global Health, The Rollins School of Public Health, Atlanta, Georgia, U.S.A.

Rachel Pessah   Department of Medicine, Mount Sinai Medical Center, New York, New York, U.S.A.

David J. Pettitt   Department of Clinical Research, Sansum Diabetes Research Institute, Santa Barbara, California, U.S.A.

Catherine Pihoker   Division of Endocrinology, Children's Hospital and Regional Medical Center, University of Washington, Seattle, Washington, U.S.A.

Orit Pinhas-Hamiel   Pediatric Endocrinology and Diabetes, Sheba Medical Center, Ramat-Gan, Israel

Arleta Rewers   Department of Pediatrics, University of Colorado at Denver and Health Sciences Center, Barbara Davis Center for Childhood Diabetes, Aurora, Colorado, U.S.A.

Melissa D. Simpson   Department of Preventive Medicine and Biometrics, University of Colorado at Denver and Health Sciences Center, Denver, Colorado, U.S.A.

Monique L. Stone   Department of Pediatric Endocrinology and Diabetes, Royal North Shore Hospital, The University of Sydney, St. Leonards, Australia

Craig E. Taplin   Barbara Davis Center for Childhood Diabetes, Aurora, Colorado, U.S.A.

Elaine M. Urbina   Department of Pediatrics, Division of Cardiology, Cincinnati Children's Hospital Medical Center, University of Cincinnati, Cincinnati, Ohio, U.S.A.

Martine Vaxillaire   CNRS UMR 8090, Institute of Biology and Pasteur Institute, Lille, France

R. Paul Wadwa   Barbara Davis Center for Childhood Diabetes, University of Colorado at Denver and Health Sciences Center, Aurora, Colorado, U.S.A.

Ram Weiss   Department of Human Nutrition and Metabolism, Hebrew University School of Medicine, Jerusalem, Israel

Terence J. Wilkin   Department of Endocrinology and Metabolism, Peninsula Medical School, Plymouth Campus, U.K.

Phil Zeitler   Department of Pediatrics, University of Colorado at Denver and Health Sciences Center, Denver, Colorado, U.S.A.

Ping Zhang   Division of Diabetes Translation, Centers for Disease Control and Prevention, Atlanta, Georgia, U.S.A.

1 Definition, Diagnosis, and Classification of Diabetes in Youth

Nancy A. Crimmins and Lawrence M. Dolan
Department of Pediatrics, Cincinnati Children's Hospital Medical Center and University of Cincinnati School of Medicine, Cincinnati, Ohio, U.S.A.

HISTORICAL PERSPECTIVE: EARLIEST DESCRIPTIONS TO 1965

Early Descriptions of Diabetes

Ancient records up to 3000 years old describe a disease in youth that was sudden in onset, resulted in acute metabolic decompensation, and culminated in death. Although this clinical picture described millennia ago was likely that of diabetes, the first accepted description of diabetes as a disorder associated with increased urine output came from ancient Egypt (the Ebers papyrus) around 1550 B.C. It was not until the second century B.C. that the term "diabetes" was used. Credit for coining "diabetes" is given to Demetrios of Apamaia who derived the term from the Greek word *diabeinein*, meaning "siphon" or "pass through."

Aretaeus of Cappadocia reported the first clinical description of the disease in the second century A.D. using the term "diabetes." Focusing on the polyuric aspect of diabetes, he wrote of the "melting down of flesh and limbs into urine" and stated that the disease was infrequent. Diabetes was recognized in Indian medicine in the fifth and sixth centuries as a disorder associated with the production of sweet urine that attracted insects. The term diabetes did not appear in an English text until 1425.

In 1674, Thomas Willis, physician to England's King Charles II, became the first European to discover the sweetness in the urine of those afflicted with diabetes. Perhaps the first English diabetes epidemiologist, Thomas, also noted the importance of lifestyle in the development of diabetes. He noted that the prevalence of diabetes was increasing because of "good fellowship and gusling down chiefly of unalloyed wine." A century later, Matthew Dobson proved that the sweetness in urine was caused by sugar and was associated with sugar in the blood. John Rollo was the first person to coin the term "diabetes mellitus" (mellitus from Latin for honey) and distinguished this disease from another disease of polyuria, "diabetes insipidus" (insipidus from Latin for tasteless) around the turn of the 18th century.

Early Recognition of Two Distinct Phenotypes of Diabetes

As early as the fifth and sixth centuries, Indian descriptions of the diabetes recognized two phenotypes: one that appeared in older, fatter people, and the other in thin people, which was more acute in presentation and quickly led to death. It was not until 1866 that this concept emerged again in a text written by George Harley. He wrote, "...I differ from my predecessors and contemporaries in believing that there are at least two different forms of the disease, requiring diametrically opposite lines of treatment.... one of which might be named *Diabetes from excessive formation*; the other *Diabetes from defective assimilation (malnutrition)*" (1). Etienne

Lancereaux, a French physician who made significant contributions in understanding the clinical spectrum of diabetes, is given much of the credit for suggesting a basis for the modern classification of diabetes. He proposed that there were two fundamental forms of presentation: "thin or pancreatic diabetes" and "fat or constitutional diabetes" (2). With the discovery and subsequent use of insulin as a therapy for diabetes, clinicians recognized insulin responsive or insulin resistant as the two main forms of diabetes. C. Wesley Dupertuis, a physical anthropologist, first suggested the terms "group I and group II diabetes" on the basis of the two main phenotypes of the disease in the 1940s; however, this classification was not widely embraced by the scientific community at that time (3).

MODERN PERSPECTIVE: 1965–2003

Definition of Diabetes Mellitus
Through the extraordinary efforts of great scientists in the 19th and 20th centuries (too vast to cover in this chapter), we now have a better understanding of the physiologic basis of diabetes mellitus. Diabetes mellitus is defined as inappropriate hyperglycemia resulting from a deficiency of insulin production, insulin action, or both with derangements in carbohydrate, protein, and lipid metabolism and subsequent long-term vascular complications.

Previous Classification Systems: WHO and ADA
An attempt to apply a universal classification system to diabetes mellitus did not occur until advances in molecular biology in the 20th century provided a better understanding of the etiology and genetics leading to the various clinical presentations of the disease. Amongst these advances were the discovery of insulitis in animal models and humans, the identification of islet cell antibodies, and histocompatibility antigens (HLA) associations with diabetes.

1965: First Report of the WHO Expert Committee on Diabetes Mellitus
The World Health Organization (WHO), in 1965, detailed the first attempt to apply a universal classification to diabetes mellitus and utilized age and insulin requirements as the main criteria for classification (4). This report written by the WHO Expert Committee on Diabetes Mellitus divided patients into one of four categories:

1. *Infantile or childhood diabetic*—onset under 14 years of age and insulin dependent
2. *Young diabetic*—onset between 15 and 24 years with most becoming insulin dependent
3. *Adult diabetic*—onset between 25 and 64 years, presenting with variable requirements for insulin
4. *Elderly diabetic*—onset after 65 years of age, frequently presenting with symptoms of diabetic complications and often controllable without insulin

Although other nomenclature was recognized in that report (i.e., juvenile-type diabetes, insulin-resistant diabetes, and gestational diabetes), it was recommended to hold to the classification terms introduced by the committee. This report also outlined criteria for diagnosis on the basis of an oral glucose challenge, although a testing standard was not provided. Diabetes was diagnosed if the venous blood glucose was ≥ 130 mg/dL two hours after a glucose load. Persons with a blood glucose between 110 and 129 mg/dL two hours after a glucose load were considered to be in a "borderline state."

1979: International Workshop of the National Diabetes Data Group

Over a decade later in 1979, the National Diabetes Data Group (NDDG) was convened in response to calls for a revised classification system for diabetes mellitus. The National Institutes of Health (NIH, which convened the group), American Diabetes Association (ADA), and WHO supported their proposal. The NDDG recommended elimination of the previous classification that was based on age at diagnosis. Instead the following subclasses were recommended, which were heavily influenced by insulin requirements (5).

1. *Insulin-dependent diabetes mellitus (IDDM), or type 1*—characterized by abrupt onset of symptoms, insulinopenia, dependence on insulin, and ketosis prone
2. *Non-insulin-dependent diabetes mellitus (NIDDM), or type 2*—presenting with few or no symptoms, in which insulin levels were variable, not ketosis prone, and did not depend on insulin to sustain life. Patients in this subclass were further divided into obese and nonobese NIDDM
3. Diabetes associated with other conditions and syndromes
4. Gestational diabetes mellitus (GDM)

The NDDG statement also outlined more specific criteria for the diagnosis of diabetes than did the previous WHO report. The diagnosis of diabetes (in nonpregnant adults) should be restricted to

1. those with classical symptoms of diabetes (polyuria, polydypsia, ketonuria, weight loss) and "gross or unequivocal hyperglycemia,"
2. those with a fasting blood glucose ≥140 mg/dL on more than one occasion, and/or
3. those who had a fasting blood glucose ≥140 mg/dL and exhibit sustained elevation of plasma glucose during a two-hour oral glucose tolerance test (OGTT, defined as a glucose ≥200 mg/dL at two hours and at least one other time interval of testing).

In addition, the category of "impaired glucose tolerance" (IGT) was introduced to encompass those individuals with a two-hour plasma glucose values between the normal and diabetic ranges.

1997: Report of the Expert Committee on the Diagnosis and Classification of Diabetes Mellitus

In 1997, the ADA invited a group of international experts in the field to examine the 1979 criteria and to determine if the diabetes classification system required alteration (6). In that report, it was recommended to abandon the terms "insulin-dependent" and "non-insulin-dependent" diabetes as they were felt to be both confusing and imprecise. The committee recommended instead that the two main subclasses of diabetes be called "type 1" and "type 2" diabetes. These terms, first proposed in the 1940s, are still in use to this day.

The committee also revised the diagnostic criteria for diabetes. Diagnostic criteria now included (1) symptoms of diabetes plus a random plasma glucose ≥200 mg/dL, or (2) a fasting glucose ≥126 mg/dL, or (3) a two-hour glucose

≥200 mg/dL during 75-g OGTT testing. Furthermore, a new category "impaired fasting glucose" (IFG) was created and defined as a fasting plasma glucose between 110 and 125 mg/dL.

1999: WHO Consultation on the Diagnosis and Classification of Diabetes Mellitus

In this report, the WHO echoed the recommendations of the ADA with one notable exception: that OGTT be used only for research and not standard clinical practice unless a random plasma glucose was in the "uncertain" range (7).

2003: Expert Committee Follow-up Report on the Diagnosis of Diabetes Mellitus

This report from the ADA suggested decreasing the lower limit for IFG from 110 mg/dL to 100 mg/dL on the basis of epidemiologic predictive data (8).

CURRENT DIAGNOSTIC CRITERIA FOR DIABETES MELLITUS

The current diagnostic criteria for diabetes mellitus are outlined in Table 1. These criteria reflect the culmination of years of epidemiologic studies in diabetes.

CURRENT DIABETES CLASSIFICATION

Type 1 Diabetes Mellitus

Type 1 diabetes mellitus (T1DM), the most common form of diabetes diagnosed in childhood (although representing only 5–10% of cases overall), is caused by immune-mediated β-cell destruction leading to insulin deficiency (Table 2). The symptoms of T1DM are usually rapid in onset and include polyuria, polydypsia, weight loss, abdominal symptoms, headaches, and ketoacidosis. Insulin is necessary for survival. Serious chronic complications can occur from long-standing disease such as nephropathy, retinopathy, cardiovascular disease, neuropathy, infection risk, and ultimately, premature death.

Insulinopenia and evidence of autoimmunity are the cornerstones to the diagnosis of T1DM. The autoimmune destruction of the β-cells is mediated by T-cells and is accompanied by the formation of autoantibodies, such as those

TABLE 1 Criteria for the Diagnosis of Diabetes Mellitus

1. Symptoms of diabetes plus casual plasma glucose concentration ≥200 mg/dL (11.1 mmol/L). Casual is defined as any time of day without regard to time since last meal. The classic symptoms of diabetes include polyuria, polydypsia, and unexplained weight loss.

OR

2. FPG ≥ 126 mg/dL (7 mmol/L). Fasting is defined as no caloric intake for at least 8 hr.

OR

3. 2-hr postload glucose ≥200 mg/dL (11.1 mmol/L) during an OGTT. The test should be performed as described by WHO, using a glucose load containing the equivalent of 75-g anhydrous glucose dissolved in water.

In the absence of unequivocal hyperglycemia, these criteria should be confirmed by repeat testing on a different day. The third measure (OGTT) is not recommended for routine clinical use.
Abbreviations: FPG, fasting plasma glucose; OGTT, oral glucose tolerance test.
Source: Adapted from Ref. 14.

TABLE 2 Etiologic Classification of Diabetes Mellitus

I. Type 1 diabetes (β-cell destruction, usually leading to absolute insulin deficiency)
   A. Immune mediated
   B. Idiopathic
II. Type 2 diabetes (may range from predominantly insulin resistance with relative insulin deficiency to a predominantly secretory defect with insulin resistance)
III. Other specific types
   A. Genetic defects of β-cell function
      1. Chromosome 12, HNF-1α (MODY3)
      2. Chromosome 7, glucokinase (MODY2)
      3. Chromosome 20, HNF-4α (MODY1)
      4. Chromosome 13, insulin promoter factor-1 (IPF-1; MODY4)
      5. Chromosome 17, HNF-1β (MODY5)
      6. Chromosome 2, NeuroD1 (MODY6)
      7. Mitochondrial DNA
      8. Others
   B. Genetic defects in insulin action
      1. Type A insulin resistance
      2. Leprechaunism
      3. Rabson-Mendenhall syndrome
      4. Lipoatrophic diabetes
      5. Others
   C. Diseases of the exocrine pancreas
      1. Pancreatitis
      2. Trauma/pancreatectomy
      3. Neoplasia
      4. Cystic fibrosis
      5. Hemochromatosis
      6. Fibrocalculous pancreatopathy
      7. Others
   D. Endocrinopathies
      1. Acromegaly
      2. Cushing's syndrome
      3. Glucagonoma
      4. Pheochromocytoma
      5. Hyperthyroidism
      6. Somatostatinoma
      7. Aldosteronoma
      8. Others
   E. Drug- or chemical-induced
      1. Vacor
      2. Pentamidine
      3. Nicotinic acid
      4. Glucocorticoids
      5. Thyroid hormone
      6. Diazoxide
      7. β-Adrenergic agonists
      8. Thiazides
      9. Dilantin
     10. α-Interferon
     11. Others
   F. Infections
      1. Congenital rubella
      2. Cytomegalovirus
      3. Others

(Continued)

TABLE 2   Etiologic Classification of Diabetes Mellitus (*Continued*)

G. Uncommon forms of immune-mediated diabetes
1. Stiff-man syndrome
2. Anti-insulin receptor antibodies
3. Others
H. Other genetic syndromes sometimes associated with diabetes
1. Down's syndrome
2. Klinefelter's syndrome
3. Turner's syndrome
4. Wolfram's syndrome
5. Friedreich's ataxia
6. Huntington's chorea
7. Laurence-Moon-Biedl syndrome
8. Myotonic dystrophy
9. Porphyria
10. Prader-Willi syndrome
11. Others
IV. GDM

Abbreviations: HNF, hepatocyte nuclear factor; MODY, maturity-onset diabetes of the young; IPF-1, insulin promoter factor-1; GDM, Gestational diabetes mellitus.
Source: Adapted from Ref. 14.

against the 65 kDa isoform of glutamic acid decarboxylase (GAD65), tyrosine phosphatase–related IA-2 molecule (IA-2), insulin autoantibodies (IAAs), and islet cell autoantibodies (ICAs). Whether these antibodies contribute to the destruction of the β-cells or are formed as a result of other immune processes are a matter of debate. What is known is that these antibodies are present prior to the appearance of clinical disease and can predict disease development (9,10). The presence of each antibody at diagnosis is dependent on the age of onset and sex of the individual. GAD65 antibodies are present in between 70% and 80% of Caucasian children diagnosed with diabetes and are less frequently found in boys. The presence of IA-2 antibodies varies with age and has been reported in 50–70% of children recently diagnosed with T1DM (11). IAAs vary the most with age, with young children having the highest prevalence at diagnosis. IAAs are found in 83% of children younger than 4 years of age, 40% of children between 7 to 13 years of age, 20% of adolescents, and 10% in adults with new-onset disease (11–13). ICAs are the most commonly found antibodies in children at diagnosis with an overall prevalence greater than 80% (11,12).

One or more of the islet cell antibodies is present during diagnosis of T1DM in 80–90% of individuals (13,14). If antibodies are present under the context of clear insulinopenia and ketosis, a diagnosis of type 1a diabetes is given. If patients have a clinical picture consistent with T1DM but no antibodies present, a diagnosis of type 1b (or idiopathic T1DM) is given. Patients with type 1b diabetes are often of African or Asian decent, tend to be older, and have a greater body mass index (BMI) than age-matched children with type 1a diabetes (13). It is not clear if these patients have a different underlying pathology to their disease or if they manifest autoantibodies that are not measured by common assays.

Of note, recent concerns have arisen regarding the lack of standardization of autoantibody assays between various laboratories. Because of these concerns, the NIH convened an international committee of experts in 2006 to ensure standardization of these assays. This standardization will be a significant step forward in ensuring correct classification of autoimmune-mediated diabetes.

The genetics underlying T1DM is complex and is covered in depth in chapter 4. T1DM has both genetic and environmental components. Specific HLA can protect or confer risk for T1DM and in fact can predict autoantibody development. HLA genes are thought to contribute up to 50% of the genetic risk for T1DM (15). Yet, studies in monozygotic twins have shown at most a 50% concordance of T1DM (16,17), proving that an environmental exposure of some kind is required for progression to disease.

Type 2 Diabetes Mellitus

Type 2 diabetes mellitus (T2DM) is primarily characterized by insulin resistance detected at the level of skeletal muscle, liver, and adipose tissues with a failure of β-cell compensation and a relative insulin deficiency. In adults, there is an established progression from insulin resistance to glucose intolerance (IFG or IGT) to T2DM. Progression through these stages can occur over many years and is often unaccompanied by symptoms of disease. The extent to which children progress through stages of obesity, insulin resistance, and glucose intolerance is not fully understood; however, it appears that the pathway to disease is much shorter and less predictable in children than in adults.

Pediatric patients with T2DM are usually overweight or obese (BMI ≥ 85th percentile for age and sex), and comorbidities such as hypertension and dyslipidemia can be present at diagnosis. Polycystic ovarian syndrome is a common comorbidity in adolescent girls diagnosed with T2DM. Often there is a strong family history in first and second degree family members. Weight loss at diagnosis is less common than in T1DM, and acanthosis is frequently identified on examination. Patients frequently present with evidence of residual β-cell function, although no standardized cutoffs exist for insulin or C-peptide levels. These patients usually lack evidence of autoimmunity. Ketosis is less common than in T1DM as individuals with T2DM usually produce enough insulin secretion to prevent lipolysis.

Diet and exercise are the mainstays of treatment for T2DM. Unlike T1DM, T2DM can successfully be treated with oral hypoglycemic agents. Insulin may or may not be required at diagnosis or for long-term treatment of hyperglycemia, but insulin is not required for survival. Because of a period of "silent" disease in adults, hyperglycemic complications can be recognized at diagnosis. In contrast, youth rarely have hyperglycemic complications at diagnosis.

Once thought to be a disease of adulthood, T2DM is becoming increasingly common in children and adolescents. T2DM now accounts for 20–50% of new-onset diabetes cases in pediatric populations within the United States (18–20). The increase in incidence in T2DM in youth is thought to be secondary to concurrent increases in obesity in children and adolescents.

Other Types of Diabetes Mellitus
Genetic Defects of β-cell function
MODY. Maturity-onset diabetes of the young (MODY) refers to monogenetic disorders of β-cell function leading to hyperglycemia and nonketotic diabetes mellitus. Onset is usually before 25 years of age. Inheritance is autosomal dominant with 80–95% penetrance (21). MODY3, the most common form of MODY, is associated with mutations in the hepatocyte nuclear factor gene HNF-1α. HNF-1α is a transcription factor important for regulation of expression of both the insulin gene and

genes that control glucose transport. The second most common form, MODY2, involves a mutation in the glucokinase gene. Glucokinase acts as a glucose sensor leading to insulin production by the β-cell. Because of the defect in glucokinase, increased glucose levels are required for insulin production and secretion to occur. Other MODY types are less common and are caused by mutations in genes encoding transcription factors, which either affect pancreas development (MODY4, MODY6) or regulate genes influencing insulin secretion (MODY1, MODY5). MODY treatment depends on the genetic lesion involved and can range from diet and exercise modification to insulin therapy (Table 3).

Mitochondrial diabetes. Mutations in mitochondrial DNA can lead to diabetes. Discrimination from MODY is based on maternal-only transmission in conjunction with bilateral hearing loss in most of the carriers (22). The most accurate way to distinguish between MODY and mitochondrial diabetes is genetic testing. The most common mitochondrial DNA mutation, which causes diabetes, is an A3243G mutation. This mutation is thought to account for 0.5–2.8% of diabetes in the general population (23). Mitochondrial diabetes as a result of the A3243G mutation presents at a mean age of 38 years of age and penetration is nearly 100% (22). Phenotypic presentations as a result of this mutation can range from a severe disorder called MELAS (mitochondrial encephalopathy, stroke-like episodes, short stature, and diabetes) to a more mild phenotype of late-onset diabetes and mild hearing loss. Deletions of mitochondrial DNA can likewise lead to diabetes mellitus. Kearns-Sayre, a syndrome of encephalomyopathy, external opthalmoplegia, retinal dystrophy, and cardiomyopathy is one such disorder.

Mitochondrial diabetes can have a presentation similar to either T1DM or T2DM depending on the degree of insulinopenia. However, the underlying pathophysiology is β-cell failure and insulin deficiency is progressive. Most patients end up requiring insulin for treatment within two to three years of diagnosis.

Neonatal diabetes. Several mutations have been identified that can lead to either transient or permanent neonatal diabetes within the first 6 to 12 months of life. Infants with neonatal diabetes mellitus can present with intrauterine growth restriction proportional to the degree of insulin deficiency in utero and failure to thrive in the postnatal period. Additional signs and symptoms of neonatal diabetes mellitus are similar to other insulin-deficient forms and can include ketoacidosis. Diabetes-related autoantibodies are not present and no HLA associations are known. Children with the transient form recover within one year of life; however, many of these patients can continue to have forms of glucose intolerance or recurrent diabetes. In fact, diabetes relapse has been reported to occur in over half of children with transient neonatal diabetes (24). It has been suggested that transient neonatal diabetes is probably a β-cell defect with variable expression during growth and development (24). Transient neonatal diabetes has been associated with uniparental disomy or parental duplications of chromosome 6q24; however, the role of this chromosomal region in causing β-cell defects is not understood (25,26). Approximately 50% of patients with neonatal diabetes mellitus have a permanent form and no one clinical feature helps distinguish the permanent and transient forms. The most common mutation leading to the permanent form is an activating mutation in the KCNJ11 gene, which encodes the Kir6.2 subunit of the potassium channel of the β-cell (24,27). Activating mutations in the ABCC8 gene,

TABLE 3 MODY-Related Genes and the Clinical Phenotypes Associated with Mutations in the Genes

MODY type	Gene	Clinical features of heterozygous state	Most common treatment	Molecular basis	Clinical features of homozygous state
MODY 1	HNF-4α	Diabetes; microvascular complications (in many cases); reductions in serum concentration of triglycerides, apolipoproteins AII and CIII, and Lp(a) lipoprotein	Oral hypoglycemic agents, insulin	Abnormal regulation of gene transcription in β-cells, leading to a defect in metabolic signaling of insulin secretion, β-cell mass, or both	
MODY 2	Glucokinase	Impaired fasting glucose, impaired glucose tolerance, diabetes, normal proinsulin-to-insulin ratio in serum	Diet and exercise	Defect in sensitivity of β-cells to glucose due to reduced glucose phosphorylation; defect in hepatic storage of glucose as glycogen	Permanent neonatal diabetes, requiring insulin treatment
MODY 3	HNF-1α	Diabetes, microvascular complications (in many cases), renal glycosuria, increased sensitivity to sulfonylurea drugs, increased proinsulin-to-insulin ratio in serum	Oral hypoglycemic agent, insulin	Abnormal regulation of gene transcription in β-cells, leading to a defect in metabolic signaling of insulin secretion, β-cell mass, or both	
MODY 4	IPF-1	Diabetes	Oral hypoglycemic agents, insulin	Abnormal transcriptional regulation of β-cell development and function	Pancreatic agenesis and neonatal diabetes, requiring insulin treatment
MODY 5	HNF-1β	Diabetes; renal cysts and other abnormalities of renal development; progressive nondiabetic renal dysfunction, leading to chronic renal insufficiency and failure; internal genital abnormalities (in female carriers)	Insulin	Abnormal regulation of gene transcription in β-cells, leading to a defect in metabolic signaling of insulin secretion, β-cell mass, or both	
MODY 6	NeuroD1, or BETA2	Diabetes	Insulin	Abnormal transcriptional regulation of β-cell development and function	

Abbreviations: MODY, maturity-onset diabetes of the young; HNF, hepatocyte nuclear factor; IPF, insulin promoter factor.
Source: Adapted from Ref. 21.

which encodes the sulfonylurea receptor (the other subunit of the potassium channel of the β-cell), have recently been described as a less common cause of this disease (28). Homozygous inactivating mutations in the pancreas duodenum homeobox 1 gene (PDX-1) and in the glucokinase gene (affecting pancreas formation and glucose sensing, respectively) have also been implicated. Of note, heterozygous mutations of these genes lead to MODY4 (PDX-1) and MODY2 (glucokinase).

Genetic Defects in Insulin Action

Mutations in the insulin receptor leading to defects in insulin action have been identified. Type A insulin resistance manifests as a severe presentation of polycystic ovary syndrome and is characterized by marked hyperandrogenism, acanthosis nigricans, and insulin resistance. Leprechaunism and Rabson-Mendenhall syndrome both present with severe insulin resistance and are diagnosed in infancy. Leprechaunism is characterized by intrauterine and postnatal growth retardation, dysmorphic facial features, severe insulin resistance and acanthosis, fasting hypoglycemia, and postprandial hyperglycemia. Most patients with this disorder die in the first year of life. Rabson-Mendenhall syndrome is associated with extreme insulin resistance and acanthosis, pineal hyperplasia, and abnormal nails and teeth. The clinical picture is not as severe as seen in those children with Leprechaunism, and most children with this disorder live beyond the first year of life.

Secondary Diabetes: Diseases of the Exocrine Pancreas, Endocrinopathies, Infections

Diabetes can occur commonly as a secondary process from either the direct effects of primary disease or as a result of the treatment of that disease. While the specific etiologies that lead to secondary diabetes are too numerous to expound on in detail (Table 2), three main categories exist according to ADA classification: (1) diseases of the exocrine pancreas (i.e., cystic fibrosis, pancreatitis), (2) endocrinopathies (i.e., Cushing's disease, acromegaly), and (3) infections (i.e., congenital rubella). These forms of diabetes can be transient and resolve as the primary disease abates or is cured such as in pancreatitis or hyperthyroidism. In some individuals, the primary disease may "unmask" developing diabetes which either continues after the primary disease resolves or reveals itself in the future. Often secondary diabetes is muddied by one or more processes. For example, cystic fibrosis–related diabetes appears to be caused by both structural pancreatic damage with subsequent insulinopenia and other complicating factors leading to insulin resistance, such as undernutrition and increases in counterregulatory hormones and inflammatory cytokines. In addition, pulmonary exacerbations are frequently treated with glucocorticoids, worsening insulin resistance in these patients.

"Stress hyperglycemia/diabetes" or "diabetes of injury" is not a separate category of diabetes according to the ADA classification system. However, this usually transient form is seen not uncommonly in pediatric critical care settings subsequent to a wide range of pathologies ranging from severe infection to head injuries. The mechanisms behind stress hyperglycemia are not fully clear and may be multifactorial. Factors involved in the pathogenesis of stress hyperglycemia include cytokine effects, hepatic and skeletal muscle insulin resistance, and unchecked counterregulatory responses (29). Yet, evidence in both adults and kids suggests that tight glucose control in stress hyperglycemia can strongly influence morbidity and mortality outcomes in these patients, and thus needs to be mentioned here as a significant form of diabetes.

Drug- or Chemical-Induced Diabetes Mellitus

Many drugs can cause hyperglycemia through either β-cell toxicity or worsening insulin resistance (Table 2). Furthermore, these drugs may not always cause diabetes in themselves, but can synergistically lead to diabetes in conjunction with the disease process they are treating (i.e., steroids in cystic fibrosis, l-asparaginase in transplant patients). In addition, drugs can increase appetite and lead to weight gain, which can accelerate diabetes development (i.e., antipsychotic medications). Once the offending agent is removed, the hyperglycemia often resolves; however, like the diseases in the last category, medications can also "unmask" developing diabetes.

Uncommon Forms of Immune-Mediated Diabetes

Two conditions exist in this category: the stiff-man syndrome and anti-insulin receptor antibodies. Stiff-man syndrome is an uncommon autoimmune disorder that leads to muscle stiffness, rigidity, and spasm involving the axial muscles, which can result in poor mobility. Other autoimmune diseases can accompany this syndrome including thyroiditis, vitiligo, and most commonly, type 1 diabetes. The autoimmune basis for this syndrome is the formation of anti-GAD antibodies, which target both GABAergic neurons and the pancreas. The onset of this disorder in childhood is rare and occurs usually between the third and seventh decades of life. Anti-insulin antibodies can block the binding of insulin to its receptor, thereby leading to decreased insulin action. These antibodies can be found in patients with other autoimmune diseases and these patients often have acanthosis. This type of diabetes has also been referred to as type B insulin resistance. Anti-insulin antibodies are rare in children.

Other Genetic Syndromes Sometimes Associated with Diabetes

Several genetic syndromes diagnosed in childhood are associated with diabetes (Table 2). Although some of these syndromes can be uncommon, collectively they make up approximately 5% of patients seen in diabetes clinics (23). Trisomy 21 is associated with an increased risk of diabetes-related antibodies and T1DM as compared with normal populations (prevalence of diabetes ranges between 1.4% and 10%) (30,31). Klinefelter's and Turner's syndromes can lead to diabetes with a predominately insulin-resistant phenotype. Some neuromuscular disorders such as Huntington's disease, Friedreich's ataxia, and myotonic dystrophy are associated with an increased risk of diabetes, which presents in adulthood. The pathophysiology behind diabetes in many of these syndromes is not fully understood.

Wolfram's syndrome (DIDMOAD, diabetes insipidus, diabetes mellitus, optic atrophy, deafness) is a rare autosomal recessive disorder characterized by β-cell loss and diabetes mellitus without evidence of autoimmunity as well as optic atrophy. Diabetes insipidus and deafness can also be associated with this syndrome. Family studies have identified the gene responsible for this syndrome as the WFS1 gene. This gene is expressed abundantly in the β-cells and encodes for a transmembrane glycoprotein in the endoplasmic reticulum. Loss of function mutations of the WFS1 gene could lead to diabetes through endoplasmic reticulum membrane instability in the β-cells (32,33).

TABLE 4 Diagnosis of GDM with a 100-g or 75-g Glucose Load

	mg/dL	mmol/L
100-g glucose load		
Fasting	95	5.3
1 hr	180	10
2 hr	155	8.6
3 hr	140	7.8
75-g glucose load		
Fasting	95	5.3
1 hr	180	10
2 hr	155	8.6

Two or more of the venous plasma concentrations must be met or exceeded for a positive diagnosis. The test should be done in the morning after an overnight fast of between 8 and 14 hours and after at least three days of unrestricted diet ($\geq$150 g carbohydrate/day) and unlimited physical activity. The subject should remain seated and should not smoke throughout the test.
Abbreviation: GDM, gestational diabetes mellitus.
Source: Adapted from Ref. 14.

Gestational Diabetes

Gestational diabetes is defined as any degree of glucose intolerance with onset or first recognition during pregnancy. Diagnostic criteria based on oral glucose tolerance testing are more stringent than the criteria used for nonpregnant individuals (Table 4). Gestational diabetes occurs in 4–7% of pregnancies (14,34). Insulin resistance is progressive during pregnancy, beginning mid-pregnancy and worsening during the third trimester. Placental hormones are thought to be, in part, responsible as insulin sensitivity improves dramatically after delivery. Like other insulin-resistance states, the β-cells of the pancreas must increase insulin secretion in order to maintain normal glucose homeostasis. If the pancreatic β-cells cannot increase insulin production accordingly, gestational diabetes results. Most women with gestational diabetes have chronic insulin resistance prior and after pregnancy, and many go on to develop diabetes later in life. The insulin-resistant state can unmask monogenic diabetes (MODY) as well.

WHERE THE CURRENT CLASSIFICATION SYSTEM FAILS: MIXED TYPES OF DIABETES

In Youth: Type 1.5 Diabetes or Double Diabetes

Although the terms "type 1.5 diabetes" (T1.5DM), "double diabetes," "latent diabetes of the young," or "mixed diabetes" are not terms found within the current recognized classification system, they are now familiar to most endocrinologists and found in well-respected journals. For over a decade, it has been recognized that obese adults and adolescents with a clinic picture suggestive of T2DM can present in ketoacidosis of varying degrees (35,36). Some of these individuals will have evidence of autoimmunity as well (37,38). If a patient is obese and insulin resistant (T2DM), yet presents in diabetic ketoacidosis and/or with positive islet cell antibodies (T1DM), it becomes difficult to assign an appropriate label according to the current method of diabetes classification. When the phenotype and presentation of disease is mixed in children and adolescents, terms such as " T1.5DM" and "double diabetes" have been used (39).

TABLE 5 Antibody Positivity in Type 1, Type 1.5, and Type 2 Diabetes Mellitus

Reference	Population	Findings[a]
37	48 with T2DM	30.3% GAD+
		34.8% IAA+
		8.1% ICA+
42	37 with T2DM	29.7% at least 1 Ab+
		8.1% GAD+
		8.1% IA-2+
		27% IAA+
40	37 T1DM, 19 with T2DM,	T1DM: 97% Ab+, 89% T-cell+
	16 Indeterminate (T1.5DM)	T2DM: 74% Ab+, 37% T-cell+
		ID: 68% Ab+, 38% T-cell+
41	21 with T1DM, 15 with	T1DM: 100% Ab+
	T2DM, 28 with T1.5DM	T2DM: 33% Ab+
		T1.5DM: 89% Ab+

[a]All Ab+ subjects with T2DM were positive for just one antibody; the majority of T1DM and T1.5DM subjects were positive for more than one.
Abbreviations: GAD, glutamic acid decarboxylase; IAA, insulin autoantibody; ICA, islet cell autoantibody; Ab+, antibody positive; T1DM, type 1 diabetes mellitus; T2DM, type 2 diabetes mellitus; T1.5DM, type 1.5 diabetes mellitus.

TABLE 6 HLA Risk by Clinically Assigned Diabetes Type

Reference	Population	High/moderate-risk DR3/DR4
40	28 with T1DM, 15 with T2DM,	T1DM: 89% (25/28)
	11 Indeterminant	T2DM: 67% (10/15)
		Indeterminant: 82% (9/11)
41	21 with T1DM, 15 with T2DM,	T1DM: 100% (21/21)
	28 with T1.5DM	T2DM: 14% (1/7)
		T1.5: 81% (23/38)

Abbreviations: HLA, histocompatibility antigens; T1DM, type 1 diabetes mellitus; T2DM, type 2 diabetes mellitus; T1.5DM, type 1.5 diabetes mellitus.

The prevalence of autoantibodies in children and adolescents diagnosed with T2DM ranges from 20% to 75% (40–42). Up to 89% of subjects with T1.5DM will demonstrate antibody positivity (41). Therefore, although the likelihood of antibody positivity is significantly less in T2DM or T1.5DM than in T1DM, it is certainly common. However, it is less likely that youth with T2DM or T1.5DM will have multiple autoantibodies compared with youth with T1DM. In a recent study, 97% of pediatric patients with T1DM had more than one antibody compared with 54% of patients diagnosed with T2DM and 57% of those with a mixed type of diabetes (40) (Table 5).

Furthermore, studies have examined the frequency of HLA risk by clinically assigned diabetes type. In one study, the frequency of high-risk DR3 and DR4 haplotypes was not significantly different when comparing type 1, type 2, and "indeterminant" diabetes (40). Another study found that T1DM and T1.5DM had similar frequencies of high and moderate HLA risk, which were significantly higher than seen in T2DM (Table 6).

Evidence suggests that the clinical outcomes for youth diagnosed with T1.5DM differ from that of those youth diagnosed with T2DM. These children are more likely to be treated with insulin at diagnosis (41). Furthermore, if initially placed on oral agents to treat hyperglycemia, it is more likely that children and adolescents with T1.5DM will require insulin earlier than their T2DM counterparts. However, little data exist that describes the differences in clinical course between youth with T1.5DM or double diabetes compared with those with T1DM and T2DM. The reasons for this are as follows: (1) only recent acknowledgment that mixed types of diabetes may exist (43), and (2) there are no accepted standards for the classification of double diabetes. Pozzilli and Buzzetti (43) recently suggested criteria for the diagnosis of double diabetes in youth. These include:

1. *The presence of clinical features of type 2 diabetes, hypertension, dyslipidaemia, increased BMI with increased cardiovascular risk as compared with children with classical type 1 diabetes. Family history for type 1 or type 2 diabetes might be present.* These criteria suggest a subjective comparison of clinical presentation as being more like T2DM than T1DM. With the increase in the obesity epidemic, about one-fourth of kids with classic T1DM have a BMI at diagnosis ≥85th percentile for age and sex (44,45). Therefore, using BMI as a criteria for classification might prove difficult. The presence of comorbidities such as hypertension and dyslipidemia are certainly more common in T2DM than T1DM, but how can one judge that there are more of these features than a type 1 but less than a type 2?

2. *The presence of a reduced number of clinical features of type 1 diabetes, such as weight loss, polyuria and polydypsia, development of ketoacidosis; insulin therapy is not the first line of therapy, by contrast to the situation in subjects with classical type 1 DM.* Presenting with ketoacidosis is not uncommon in patients diagnosed with T2DM so it would be difficult to use the lack of ketoacidosis to define double diabetes. In addition, a significant portion of these individuals do require insulin at diagnosis (39,41).

3. *The presence of autoantibodies to islet cells, although with a reduced number and titre compared with type 1 diabetes and probably a reduced risk associated with the MHC locus compared with subjects with type 1 diabetes. As compared with T1DM, where insulin resistance and obesity are not common features, double diabetes is always characterized by an obese phenotype, with the additional coexistence of β-cell autoimmunity.* Ultimately, categorizing the degree of autoimmunity, insulin-resistance, and β-cell failure at diagnosis will be the cornerstones to a diagnosis of double diabetes. More work needs to be done in this regard. Currently, a multicenter study called "SEARCH for Diabetes in Youth" is addressing many of these questions.

In Adults: Latent Autoimmune Diabetes in Adulthood

In the adult population, the term latent autoimmune diabetes in adulthood (LADA) is assigned to patients with a slowly progressive autoimmune form of diabetes (46). It is estimated that 10% of adults who present with non-insulin-requiring diabetes have LADA (47). The clinical presentation of LADA is more similar to T2DM than T1DM. Patients can either be lean or obese. The term T1.5DM has also been used as a label for this type of diabetes.

The Immunology of Diabetes Society has attempted to establish criteria for the diagnosis of LADA (38,48). These criteria include: (1) adult age at diagnosis (≥30 years), (2) evidence of autoimmunity (at least one diabetes-associated anti-body positive), and (3) non-insulin requiring at diagnosis for ≥ six months (49). The third criterion is meant to distinguish patients with adult-onset T1DM and LADA. Patients with LADA have reduced fasting and stimulated C-peptide levels as compared with patients with T2DM; however, the C-peptide levels are higher and demonstrate a slower decline than in T1DM. In one study, 94% of patients with LADA required insulin within six years as compared with 14% of those diagnosed with T2DM and no evidence of autoimmunity (47). Oral hypoglycemic agents are initially effective in LADA; however, ultimately β-cell failure progresses to the point at which insulin is required.

ICAs and GAD antibodies are common in LADA, whereas IAAs and IA-2 antibodies are less common (49). Patients with LADA are most often positive for only one antibody in contrast to T1DM patients who often present with multiple antibody positivity. Like T1DM, LADA shows HLA genetic susceptibility (50,51). These findings suggest that LADA is an autoimmune disease like T1DM; however, there are some differences in antibody positivity and T-cell responses that lead to different tempo of β-cell failure in the two disorders.

DIABETES AS A SPECTRUM OF DISEASE

The more we learn about the pathophysiology and clinical heterogeneity of diabetes mellitus, the more it appears to be a spectrum of disease. The remainder of this chapter summarizes data that in addition to the mixed types of diabetes support the concept of diabetes as a spectrum of disease.

The Accelerator Hypothesis

Wilkin, in 2001, initially proposed the accelerator hypothesis that outlines how a spectrum of diabetes phenotypes could occur (see chap. 7 for a full discussion). The accelerator hypothesis proposes that T1DM and T2DM are the same disease and are only distinguishable by the rate of β-cell loss and the "accelerators" responsible (52). The three accelerators are: (1) an intrinsically high rate of β-cell apoptosis, (2) weight gain and subsequent insulin resistance, and (3) the development of β-cell autoimmunity. Accelerators 1 and 2 are common to both T1DM and T2DM. Only the addition of accelerator 3—autoimmunity—leads to the more acute and severe presentation seen in T1DM.

In fact, the prevalence of T1DM has been increasing over the last several years in various populations. Since the underlying genetic structure of the population is unlikely to change drastically within a generation, it is likely that some change in the environment has led to the increase. The rise in the prevalence of obesity in children and adolescents over the same time frame has been suggested as a possible culprit and is one of the proposed accelerators. In fact, insulin resistance has been shown to be associated with progression to diabetes in antibody positive first degree relatives of individuals with T1DM (53). In addition, weight gain in infancy may be associated with increased risk of developing T1DM later in childhood (54,55).

Family Studies

Family studies suggest that there might be overlap in the pathophysiologic processes that underlie T1DM and T2DM. Studies have reported an increased frequency of T2DM in families with T1DM, and a parental history of T2DM was associated with an increased risk of T1DM in siblings of type 1 diabetic patients (56). In addition, evidence suggests that there might be an increased risk of diabetes-related complications such as cardiovascular disease and nephropathy in individuals with T1DM and a family history of T2DM (57–59). Interestingly, a family history of T1DM appears to convey less risk of cardiovascular disease in individuals with T2DM (60,61).

Basic Science Studies

Epidemiologic studies provided much of the fuel for the argument of overlapping pathophysiology of T1DM and T2DM. However, basic science has also provided some clues in this regard. Recently, Chaparro et al. reported that many genes differentially regulated in the NOD mouse (a murine model of T1DM) are more commonly associated with T1DM than T1DM (62). The authors suggest that the NOD mouse is a better model for T1.5DM in humans than for T1DM. Furthermore, factors leading to β-cell failure are similar in T1DM and T2DM, and recent studies have shown immune processes in the islets of patients with T2DM (63).

SUMMARY: COMING FULL CIRCLE IN CLASSIFYING DIABETES MELLITUS

The diabetes classification system endorsed by the ADA and WHO clearly has limitations. These limitations include arbitrary cutoffs for antibody positivity, no specific guidelines for what constitutes insulin deficiency or insulin resistance, and considerable overlap between phenotypes of disease. As a result, "mixed" types of diabetes are difficult to classify.

So why classify at all? As Gale stated in an editorial entitled "Declassifying Diabetes," a classification system provides a "construct—or paradigm—that encapsulates current scientific understanding of a disease, and offers guidance as to how this might translate into clinical practice" (64). Currently, the diabetes classification system approaches diabetes as a categorical disease. This approach provides clinicians, parents, and scientists a common ground for communication. Physicians offer prognostic guidance and patients develop expectations on further treatment based on diabetes type. However, different types of diabetes frequently require similar treatments, monitoring, metabolic derangements, and long-term vascular complications. Furthermore, research into the pathophysiologic mechanisms by type of diabetes has led to a common and unifying theme of a balance between insulin resistance and β-cell compromise in all diabetes types. As Dr. Gale also states, "Above all, we need to avoid the humiliation of being taken prisoner by constructs invented for our own convenience" (64). Although the classification of diabetes is an important tool for practitioners, its limitations secondary to gaps in current knowledge need to be recognized.

Over the past 40 years, the diabetes community appears to have come full circle. Prior to the first proposed classification system in 1965, diabetes mellitus was largely considered a single entity. As the science and treatment of diabetes advanced, categories of diabetes were created on the basis of age at diagnosis and the need for insulin. By 1997, clinicians and investigators recognized that neither age nor insulin requirements were accurate bases for classification. Instead, pathophysiology was used to attempt to better classify disease. Recently, mixed types of diabetes have been recognized that challenge the current classification system. Thus, we have moved from the concept of diabetes as a single entity to treatment and pathophysiology-based classifications, to most recently considering diabetes as a spectrum of disease. In some respects, the debate over classification has divided the diabetes community. In our view, challenging the current classification of diabetes should not be devised. Rather, this process is a natural, ongoing consequence of scientific investigation.

REFERENCES

1. Harley G. Diabetes: Its Various Forms and Different Treatments. London: Walton and Mabberly, 1866.
2. Master Series: Etienne Lancereaux. Diabetologia 2005; 48(11).
3. Gale EA. The discovery of type 1 diabetes. Diabetes 2001; 50(2):217–226.
4. World Health Organization. Diabetes Mellitus: Report of a WHO Expert Committee. World Health Organization Technical Support Series 1965(310).
5. National Diabetes Data Group. Classification and diagnosis of diabetes mellitus and other categories of glucose intolerance. Diabetes 1979; 28(12):1039–1057.
6. The Expert Committee on the Diagnosis and Classification of Diabetes Mellitus. Report of the Expert Committee on the Diagnosis and Classification of Diabetes Mellitus. Diabetes Care 1997; 20(7):1183–1197.
7. World Health Organization. Definition, Diagnosis, and Classification of Diabetes Mellitus and Its Complications. Report of a WHO Consultation. Part 1: Diagnosis and Classification of Diabetes Mellius. World Health Organization, 1999.
8. American Diabetes Association. Follow-up report on the diagnosis of diabetes mellitus. Diabetes Care 2003; 26(11):3160–3167.
9. Riley WJ, Maclaren NK, Krischer J, et al. A prospective study of the development of diabetes in relatives of patients with insulin-dependent diabetes. N Engl J Med 1990; 323 (17):1167–1172.
10. Srikanta S, Ganda OP, Eisenbarth GS, et al. Islet-cell antibodies and beta-cell function in monozygotic triplets and twins initially discordant for Type I diabetes mellitus. N Engl J Med 1983; 308(6):322–325.
11. Pihoker C, Gilliam LK, Hampe CS, et al. Autoantibodies in diabetes. Diabetes 2005; 54 (suppl 2):S52–S61.
12. Graham J, Hagopian WA, Kockum I, et al. Genetic effects on age-dependent onset and islet cell autoantibody markers in type 1 diabetes. Diabetes 2002; 51(5):1346–1355.
13. Wang J, Miao D, Babu S, et al. Prevalence of autoantibody-negative diabetes is not rare at all ages and increases with older age and obesity. J Clin Endocrinol Metab 2007; 92 (1):88–92.
14. American Diabetes Association. Diagnosis and classification of diabetes mellitus. Diabetes Care 2007; 30(suppl 1):s42–s47.
15. Achenbach P, Bonifacio E, Koczwara K, et al. Natural history of type 1 diabetes. Diabetes 2005; 54(suppl 2):s25–s31.
16. Kyvik KO, Green A, Beck-Nielsen H. Concordance rates of insulin-dependent diabetes mellitus: a population based study of young Danish twins. BMJ 1995; 311(7010):913–917.
17. Redondo MJ, Rewers M, Yu L, et al. Genetic determination of islet cell autoimmunity in monozygotic twin, dizygotic twin, and non-twin siblings of patients with type 1 diabetes: prospective twin study. BMJ 1999; 318(7185):698–702.
18. Hannon TS, Rao G, Arslanian SA. Childhood obesity and type 2 diabetes mellitus. Pediatrics 2005; 116(2):473–480.
19. Diabetes in Children Adolescents Work Group of the National Diabetes Education Program. An update on type 2 diabetes in youth from the national diabetes education program. Pediatrics 2004; 114:259–263.
20. Duncan G. Prevalence of diabetes and impaired fasting glucose levels among US adolescents: National Health and Nutrition Examination Survey, 1999–2002. Arch Pediatr Adolesc Med 2006; 160(5):523–528.
21. Fajans SS, Bell GI, Polonsky KS. Molecular mechanisms and clinical pathophysiology of maturity-onset diabetes of the young. N Engl J Med 2001; 345(13):971–980.
22. Maassen JA, Lm TH, Van Essen E, et al. Mitochondrial diabetes: molecular mechanisms and clinical presentation. Diabetes 2004; 53(suppl 1):S103–S109.
23. Barrett TG. Mitochondrial diabetes, DIDMOAD and other inherited diabetes syndromes. Best Pract Res Clin Endocrinol Metab 2001; 15(3):325–343.

24. Polak M. Neonatal diabetes mellitus: a disease linked to multiple mechanisms. Orphanet J Rare Dis 2007; 2(1):12.
25. Hermann R, Laine AP, Johansson C, et al. Transient but not permanent neonatal diabetes mellitus is associated with paternal uniparental isodisomy of chromosome 6. Pediatrics 2000; 105(1 pt 1):49–52.
26. Temple IK, Gardner RJ, Mackay DJ, et al. Transient neonatal diabetes: widening the understanding of the etiopathogenesis of diabetes. Diabetes 2000; 49(8):1359–1366.
27. Pearson ER, Flechtner I, Njolstad PR, et al. Switching from insulin to oral sulfonylureas in patients with diabetes due to Kir6.2 mutations. N Engl J Med 2006; 355(5):467–477.
28. Babenko AP, Polak M, Cave H, et al. Activating mutations in the ABCC8 gene in neonatal diabetes mellitus. N Engl J Med 2006; 355(5):456–466.
29. Van den Berge G. How does blood glucose control with insulin save lives in intensive care? J Clin Invest 2004; 114(9):1187–1195.
30. Anwar AJ, Walker JD, Frier BM. Type 1 diabetes mellitus and Down's syndrome: prevalence, management and diabetic complications. Diabet Med 1998; 15(2):160–163.
31. Gillespie KM, Dix RJ, Williams AJ, et al. Islet autoimmunity in children with Down's syndrome. Diabetes 2006; 55(11):3185–3188.
32. Fonseca SG, Fukuma M, Lipson KL, et al. WFS1 is a novel component of the unfolded protein response and maintains homeostasis of the endoplasmic reticulum in pancreatic beta-cells. J Biol Chem 2005; 280(47):39609–39615.
33. Hofmann S, Bauer MF. Wolfram syndrome-associated mutations lead to instability and proteasomal degradation of wolframin. FEBS Lett 2006; 580(16):4000–4004.
34. Buchanan TA, Xiang AH. Gestational diabetes mellitus. J Clin Invest 2005; 115 (3):485–491.
35. Pinhas-Hamiel O, Dolan LM, Zeitler PS. Diabetic ketoacidosis among obese African-American adolescents with NIDDM. Diabetes Care 1997; 20(4):484–486.
36. Umpierrez GE, Casals MM, Gebhart SP, et al. Diabetic ketoacidosis in obese African-Americans. Diabetes 1995; 44(7):790–795.
37. Hathout EH, Thomas W, El-Shahawy M, et al. Diabetic autoimmune markers in children and adolescents with type 2 diabetes. Pediatrics 2001; 107(6):E102.
38. Leslie R, Wiliams R, Pozzilli P. Type 1 diabetes and latent autoimmune diabetes. J Clin Endocrinol Metab 2006; 91(5):1654–1659.
39. Libman IM, Becker DJ. Coexistence of type 1 and type 2 diabetes mellitus: "double" diabetes? Pediatr Diabetes 2003; 4(2):110–113.
40. Brooks-Worrell BM, Greenbaum CJ, Palmer JP, et al. Autoimmunity to islet proteins in children diagnosed with new-onset diabetes. J Clin Endocrinol Metab 2004; 89 (5):2222–2227.
41. Gilliam LK, Brooks-Worrell BM, Palmer JP, et al. Autoimmunity and clinical course in children with type 1, type 2, and type 1.5 diabetes. J Autoimmun 2005; 25(3):244–250.
42. Umpaichitra V, Banerji MA, Castells S. Autoantibodies in children with type 2 diabetes mellitus. J Pediatr Endocrinol Metab 2002; 15(suppl 1):525–530.
43. Pozzilli P, Buzzetti R. A new expression of diabetes: double diabetes. Trends Endocrinol Metab 2007; 18(2):52–57.
44. Scott CR, Smith JM, Cradock MM, et al. Characteristics of youth-onset noninsulin-dependent diabetes and insulin-dependent diabetes mellitus at diagnosis. Pediatrics 1997; 100(1):84–91.
45. Lipton RB, Drum M, Burnet D, et al. Obesity at the onset of diabetes in an ethnically diverse population of children: what does it mean for epidemiologists and clinicians? Pediatrics 2005; 115(5):e553–e560.
46. Tuomi T, Groop LC, Zimmet PZ, et al. Antibodies to glutamic acid decarboxylase reveal latent autoimmune diabetes mellitus in adults with a non-insulin-dependent onset of disease. Diabetes 1993; 42(2):359–362.
47. Turner R, Stratton I, Horton V, et al. UKPDS 25: autoantibodies to islet-cell cytoplasm and glutamic acid decarboxylase for prediction of insulin requirement in type 2 diabetes. UK Prospective Diabetes Study Group. Lancet 1997; 350(9087):1288–1293.
48. Fourlanos S, Dotta F, Greenbaum CJ, et al. Latent autoimmune diabetes in adults (LADA) should be less latent. Diabetologia 2005; 48(11):2206–2212.

49. Palmer JP, Hampe CS, Chiu H, et al. Is latent autoimmune diabetes in adults distinct from type 1 diabetes or just type 1 diabetes at an older age? Diabetes 2005; 54(suppl 2): S62–S67.
50. Hosszufalusi N, Vatay A, Rajczy K, et al. Similar genetic features and different islet cell autoantibody pattern of latent autoimmune diabetes in adults (LADA) compared with adult-onset type 1 diabetes with rapid progression. Diabetes Care 2003; 26(2):452–457.
51. Vatay A, Rajczy K, Pozsonyi E, et al. Differences in the genetic background of latent autoimmune diabetes in adults (LADA) and type 1 diabetes mellitus. Immunol Lett 2002; 84(2):109–115.
52. Wilkin T. The accelerator hypothesis: weight gain as the missing link between type I and type II diabetes. Diabetologia 2001; 44(7):914–922.
53. Fourlanos S, Narendran P, Byrnes GB, et al. Insulin resistance is a risk factor for progression to type 1 diabetes. Diabetologia 2004; 47(10):1661–1667.
54. Baum JD, Ounsted M, Smith MA. Letter: weight gain in infancy and subsequent development of diabetes mellitus in childhood. Lancet 1975; 2(7940):866.
55. Johansson C, Samuelsson U, Ludvigsson J. A high weight gain early in life is associated with an increased risk of type 1 (insulin-dependent) diabetes mellitus. Diabetologia 1994; 37(1):91–94.
56. Tuomi T. Type 1 and type 2 diabetes: what do they have in common? Diabetes 2005; 54 (suppl 2):S40–S45.
57. Erbey JR, Kuller LH, Becker DJ, et al. The association between a family history of type 2 diabetes and coronary artery disease in a type 1 diabetes population. Diabetes Care 1998; 21(4):610–614.
58. Fagerudd JA, Pettersson-Fernholm KJ, Gronhagen-Riska C, et al. The impact of a family history of Type II (non-insulin-dependent) diabetes mellitus on the risk of diabetic nephropathy in patients with Type I (insulin-dependent) diabetes mellitus. Diabetologia 1999; 42(5):519–526.
59. Makimattila S, Ylitalo K, Schlenzka A, et al. Family histories of Type II diabetes and hypertension predict intima-media thickness in patients with Type I diabetes. Diabetologia 2002; 45(5):711–718.
60. Forsblom CM, Sane T, Groop PH, et al. Risk factors for mortality in Type II (non-insulin-dependent) diabetes: evidence of a role for neuropathy and a protective effect of HLA-DR4. Diabetologia 1998; 41(11):1253–1262.
61. Li H, Isomaa B, Taskinen MR, Groop L, et al. Consequences of a family history of type 1 and type 2 diabetes on the phenotype of patients with type 2 diabetes. Diabetes Care 2000; 23(5):589–594.
62. Chaparro RJ, Konigshofer Y, Beilhack GF, et al. Nonobese diabetic mice express aspects of both type 1 and type 2 diabetes. Proc Natl Acad Sci U S A 2006; 103(33):12475–12480.
63. Donath M, Ehses J. Type 1, type 1.5, and type 2 diabetes: *NOD* the diabetes we thought it was. Proc Natl Acad Sci U S A 2006; 103(33):12217–12218.
64. Gale EA. Declassifying diabetes. Diabetologia 2006; 49(9):1989–1995.

2 Descriptive Epidemiology of Type 1 Diabetes in Youth: Incidence, Mortality, Prevalence, and Secular Trends

Anders Green
Department of Epidemiology, Institute of Public Health, University of Southern Denmark and Department of Applied Research and Health Technology Assessment, Odense University Hospital, Odense, Denmark

INTRODUCTION

Diabetes mellitus with onset in childhood represents one of the most frequent chronic diseases in children and young adults. The disease is associated with a significant burden to society and patients because most cases require lifelong treatment with insulin as well as access to day-to-day monitoring and treatment of complications and because the disease confers increased risk of severe late complications such as renal failure, blindness, amputations, heart disease, and stroke. Even in societies with unrestricted access to the treatment of diabetes and its complications, the disease is associated with the risk of premature death.

This chapter concerns the contemporary epidemiological characteristics of type 1 diabetes with onset in the age group 0–14 years, with a particular focus on the projected future trends in the global epidemiology of the disease. Only type 1 diabetes with onset in childhood will be considered. Even though the clinical presentation of type 2 diabetes represents a growing problem in childhood and adolescence, the available epidemiological information suggests that so far patients with type 2 diabetes in childhood are outnumbered by cases with classical type 1 diabetes (1,2). Type 2 diabetes with onset in childhood will be dealt with elsewhere in this volume.

The etiology and pathogenesis of childhood-onset type 1 diabetes are reviewed from various perspectives elsewhere in this volume and will only be commented upon sporadically. It is, however, important to note that it is generally accepted that type 1 diabetes develops as a consequence of interaction(s) between susceptibility genotypes and environmental factors.

THE EPIDEMIOLOGY OF TYPE 1 DIABETES IN CHILDREN

During the last decades large international collaborative studies, using standardized ascertainment schemes, such as the Diabetes Epidemiology Research International (DERI) studies (3), WHO Diabetes Mondiale (WHO DiaMond) Project (4), and studies on the childhood-onset type 1 diabetes as part of the Concerted Action EURODIAB (Europe and Diabetes) Program (5), have offered significant contributions to our knowledge of the global epidemiology of the disease. Yet, epidemiological data on type 1 diabetes are still lacking for the major part of the global population of children, especially in Africa, Asia, and South America (4).

Incidence

The measure of incidence represents an enumeration of new cases of a disease in a well-defined population. Incidence may be expressed in absolute numbers and in rates (where the absolute numbers are expressed relative to the background population at risk of developing the disease). It is important to stress that incidence is specific for the calendar time period during which new cases are accumulated. Even though the incidence level may be constant over a period, any changes in the demography of the background risk population will lead to changes in the *absolute* number of incident cases over time.

Type 1 diabetes in children typically has a rather abrupt onset with a few weeks of specific symptoms and may be even diagnosed on the background of severe ketoacidosis. This consideration, combined with the fact that the health care of sick children is often centralized in societies with well-established health care systems, makes regional incidence-based registration systems feasible. On the other hand, in societies without a well-organized health care service and with limited access to treatment and care, it is difficult to establish a valid incidence registration system, and even the diagnosis of type 1 diabetes may be missed.

Geography

The incidence of childhood-onset type 1 diabetes exhibits huge geographical variation. The recent account from the DiaMond studies covers incidence registrations from year 1990 until year 2000 and has demonstrated a >350-fold variability in incidence level across the populations studied (4). Finland has a record high incidence level at more than 40 new cases per 100,000 children at risk, whereas regions in China have the lowest recorded incidence level at about 0.1 cases per 100,000 children at risk. Europe, particularly Finland and the Scandinavian countries, is generally considered the continent with the highest risk level, but even within Europe a substantial variability has been demonstrated between populations (6) with a range from the record high incidence in Finland to a level at some 4.2 cases per 100,000 in the Former Yugoslavian Republic of Macedonia (6). In the American continent, the incidence level is relatively high in the Caucasian populations of the United States and Canada with an incidence level approaching that of Norway and Sweden (4). Africa and particularly Asia represent continents where the incidence level is low, but the estimates are affected by some uncertainties due to possible underreporting in societies with less developed health care systems (4). In terms of population size, Oceania is dominated by Australia and New Zealand where the incidence level is comparable to that seen in Central and Western Europe (4).

Ethnicity

The incidence of childhood-onset type 1 diabetes by ethnicity correlates strongly with the variability in incidence across countries. In general, Caucasian populations, in particular of Northern European ancestry, have the highest incidence levels (4). As mentioned above, the incidence levels in the Scandinavian countries parallel those of Canada, the United States (non-Hispanic whites), and New Zealand and Australia. Even within Europe, remarkably sharp contrasts are found between neighboring countries and populations (6). Thus, Sardinia represents a ''hot spot'' with an incidence level approaching that of Finland, which is several times higher than the surrounding Italian and other neighboring populations. Estonia, with its ethnic and cultural similarities with Finland, has an incidence level that is several times less than in Finland. Iceland, founded many centuries ago by migration from Western Norway, has an incidence level much less than the level in Norway and even smaller rates than in the United Kingdom from where there may have been genetic admixture to the Icelandic population.

It seems that non-Caucasian populations generally have low or very low incidence levels of childhood-onset type 1 diabetes. In the native populations of the Pacific region and in Inuit, the incidence is considered extremely low. All Asian populations studied so far have very low incidence levels and the same apply to sub-Saharan Africa. However, incidence estimates from rural populations in Asia and sub-Saharan Africa with less advanced health care services are difficult to obtain and afflicted with considerable uncertainty due to a high probability of misdiagnosis and underreporting of childhood-onset type 1 diabetes.

Temporal Variation

The incidence of childhood-onset type 1 diabetes exhibits remarkable temporal variation concerning seasonality at onset and secular trends.

It has been found repeatedly that the clinical onset of the disease occurs relatively more frequently in the winter months in both the northern and southern hemispheres (7,8). Possibly, this pattern of seasonality is most pronounced for children with diagnosis around puberty and less pronounced for those with onset within the first years of life (6).

For the last few decades it has been known that the incidence of childhood-onset type 1 diabetes has been on a steady rise since about World War II (4,6,9–11). Because the contemporary incidence level is rather low in most non-Caucasian populations, this trend in increasing incidence has been most pronounced for Caucasian populations. In fact, on the basis of a compilation of the old literature and clinical reports, it has been found plausible that in Scandinavia the incidence level was five- to sixfold less than the contemporary level in the pre–World War II era (12). Reports from the cumulative data from the large international collaborative incidence registration systems have consistently found that since about 1990 the incidence of childhood-onset type 1 diabetes has been rising about 3% annually (4,6). This applies to European populations as well as globally, with the possible exemption of Central America and West Indies where the incidence seems to decrease (4). It remains unknown whether the increase in incidence in low-risk populations represents a recent phenomenon. For European populations it has been found that the absolute annual increment in the incidence level is similar for the age groups 0–4, 5–9, and 10–14 years. Since the incidence level is lowest in the younger age groups, the relative increase in incidence may appear larger for these age groups as compared with the older age groups (6).

The Incidence of Type 1 Diabetes in Children: Implications for Understanding the Etiology

Descriptive epidemiological data support the generation of hypotheses concerning disease etiology and pathogenesis, but in general, evidence from specifically designed studies will be needed to reach conclusions that are more firm. This strategy also applies to a lifelong disease like childhood-onset type 1 diabetes. Since aspects related to the etiology and pathogenesis of childhood-onset type 1 diabetes will be dealt with elsewhere in this volume, only a few highlights of the inference made from descriptive epidemiology concerning these aspects will be reviewed here.

The increasing trend in incidence of childhood-onset type 1 diabetes seems to represent a global phenomenon, regardless of whether the general background population-risk level is low or high. It is also well established that the disease develops as a consequence of interaction(s) between genetic susceptibility and environmental factors. There is no possible way to explain the increasing trend, taking place over a few generations' time, by major changes in the distribution of susceptibility genes in the respective background populations across the world. Even today, in high-risk population, by far the most cases of child-onset type 1 diabetes will appear in families where the disease is unknown among the close relatives. This means that the pool of susceptibility genes is maintained most of all by subjects without the disease and thereby unaffected by changes in the prognosis and reproduction capacity of the patients. The only possible implication is that either subjects carrying susceptibility genes are to an increasing extent being more susceptible to precipitate type 1 diabetes because of influences within their environment and/or that new environmental agents are being introduced in the society, with the development of new disease-promoting genotype-environment interactions as a consequence.

Another, and correlated, issue relates to the question whether the increase in incidence, as documented for childhood-onset type 1 diabetes, generalizes to the age classes above childhood. If this is not the case, the increasing incidence seen in childhood-onset type 1 diabetes may simply reflect a situation with "anticipation," i.e., in modern societies, subjects carrying susceptibility genotypes eventually develop the type 1 diabetes phenotype at an earlier age than previously, implying that the lifetime risk (assuming survival from other causes independent from type 1 diabetes) may be unchanged over time. So far, empirical studies from both populations with high and with low background incidence levels, where it has been possible to monitor incidence trends in age groups up to 40 years of age, have been inconclusive (13,14). The distinct feature that the clinical onset of type 1 diabetes in children occurs more frequently in winter months must relate to factors influencing the last stages of the pathogenic process that by immune-mediated mechanisms destroys the insulin-producing β-cells of the pancreas. Because immune markers of preclinical type 1 diabetes may appear for a long time, maybe even years, before type 1 diabetes develops clinically, it is difficult to imply from the patterns of seasonality at diagnosis to etiological mechanisms.

Mortality

Without insulin treatment, patients with type 1 diabetes will die within one to two years after clinical onset. Even in societies with unrestricted access to insulin treatment and well-organized health care systems, type 1 diabetes confers a considerable risk of premature death due to acute and late complications as well as accompanying diseases of the heart, vessels, and nervous system.

Valid reports on mortality in children with type 1 diabetes are rare. Nevertheless, studies from developed countries have consistently reported that the relative mortality (all causes considered) in type 1 diabetes is of the magnitude of about 3, corresponding with a mortality rate at about 1/1000 patient-years at risk in children aged 0 to 14 years (15–17). The excess mortality in children is predominantly attributable to acute complications (mainly ketoacidosis), infections, external causes, and unexplained deaths (15–19). The studies have also indicated that the mortality may be higher in countries with lower incidence levels (18–21), suggesting that awareness and knowledge of managing type 1 diabetes in children may be an important factor (22).

Children with type 1 diabetes in societies without access to insulin, blood-glucose monitoring, and health care services face a very high risk of dying in connection with the diagnosis of type 1 diabetes or soon after disease onset due to acute complications. In many such children it is likely that type one diabetes may have remained undiagnosed, being masked by the clinical picture of competing infectious diseases and malnutrition (23). The situation for the children with type 1 diabetes in these societies is similar to the children in the developed part of the world before the introduction of insulin treatment and modern diabetes care.

Prevalence

Prevalence as a measure is defined as the size (in absolute number or as a proportion) of the patient population in a well-defined general population at a given point of time. It is important to realize that the prevalence is a consequence of the number of new cases (incidence) and the number of deaths (regardless of cause of death) among the patients and the number of cured patients that have occurred prior to the point of time the prevalence estimate refers to. In this context, migrations across the borders delineating the population concerned have been ignored. Thus, the prevalence at a given point of time depends not only on past incidence levels and secular trends in incidence but also on mortality and changes in mortality. Another determinant of the prevalence is past changes in the size of the population at risk of developing the disease since such trends affect the accumulated absolute number of incident cases. Because type 1 diabetes is a lifelong disease, currently without the possibility of a cure, the only possible mode of exit from the prevalence population of patients is death (again, ignoring migrations to and from the population). However, when restricting the scope to the population of children aged 0 to 14 years, transitions to age 15 years represent another mode of exit from the prevalence population of affected children.

Empirical estimates of the prevalence of type 1 diabetes in children are relatively rare. In areas with no or restricted access to treatment and care, it must be assumed that the prevalence of type 1 diabetes in children is low and mainly determined by the incidence level, since the patients will most likely die shortly after diagnosis. In societies with well-developed system for treatment and care of children with the disease, it is reasonable to assume that only few children with the disease will die before reaching the age of 15 years, even in spite of the increased relative mortality (see above). In these societies, the prevalence of type 1 diabetes in children will depend largely on past accumulated numbers of incident cases incidence as well as of upgrades to 15 years of age.

The Diabetes Atlas, updated by the International Diabetes Federation every third year since year 2000, presents global estimates of the incidence and prevalence of type 1 diabetes in children (1,24,25). These estimates have been produced by combining known or assumed incidence numbers with expected mean duration of the disease from the time of diagnosis until death or reaching the age of 15 years. The estimates have been established for each country in the World, with subsequent grouping into global regions. Estimates of the contemporary and future prevalence of type 1 diabetes in children will be presented below.

EPIDEMIOLOGICAL PROJECTIONS OF TYPE 1 DIABETES IN CHILDREN

Methodology

Epidemiological projections of type 1 diabetes in children involve estimation of the future incidence, mortality, and prevalence of the disease. This procedure requires knowledge (or, at least, reasonably valid estimates) of the prevalence of the disease, size of the background population, mortality level, and incidence level at a specified starting point in calendar time as well as assumptions concerning any future trends in background population demography, incidence, and mortality. Thus, the future prevalence will depend on the current prevalence level and any future changes in demography, incidence, and prognosis.

For the present purpose, epidemiological projections for type 1 diabetes in children aged 0 to 14 years are made for the period 2000–2025. This has been achieved by applying epidemiological modeling techniques previously described (26) and consists of building up year by year the future prevalence under assumptions concerning baseline estimates of prevalence, incidence, mortality, and background population size as well as the future annual levels of incidence, mortality, and population size. Formally, this estimate may be expressed as follows:

Number of prevalent cases$_{\text{end of year } t+1}$ = Number of prevalent cases$_{\text{end of year } t}$ + number of incident cases$_{\text{during year } t}$ − number of deaths$_{\text{during year } t}$ − number of upgrades to age 15 years$_{\text{during year } t}$.

The projections have been made at the level of the five continents, i.e., for Europe, Asia, America, Africa, and Oceania, with summary aggregation at global level.

Information on the size of the population of children in the age group 0–14 years has been obtained similarly to that used for the Diabetes Atlas 2000, with estimates of annual growth in the population size obtained from information available with the World Bank (27).

The prevalence estimates (in absolute numbers) of type 1 diabetes in children aged 0 to 14 years at the end of year 1999 follow those published with the Diabetes Atlas 2000 (24).

The estimated numbers of incident cases and corresponding incidence rates for year 2000 also follow those published with the Diabetes Atlas 2000 (24). Concerning the incidence rates during the period 2000 through 2024, it is assumed that for each continent the incidence will increase with an increment corresponding to 3% of the incidence rate by year 2000. Using increments rather than proportional annual increases is considered more realistic since it will lead to a linear increase rather than an exponential increase in the incidence rates during the period concerned. The mortality rates in children with type 1 diabetes have been assumed as follows: For well-established societies with optimal facilities for managing treatment and care of children with type 1 diabetes, a mortality rate at 0.09 deaths per 100 patient-years has been used. In contrast, in less developed societies the mortality rate is assumed to be much higher, representing an average with a range from an extremely high value at some 65 deaths per 100 patient-years (assuming that the patients die within 1.5 years) to the mortality level seen in well-established societies (assuming that some population segments in the less developed countries have access to optimal treatment and care). It is globally assumed that the mortally rate is decreasing by 2% annually from year 2000 under the expectation of continuous improvements in the access to insulin and diabetes care in less developed societies.

In the modeled projections, it is a delicate issue how to adjust for the children with childhood-onset type 1 diabetes that live beyond the age of 15 years and thus disappear from the universe of patients concerned. For the present purpose, it has been assumed that globally the mean age at diagnosis of type 1 diabetes among children aged 0 to 14 years is 8 years. This means that for patients who do not die before reaching the age of 15 years, the mean length of stay in the population of children with type 1 diabetes is 7 years. Accordingly, the annual number of children who upgrade from childhood to age 15 years has been estimated with a rate of upgrading at $1/7 = 14.3/100$ patient-years. The rate of upgrading has, for a given year, been applied to the size of the prevalent population the year before minus the estimated number of deaths for the year before.

Baseline Characteristics Year 2000

Table 1 (upper panel) summarizes the key baseline data estimated for year 2000. Concerning incidence, about 100,000 children aged 0 to 14 years developed diabetes within year 2000. In spite of a low incidence level in Asia, this continent contributed with almost half of the incident cases because of the huge population of children in Asia. In contrast, Europe together with Oceania contributed with less than 20% to the global incidence in spite of high incidence levels. America, representing a high incidence level in North America and lower incidence levels in Central and South America, contributed with 20–25% of the global incidence. The African continent, representing about 19% of the global population of children, contributed with less than 10% because of the assumed low incidence level.

The mortality rate varies considerably between continents as reviewed above. Oceania has the lowest assumed mortality rate because this continent is, in terms of prevalence of type 1 diabetes in children, completely dominated by Australia and New Zealand, and the patients here are assumed to have close to optimal living conditions with type 1 diabetes. The mortality rate in Europe is assumed to be slightly lower because Europe also represents populations that may not yet have reached a level of optimal treatment and care of children with type 1 diabetes. America is considered to have a somewhat higher mortality level because of the inclusion of patients from less developed countries in South America. Asia and, in particular, Africa are continents in which the mortality rate must be considered high and in certain societies at the level seen in the developed societies before insulin treatment was introduced. The mortality rates applied in Asia and Africa for year 2000 represent weighted averages across subregions by socioeconomic development within each of these continents. Regarding worldwide prevalence of type 1 diabetes, it is estimated that among some 2 billion children aged 0 to 14 years almost 400,000 (0.2 per 1000) had type 1 diabetes at the end of year 1999. In spite of low incidence level and high mortality level, Asia has the largest contribution ($\sim 43\%$) to the global prevalence because of its huge background population of children. On the relative scale, Europe and Oceania have the highest prevalence level because of high incidence level and low mortality level. In America, representing a mixture of the well-developed societies in North America and less developed societies in South America, the prevalence proportion is slightly less than those of Europe and Oceania because of slightly lower incidence and slightly higher mortality level. The prevalence proportion is considered to be very low in Africa because of a combination of low incidence and high mortality levels.

Table 1 (lower panel) specifies the annual changes that have been considered in the epidemiological projections concerning background population size, incidence rate, and mortality rate as discussed above.

TABLE 1 Baseline Data (Year 2000) and Parameters for Projecting Epidemiological Indicators of Type 1 Diabetes

	Europe	Asia	America	Africa	Oceania	World
Baseline data for year 2000						
Population size (number in 1000s)	147,465	1,234,896	248,141	376,928	7,447	2,014,877
Incidence rate (per 100,000)	11.96	3.91	9.20	2.59	10.35	4.93
Incidence (number)	17,637	48,284	22,829	9,753	771	99,274
Mortality rate (per 100 patient-years)	0.11	9.04	0.27	11.30	0.09	4.86
Mortality in patient population (numbers)	93	15,291	282	3,498	4	19,167
Prevalence (number)	85,985	169,159	103,920	30,956	4,248	394,269
Prevalence proportion (per 1000)	0.58	0.14	0.43	0.08	0.57	0.20
Parameters for projection, years 2000–2025						
Annual growth rate (%) in population size	0.07	1.70	1.50	2.90	0.10	1.77
Annual increment in incidence rate (per 100,000)	0.312	0.102	0.240	0.068	0.270	0.246
Annual reduction (%) in mortality rate	0.02	0.02	0.02	0.02	0.02	0.02

All quantities refer to the population restricted to age group 0–14 years.

Scenario Building

For the epidemiological projection of the epidemiology of childhood-onset type 1 diabetes over the period 2000–2025, various scenarios have been established. The key *reference scenario* represents the situation where population growth, increase in incidence, and reduction in mortality from baseline in year 2000 are controlled by the parameters listed in Table 1 (lower panel).

In order to estimate the effects of population growth and changes in the incidence and mortality levels, alternative scenarios have been established. The most simplistic scenario represents the situation where it is assumed that there is no growth in the population at risk of childhood-onset type 1 diabetes and changes in neither incidence level nor mortality level. This scenario explores the effects of epidemiological equilibrium: If the demographic composition and size of the background population remains unchanged and if there are no trends in incidence and mortality, a disease will reach a state of epidemiological equilibrium, i.e., the prevalence remains stable and the annual incidence equals annual mortality. If, on the other hand, one or more of these quantities exhibit trends over time, the disease will be in a state of epidemiological disequilibrium and the prevalence will change over time because of imbalance between annual incidence and annual mortality. Currently, it is reasonable to assume that childhood-onset type 1 diabetes is in a state of epidemiological disequilibrium with increasing prevalence because of the increasing incidence, increasing size of the population, and assumed improving prognosis in a substantial part of the world.

Another scenario reflects the situation where the background population at risk is assumed to grow but where changes in incidence and mortality are not allowed. The difference between the result of this scenario and the scenario representing no changes at all estimates the part of the change in the future prevalence that is attributable to changes in the demography of the background population. The impact on the future prevalence resulting from future changes in incidence is explored similarly in a scenario where changes in population size and incidence level are allowed for, but the future mortality is kept constant.

Finally, the impact on the future prevalence resulting from future changes in the mortality level is estimated by contrasting the key reference scenario with that characterized by changes in demography and incidence only.

WORLDWIDE INCIDENCE AND PREVALENCE OF TYPE 1 DIABETES IN CHILDREN 2000–2025

Projection of Incidence

The projected annual global numbers of incident cases are illustrated in Figure 1 within three contrasting scenarios. Under the assumptions of growth in the size of the population of children and increasing incidence rates as specified in Table 1, the annual number of incident cases will increase from almost 100,000 in year 2000 to some 240,000 in year 2025. Almost half of this increase during the period is accounted for solely by the expected growth in the population of children, since assuming constant incidence rates across continents from year 2000, the annual number of new cases is expected to rise to some 145,000 by year 2025.

Projection of Prevalence

Figure 2 shows the future projected global prevalence in absolute numbers of type 1 diabetes in children aged 0 to 14 years. Even assuming no growth in the

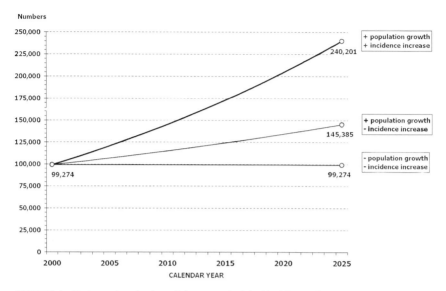

FIGURE 1 Estimated projection of the annual global incidence (in absolute numbers) of type 1 diabetes with onset in age group 0–14 years by contrasting scenarios. For specification of scenarios, see Table 1 and text.

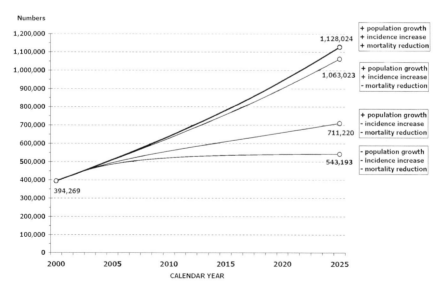

FIGURE 2 Estimated projection of the annual global prevalence (in absolute numbers) of type 1 diabetes in age group 0–14 years by contrasting scenarios. For specification of scenarios, see Table 1 and text.

background population at risk and unchanged incidence and mortality rates from year 2000 onward, the prevalence is expected to rise from almost 400,000 children in year 2000 to almost 550,000 by year 2025. This rise is an effect of the epidemiological disequilibrium that characterizes childhood-onset type 1 diabetes. Allowing for growth in the background population but no changes in incidence and mortality rates will result in a prevalence number at more than 710,000 by year 2025. If future increases in incidence (as specified in Table 1) but no further improvements in the prognosis are also allowed for, the expected prevalence number will be more than 1,000,000. Finally, in the key reference scenario, also allowing for future improvements in prognosis, the projected prevalence number by year 2025 is expected to be almost 1,130,000 children. Since it is unrealistic to assume no increase in the global population of children and no further increase in the incidence rate, it seems reasonable to assume that the prevalence by year 2025 will comprise at least some 1,000,000 children aged 0 to 14 years.

The upper part of Table 2 enumerates the estimated prevalence under the key reference scenario for the end of year 2024 globally as well as by continent. Worldwide, the expected increase in prevalence since the end of year 1999 corresponds with 186%. However, the increase varies considerably across the continents, with the relatively smallest increases expected in Oceania and Europe and the largest increases expected in America, Asia, and particularly Africa.

Drivers of the Future Prevalence
The lower part of Table 2 quantifies the components that drive the future prevalence increase. Globally, almost half of the increase in prevalence is estimated to be caused by the assumed increasing incidence; some 20% may be ascribed to the effect of epidemiological disequilibrium and about 23% will be accounted for by demographical evolution. The assumed improvement in prognosis accounts for only 9% of the expected increase in prevalence.

The drivers of the prevalence increase vary markedly across the continents. Thus, the effect of assumed improvement in prognosis is relatively largest in Asia and Africa where the current mortality level supposedly is considerably higher than elsewhere. In the more developed continents like Oceania, Europe, and partly America, the effect of epidemiological disequilibrium is relatively largest and the effects of demographical changes and improved prognosis are very modest (with the exemption of America concerning population growth).

COMMENTS

Childhood-onset type 1 diabetes represents a global health problem and is a disease undergoing dramatic epidemiological changes, with marked differences in the epidemiological characteristics between the continents. Inevitably, projections of the future incidence and prevalence will depend on the assumptions made in the epidemiological modeling. In the analysis presented here, most uncertainty must be attached to the assumptions regarding current and future mortality. However, the projections also suggest that the effects on the future prevalence from future changes in mortality are modest only. It is therefore reasonable to assume that the prevalence of type 1 diabetes will increase dramatically and reach a level about 1,000,000 children by year 2025, against a level at less than 400,000 by year 2000. The prevalence will increase most in the less developed part of the world, even

TABLE 2 Estimated Global Prevalence of Type 1 Diabetes in Children Aged 0 to 14 Years for Year 2025 by Continent, with Estimated Increase in Prevalence Numbers Since Year 2000 and the Break Down of the Increase by Contributable Components

	Europe	Asia	America	Africa	Oceania	World
Estimated population size by year 2025 (number in 1000's)	150,067	1,882,150	360,038	770,269	7,636	3,170,160
Estimated prevalence (number) by end of year 2024	179,519	516,540	298,688	125,374	7,903	1,128,024
Estimated increase in prevalence (number) since year 2000	93,534	347,381	194,768	94,418	3,654	733,755
Increase (in %)	109	205	187	305	86	186
Estimated increase in prevalence (numbers) attributable to						
Epidemiological disequilibrium	35,909	49,934	52,258	9,728	1,094	148,924
Growth in population at risk	1,488	87,442	46,868	32,137	93	168,028
Increase in incidence	55,840	160,085	94,504	38,917	2,456	351,803
Reduced mortality	297	49,920	1,137	13,636	11	65,001
Proportion of increase in prevalence attributable to (in %)						
Epidemiological disequilibrium	38.4	14.4	26.8	10.3	29.9	20.3
Growth in population at risk	1.6	25.%	24.1	34.0	2.6	22.9
Increase in incidence	59.7	46.1	48.5	41.2	67.2	47.9
Reduced mortality	0.3	14.4	0.6	14.4	0.3	8.9

though the incidence level is lowest here. The future expected increase in the prevalence of type 1 diabetes in children represents an increasing burden to society and health care systems that must be acknowledged and managed appropriately to ensure treatment and access to care for the increasing number of patients.

REFERENCES

1. International Diabetes Federation. Diabetes Atlas. 3rd ed. Brussels: The International Diabetes Federation, 2006.
2. Writing Group for the SEARCH for Diabetes in Youth Study Group. Incidence of diabetes in youth in the United States. The SEARCH for Diabetes in Youth Study. JAMA 2007; 297:2716–2724.
3. Diabetes Epidemiology Research International Group. Geographic patterns of childhood insulin-dependent diabetes mellitus. Diabetes 1988; 37:1113–1119.
4. The DIAMOND Project Group. Incidence and trends of childhood type 1 diabetes worldwide 1990–1999. Diabet Med 2006; 23:857–866.
5. Green A. The EURODIAB studies on childhood diabetes 1988–1999. Diabetologia 2001; 44(suppl 3):B1–B2.
6. Green A, Patterson CC on behalf of the EURODIAB TIGER Study Group. Trends in the incidence of childhood-onset diabetes in Europe 1989–1998. Diabetologia 2001; 44 (suppl 3):B3–B8.
7. Fishbein HA, LaPorte RE, Orchard TJ, et al. The Pittsburgh insulin-dependent diabetes mellitus registry: seasonal incidence. Diabetologia 1982; 23:83–85.
8. Durruty P, Ruiz F, Garcia de los Rios M. Age at diagnosis and seasonal variation in the onset of insulin-dependent diabetes in Chile (southern hemisphere). Diabetologia 1979; 17:357–360.
9. Patterson CC, Thorogood M, Smith PG, et al. Epidemiology of type 1 (insulin-dependent) diabetes in Scotland 1968–1976: evidence of an increasing incidence. Diabetologia 1983; 24:238–243.
10. Green A, Andersen PK. Epidemiological studies of diabetes mellitus in Denmark: 3. Clinical characteristics and incidence of diabetes among males aged 0 to 19 years. Diabetologia 1983; 25:226–230.
11. Bingley PJ, Gale EAM. Rising incidence of IDDM in Europe. Diabetes Care 1989; 12: 289–295.
12. Gale EAM. The rise of childhood type 1 diabetes in the 20th century. Diabetes 2002; 51:3353–3361.
13. Feltbower RG, McKinney PA, Parslow RC, et al. Type 1 diabetes in Yorkshire, UK: time trends in 0–14 and 15–29-year-olds, age at onset and age-period-cohort modelling. Diabet Med 2003; 20:437–441.
14. Kyvik KO, Nystrom L, Gorus F, et al. The epidemiology of type 1 diabetes is not the same in young adults as in children. Diabetologia 2004; 47:377–384.
15. Laron-Kenet T, Shamis I, Weitzman S, et al. Mortality of patients with childhood onset (0–17 years) type I diabetes in Israel: a population-based study. Diabetologia 2001; 44 (suppl 3):B81–B86.
16. Dahlquist G, Källen B. Mortality in childhood-onset type 1 diabetes. Diabetes Care 2005; 28:2384–2387.
17. Skrivarhaug T, Bangstad H-J, Stene LC, et al. Long-term mortality in a nationwide cohort of childhood-onset type 1 diabetic patients in Norway. Diabetologia 2006; 49:298–305.
18. Podar T, Solntsev A, Reunanen A, et al. Mortality in patients with childhood-onset type 1 diabetes in Finland, Estonia, and Lithuania. Follow-up of nationwide cohorts. Diabetes Care 2000; 23:290–294.
19. Barcelo A, Bosnyak Z, Orchard T. A cohort analysis of type 1 diabetes mortality in Havana and Allegheny County, Pittsburgh, PA. Diabetes Res Clin Pract 2007; 75: 214–219.

20. Urbonaite B, Zalinkevicius R, Green A. Incidence, prevalence, and mortality of insulin-dependent (type 1) diabetes mellitus in Lithuanian children during 1983–98. Pediatr Diabetes 2002; 3:23–30.
21. Asa K, Sarti C Forsen T, et al. Long-term mortality in nationwide cohorts of childhood-onset type 1 diabetes in Japan and Finland. Diabetes Care 2003; 26:2037–2042.
22. Levy-Marchal C, Patterson CC, Green A on behalf of the EURODIAB ACE Study Group. Geographical variation of presentation at diagnosis of Type I diabetes in children: the EURODIAB study. Diabetologia 2001; 44(suppl 3):B75–B80.
23. Beran D, Yudkin JS. Diabetes care in sub-Saharan Africa. The Lancet 2006; 368: 1689–1695.
24. International Diabetes Federation. Diabetes Atlas 2000. Brussels: The International Diabetes Federation, 2000.
25. International Diabetes Federation. Diabetes Atlas 2003. Brussels: The International Diabetes Federation, 2003.
26. Green A, Sjølie AK, Eshøj O. Trends in the epidemiology of IDDM during 1970–2020 in Fyn County, Denmark. Diabetes Care 1996; 19:801–806.
27. http://web.worldbank.org. Accessed May 2007.

3 | Genetic Epidemiology of Type 1 Diabetes

George S. Eisenbarth and Theresa A. Aly
Barbara Davis Center for Childhood Diabetes and Human Medical Genetics Program,
University of Colorado at Denver and Health Sciences Center, Aurora, Colorado, U.S.A.

INTRODUCTION

Diabetes mellitus results from multiple genetic and pathologic processes in human and animal models. The current nomenclature from the American Diabetes Association Expert Committee classifies diabetes into broad groups on the basis of the etiological causes of diabetes. This review focuses on type 1A diabetes, which is caused by the immune-mediated destruction of β cells. Type 1A diabetes is a genetically heterogeneous disorder with certain well-defined rare syndromes. In particular, both the neonatal diabetes of the immunodysregulation, polyendocrino-pathy, enteropathy, X-linked (IPEX) syndrome and the diabetes of approximately 15% of patients with autoimmune polyendocrine syndrome type 1 (APS-1) are determined by major "monogenic" mutations (IPEX: *FOXP3* gene and APS-1: *AIRE* gene) (1–3). In contrast, type 1A diabetes is more typically associated with a polygenic pattern of inheritance (typical type 1A diabetes), with risk predominantly determined by genes within or linked to the major histocompatibility complex (MHC) on chromosome 6. The rare monogenic syndromes provide important and precise information as to the pathologic processes that can cause immune-mediated diabetes when mechanisms of self-tolerance fail. It is likely that mutations of the *FOXP3* gene lead to diabetes by eliminating a major class of regulatory T lymphocytes (CD4+CD25+), while mutations of the *AIRE* gene contribute to diabetes by decreasing the expression of "peripheral" antigens within the thymus, such as insulin, and thereby reduce the negative selection of T cells within the thymus (4).

It is likely that just as critical but less dramatic failures of mechanisms of maintenance of self-tolerance cause typical type 1A diabetes. In addition, the genes associated with typical type 1A diabetes have a lower penetrance than the genes associated with the monogenic forms of type 1A diabetes, and typical type 1A diabetes is more likely to be influenced by environmental factors. A general hypothesis is that type 1A diabetes is mediated by autoreactive T lymphocytes and that polymorphic HLA alleles (e.g., *HLA-DP, HLA-DQ, HLA-DR, HLA-A*, and *HLA-B*), which influence the targeting of islet β-cell antigens in combination with polymorphisms of genes, which in turn influence T-cell receptor signaling (e.g., *PTPN22, CTLA4*) or expression of major islet autoantigens (e.g., *INS* gene), determine the probability that an individual will develop type 1A diabetes. To date, genetic loci/genes associated with type II diabetes (e.g., *TCF7L2*) do not appear to contribute to the genetic risk of type 1A diabetes (5), and insulin resistance is likely not crucial to genetic susceptibility of type 1A diabetes, although it can influence when an individual will present with hyperglycemia.

PATHOPHYSIOLOGY: GENES AND THE ENVIRONMENT

The onset of type 1A diabetes occurs when the destruction of pancreatic β cells by the immune system has progressed to a level where not enough insulin is being produced to regulate glucose levels in the blood. The onset of diabetes in both humans and animal models is associated with insulitis, an infiltrate of CD8 and CD4 T lymphocytes, B lymphocytes, and macrophages (6). Whereas the etiology of the autoimmune attack on the β cells is not fully understood, evidence suggests that an environmental exposure, such as an infection (7) or a food introduction (e.g., cereal exposure prior to 3 months of age) (8), may lead to autoimmunity in individuals with an underlying genetic predisposition for diabetes. Vitamin D deficiency might also contribute to risk for diabetes (9).

Interestingly, the infection of a colony of diabetes resistant BB (DR-BB) rats with the Kilham rat virus led to the spontaneous development of diabetes (10). Extensive studies of this spontaneous animal model suggest that the Kilham rat virus does not infect the islets, but rather activates innate immunity in a genetically susceptible animal leading to T-cell mediated islet β-cell destruction. Similarly, activation of the innate immune system with inosinic cytidylic acid (poly-IC), a mimic of double-stranded RNA, can induce diabetes. For diabetes to develop with poly-IC injection, a rat strain must have high-risk MHC alleles, such as RT1-U (11). In a similar poly-IC mouse model, the induction of interferon alfa expression following poly-IC injection is essential for the triggering of diabetes (12). Thus, relatively nonspecific activation of innate immunity by viruses in genetically susceptible individuals may relate to diabetes induction.

The one viral infection clearly associated with type 1A diabetes in humans is congenital rubella infection, but only congenital (resulting from rubella exposure in utero). Predominantly, individuals with higher genetic susceptibility (i.e., with higher risk HLA alleles) develop diabetes following congenital rubella (13), and the onset of diabetes often occurs decades after birth. These individuals are also at a higher risk for a series of other autoimmune disorders, in particular, thyroiditis. One possible explanation for the clinical course of these individuals is that the rubella virus induces long-term changes in T-cell function that leads to an increase in diabetes risk (14).

POPULATION STUDIES

Type 1A diabetes affects approximately 1.4 million people in the United States, with siblings at a higher risk than offspring, and both with a higher risk than the general population (sibling risk relative to population risk, $\lambda_s = 6/0.4 = 15$) (15–17). Approximately half of the newly diagnosed cases of type 1A diabetes occur in adults and the condition is one of the most common chronic diseases diagnosed in youth (15). Approximately 160,000 children in the United States under the age of 15 years have type 1A diabetes (15). The SEARCH for Diabetes in Youth study found a crude prevalence of 2.8 cases out of 1000 children at ages 10 through 19 years, with the highest prevalence in non-Hispanic white children (3.2 per 1000) (18). The incidence of type 1A diabetes is increasing in most countries around the world; the EURODIAB study has reported an increased incidence of approximately 3–4% each year in Europe (19). Interestingly, there is a large amount of variation of disease incidence by country, with a child in Finland at 100 times the risk for type 1A diabetes than a child in the Zunyi region of China (19).

The incidence of type 1A diabetes is particularly increasing in developed countries around the world, and it is postulated that the increased risk of diabetes is caused by a change (an increase or a decrease) in environmental exposures in these countries. Given a genetically susceptible host, one or more environmental exposures may help to protect against the development of immune-mediated diabetes (20). One hypothesis (the "hygiene hypothesis") for the increasing incidence of type 1A diabetes in developed countries is that potentially protective environmental exposures, such as infectious agents, are decreasing in these countries (21). An interesting observation is the unusually high incidence rate of type 1A diabetes in Jewish children from Yemen living in Israel (as high as in Finland), with the highest risk associated with the DR3-DQ2/DR4-DQ8 genotype (22). By oral history, this Jewish population was not aware of any cases of childhood diabetes in their population until they were transplanted from Yemen to Israel. This "anecdote" may well reflect a lower risk of type 1A diabetes in populations that carry major burden of chronic infections (such as in Yemen) and suggests that a major increase in diabetes risk can occur within one generation with a change in environmental exposures (such as with a reduced exposure to pathogens).

TWIN STUDIES

The genetic liability for diabetes has been investigated by comparing concordance rates for diabetes in monozygotic (identical) twins versus dizygotic twins. In a study of 187 initially discordant monozygotic twins in Great Britain and the United States, the nondiabetic monozygotic twin of a proband diagnosed with diabetes prior to six years of age had a 60% risk for developing diabetes within 40 years of follow-up (23). The risk for initially discordant dizygotic twins was reported as being similar to the risk of non-twin siblings (with a risk of 5–10% for diabetes) (24,25). A study of 228 Finish twin pairs with diabetes suggested that 88% of the phenotypic variance was due to genetic factors, and a model with additive genetic and individual environmental effects was the best-fitting liability model (26).

THE MAJOR HISTOCOMPATIBILITY COMPLEX

Although type 1A diabetes is a complex genetic disorder, it is linked more with the MHC region on chromosome 6p21.3 (LOD score ~ 116, $p = 1.9 \times 10^{-52}$) (27) than any other chromosomal region. The *HLA-DR* and *HLA-DQ* genes are established as being associated with diabetes risk by genetic, functional, structural, and animal model studies (28–31). The heterozygous DR3-DQ2/DR4-DQ8 genotype represents the highest risk combination of *HLA-DR* and *HLA-DQ* alleles (with the *HLA-DRB1*03-DQA1*0501-DQB1*0201* and *HLA-DRB1*04-DQA1*0301-DQB1*0302* haplotypes). Only 2.4% of the general population have the high-risk DR3-DQ2/DR4-DQ8 genotype, whereas almost 50% of children developing anti-islet autoimmunity by the age of five years have the DR3-DQ2/DR4-DQ8 genotype (17). Moderate-risk *HLA-DR-DQ* genotypes include the *HLA-DR3-DQ2/DR3-DQ2*, the *HLA-DR4-DQ8/DR4-DQ8*, and the *HLA-DR4-DQ8/X* genotypes (where X is not *DQ2*, *DQ8*, or *DQB1*0602*). Lower-risk genotypes have protective alleles such as *HLA-DQB1*0602*, *HLA-DQB1*0503* (with *HLA-DRB1*1401*), and *HLA-DQB1*0303* (with *HLA-DRB1*0701*). Other *HLA-DQ* genotypes are associated with neutral risk. *HLA-DRB1*04* subtypes can change the risk associated with the *HLA-DR4-DQ8* haplotype. The *HLA-DRB1*0405* and *HLA-DRB1*0401* subtypes are associated with higher risk, the *HLA-DRB1*0402* and *HLA-DRB1*0404* subtypes are predisposing, and the *HLA-DRB1*0403* subtype is protective.

Each class II HLA molecule (DR, DQ, and DP) is composed of an α chain and a β chain with the *HLA-DQA* loci coding for DQ-α subunits and the *HLA-DQB* loci coding for DQ-β subunits. Class II HLA dimers present peptide antigens to the

T-cell receptors (TCR) to generate an immune response to the peptide. It is interesting that the heterozygous genotype (DR3-DQ2/DR4-DQ8) for the *HLA-DR3-DQ2* and *HLA-DR4-DQ8* haplotypes has a higher risk than the homozygous genotypes (*DR3-DQ2/DR3-DQ2* and *DR4-DQ8/DR4-DQ8*). One explanation for this is that the DQ-α subunit encoded by the *HLA-DQA1*0301* allele (associated with the DR4-DQ8 haplotype) may combine with the DQ-β subunit encoded by the *HLA-DQB1*0201* allele (associated with the DR3-DQ2 haplotype) to form a hybrid HLA *trans*-dimer that confers particularly high risk (32). High-performance liquid chromatography (HPLC) peptide-map analysis has confirmed the existence of hybrid HLA dimers in individuals with the DR3-DQ2/DR4-DQ8 genotype (33).

Even though linkage disequilibrium in the MHC region complicates efforts to identify non-*HLA-DR-DQ* determinants of diabetes in or linked to the MHC (34), there have been reports of independent non-*HLA-DR-DQ* diabetes-associated loci in the MHC region, including the *HLA-DPB1*, *MICA*, and *HLA-A* loci (35–38). Also, linkage and haplotype mapping studies performed by Johansson et al. suggest that there is at least one diabetes susceptibility locus telomeric of the MHC that contributes risk independently of the *HLA-DR-DQ* loci (39).

Although it is estimated that 50–60% of the familial aggregation of diabetes risk results from polymorphisms of non-MHC alleles (40), the observed contribution of risk from individual non-MHC alleles on chromosomes other than chromosome 6 is lower [odds ratio (OR) < 2] than the diabetes risk attributable to MHC polymorphisms on chromosome 6 (OR $\cong$ 30). The studies that suggest the approximately 50–50 division of risk between MHC and non-MHC loci are dependent on the percentage of sib pairs (both children with diabetes) who share zero MHC haplotypes in common (41). A major assumption underlying the estimate that non-MHC genes contribute such a high portion (50–60%) of the genetic risk of type 1A diabetes is that there is negligible recombination between contributing MHC linked loci. This assumption may not be met if genes linked to, but located several million base pairs away from, the class II region of the MHC (e.g., genes telomeric of *HLA-F* or centromeric of *HLA-DP*) are major contributors to genetic risk in addition to the HLA class II alleles (*HLA-DR*, *HLA-DQ*, and *HLA-DP*). In particular, evidence from the Diabetes Autoimmunity Study of the Youth (DAISY) suggests that risk of type 1A diabetes-associated autoimmunity may be as high as 85% for DR3-DQ2/DR4-DQ8 siblings sharing both MHC regions identical by descent with their proband sibling (42). This evidence suggests that a higher portion of the risk is caused by MHC or MHC-linked polymorphisms than previously reported.

If the known *HLA-DR-DQ* sequences were the only major MHC risk loci for diabetes, one would expect a similar risk for diabetes between DR3-DQ2/DR4-DQ8 siblings, DR3-DQ2/DR4-DQ8 offspring, and DR3-DQ2/DR4-DQ8 general population children with no family history of diabetes. However, in the DAISY, the risk by the age of seven years for DR3-DQ2/DR4-DQ8 siblings differed dramatically from the risk in the DR3-DQ2/DR4-DQ8 offspring and the DR3-DQ2/DR4-DQ8 general population children (45%, 15%, and 7%, respectively, the "relative paradox"). The simplest hypothesis to explain the relative paradox is that all *HLA-DR3-DQ2* and *HLA-DR4-DQ8* haplotypes do not have identical risk of diabetes, and that polymorphisms of genes linked to the *HLA-DR* and *HLA-DQ* genes contribute to diabetes risk. With this hypothesis, the higher risk in the DR3-DQ2/DR4-DQ8 siblings is explained by their potential to share both of their MHC haplotypes identical by descent with their proband, whereas DR3-DQ2/DR4-DQ8 offspring can inherit only one MHC haplotype

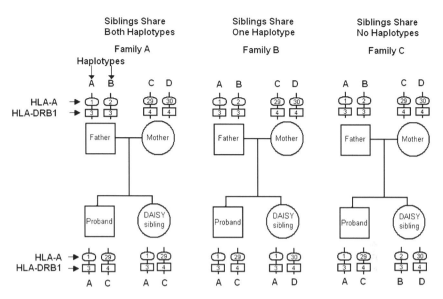

FIGURE 1 Illustration of haplotype sharing analysis. Haplotype sharing is illustrated in three representative families in which the DR3-DQ2/DR4-DQ8 DAISY sibling shares both (family A), one (family B), or no haplotypes (family C) with the diabetic proband. *Source*: From Ref. 41.

from their diabetic parent. In accordance with this hypothesis, DR3-DQ2/DR4-DQ8 children from the general population might have lower-risk MHC haplotypes than the siblings and offspring because they have fewer additional diabetes-associated polymorphisms on their *HLA-DR3-DQ2* and *HLA-DR4-DQ8* haplotypes.

Figure 1 portrays the determination of haplotype sharing in three representative DAISY families. In each family, a DAISY sibling with the DR3-DQ2/DR4-DQ8 genotype is prospectively monitored for islet autoimmunity and development of diabetes; the proband sibling is not selected based on HLA genotype (42). Despite all the DAISY children having DR3-DQ2/DR4-DQ8 genotype, the number of identical-by-descent haplotypes shared with their proband ranges between 0 and 2. The sharing of *HLA-DR3-DQ2* and *HLA-DR4-DQ8* haplotypes identical by descent with diabetic siblings dramatically correlated with higher diabetes risk in the prospectively followed DAISY siblings (Fig. 2) (42). DR3-DQ2/DR4-DQ8 siblings sharing both HLA haplotypes with their diabetic proband sibling had a 63% [±11% (SEM)] risk of developing persistent anti-islet autoantibodies by age 7 and an 85% (±12%) risk by age 15 and also had an increased risk of progression to diabetes [55% (±13%) by the age of 12]. The higher risk in DR3-DQ2/DR4-DQ8 siblings associated with MHC haplotype sharing by descent indicates that variants on MHC haplotypes in addition to known variants at the DR-DQ loci contribute major risk for type 1A diabetes.

The DAISY analysis of siblings at this time is limited to evaluation of families in which the proband has a very young age of onset. The younger ages of the proband sibling combined with analysis of the most common HLA high-risk genotype, DR3-DQ2/DR4-DQ8, may contribute to the observation of extremely high risk in the prospectively followed siblings. If such a high risk is, however,

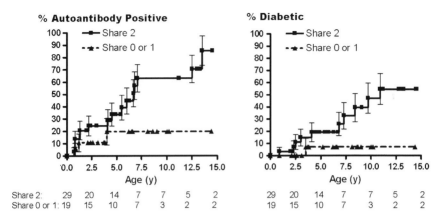

FIGURE 2 Haplotype sharing survival curves. Progression to anti-islet autoimmunity (*left panel*) and type 1A diabetes (*right panel*) in DR3-DQ2/DR4-DQ8 siblings stratified by the number of HLA haplotypes shared with their proband siblings. *N* = 48 for both panels; error bars for all panels represent the SEM. *Abbreviation*: SEM, standard error of the mean. *Source*: From Ref. 41.

confirmed in other studies, it suggests that the genetic factors associated with risk of type 1A diabetes autoimmunity is very high, at least for siblings, and rare triggering environmental factors are unlikely. Common environmental factors may, however, still be present and essential for disease.

It will be important to predict extreme type 1A diabetes risk not only for siblings of patients but also in the general population because the great majority (over 85%) of individuals with type 1A diabetes do not have a first-degree relative with type 1A diabetes. A recent analysis using *HLA-DPB1* and *HLA-DRB1* subtyping indicates a lower risk for type 1A diabetes in DR3-DQ2/DR4-DQ8 children that have the protective *HLA-DPB1*0402* or *HLA-DRB1*0403* allele (43). Prospectively followed children from the general population had a 19% (±5%) risk for expression of persistent anti-islet autoantibodies if they had the DR3-DQ2/DR4-DQ8 genotype but did not have the *HLA-DPB1*0402* or *HLA-DRB1*0403* allele (Fig. 3). The identification and localization of additional genetic determinants that

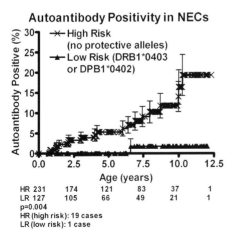

FIGURE 3 Progression to anti-islet autoantibody positivity in prospectively followed newborns with the HLA-DR3-DQ2/DR4-DQ8 genotype from the general population (NEwborn Cohort, NECs). Children with the DR3-DQ/DR4-DQ8 genotype that did not have either a *DRB1*0403* or a *DPB1*0402* allele had a 19% (± 5%) risk for anti-islet autoantibody positivity by age 12 versus a 2% (±2%) risk if the DR3-DQ2/DR4-DQ8 children did have a *DRB1*0403* or a *DPB1*0402* allele. *Source*: From Ref. 42.

cause the risk observed with MHC haplotype sharing may further improve prediction of risk in children from the general population.

EXTENDED MHC HAPLOTYPES

Given the evidence for diabetes-associated loci in or linked to the MHC in addition to classical HLA alleles, a major effort is underway to identify such loci. The localization of MHC and MHC-linked loci is complicated by the extensive linkage disequilibrium (the nonrandom association between alleles of linked genes) in the MHC (44,45). For instance, HLA-A1, HLA-B8, and HLA-DR3 each occur on approximately 17%, 11%, and 12% of chromosomes in the United States population (www.allelefrequencies.net). If random "equilibrium" existed between these alleles, one would predict that chromosomes with the HLA-A1, HLA-B8, HLA-DR3 combination would be present on 0.2% (17% x 11% x 12%) of the chromosomes. Since approximately 9% of Caucasian chromosomes have this combination of alleles (44) (much more than 0.2%), there is linkage disequilibrium between the HLA-A1, HLA-B8, and HLA-DR3 alleles and this combination of the HLA-A, HLA-B, and HLA-DRB1 alleles is a haplotype (series of alleles at linked loci on a chromosome). Such disequilibrium could be present due to founder effects in the population or selection for the specific haplotype.

The *HLA-A1-B8-DR3-DQ2* extended haplotype (8.1 haplotype) is common (in ~18% of individuals in Caucasian populations), extended, and extremely conserved (45,46). It is associated with multiple autoimmune diseases, including type 1A diabetes, celiac disease, systemic lupus erythematosus, common variable immunodeficiency, myasthenia gravis, and accelerated human immunodeficiency virus (HIV) disease (47,48). Although this haplotype is associated with diabetes, it is less associated than at least another *HLA-DR3-DQ2* haplotype (46,49). The *HLA-A30-B18-DR3-DQ2* haplotype has a high frequency in the Basque population, is more strongly associated with diabetes than the 8.1 haplotype, and is also highly conserved (49). Comparison of 8.1 haplotypes from unrelated individuals indicates that they can be identical for greater than 99% of single nucleotide polymorphisms (SNPs) for as long as 9 million nucleotides (the MHC is less than 4 million nucleotides long) (50). Thus, for extended haplotypes, such as the 8.1 and Basque haplotypes, SNPs anywhere on the haplotype will be "overtransmitted" to children with type 1A diabetes, even if the overtransmission is only caused by linkage disequilibrium with the high-risk *HLA-DRB1*0301* allele. We believe it is likely that better characterization of such haplotypes in populations of patients with type 1A diabetes will contribute to identifying additional MHC or MHC-linked type 1A diabetes relevant genes.

NON-MHC LOCI

There are a large number of reported putative non-MHC type 1A diabetes–associated loci in addition to the MHC loci (Table 1). Analysis of polymorphisms of the insulin (*INS*) and *PTPN22* genes identified these genes as candidate genes for type 1A diabetes prior to the current era of "genome" wide linkage and association studies. The genome-wide linkage and association studies have not found any major loci with effect sizes similar to the MHC for type 1A diabetes risk. It appears that most of the original reported insulin-dependent diabetes mellitus loci identified with linkage analysis are non-reproducible in large studies of different populations and were likely "false

TABLE 1 Selected Gene Associations with Type 1A Diabetes

Locus	Chromosome	Higher risk variants	Lower risk variants	Odds ratio	Reference
FOXP3	Xp11.23-q13.3	Various mutations			1
AIRE	21q22.3	Various mutations			2
HLA-DR/DQ	6p21.3, Class II region	DRB1*03–DQB1*0201 DRB1*04–DQB1*0302 DRB1*0405, DRB1*0401	DRB1*1501–DQB1*0602, DRB1*0403	≅ 30	27,54
HLA-DP	6p21.3, Class II region	DPB1*0301	DPB1*0402		55,43
ITPR3	6p21 (MHC, centromeric)	rs2296336, G allele	rs2296336, C allele	2.5	56
HLA-A	6p21.3, Class I region	A*2402 (earlier onset)			35
MICA	6p21.3, Class III region	Differs by population	MICA*A6	0.73 (*A6)	57
INS	11p15.5	Class I VNTR (short), (−23) HphI A allele	Class III VNTR (long), (−23) HphI T allele	1.9	53,27
CTLA4	2q33	+6230G > A, CT60		1.2	58
PTPN22	1p13	1858C > T, Arg620Trp (TT and CT genotypes)	(CC genotype)	1.7	27,59
IFIH1	2q24.3	rs1990760, A allele	rs1990760, G allele	1.2	60
SUMO4	6q25	163A > G, M55V		1.3	61
IL2RA/CD25	10p15.1	rs3118470, C allele	rs3118470, T allele	1.3	52,51

positives''. Recent studies analyzing large populations with extensive panels of SNPs for the association of alleles with diabetes are identifying additional loci, and presumed diabetes-associated genes with strong statistical evidence, but weak effects. In particular, the *CTLA4* locus and to a lesser extent polymorphisms of the *CTLA4* gene contribute to diabetes risk. A weak association (OR = 1.3) between the *IL2RA* locus and type 1A diabetes has also been reported (51,52). The *IL2RA* gene is an interesting candidate gene because IL2RA mediates the IL-2 signaling that is important for regulatory T-cell growth and survival. In a recent report, polymorphisms of the interferon induced with helicase C domain 1 (*IFIH1*) gene were also associated with diabetes (OR = 1.2). However, it required the study of thousands of individuals to demonstrate such an association, and analysis of additional large populations for confirmation will be a major task. With the advent of whole genome analysis, undoubtedly other loci with similarly weak associations with diabetes will be identified.

Of the non-MHC candidate genes for diabetes, the insulin gene is most strongly associated with an allelic odds ratio of 1.9 (27). Even this odds ratio is relatively small compared to the MHC and at the border of where contribution to the prediction of diabetes is measurable. Nevertheless, the pathophysiological pathway that is illuminated by the diabetes association with the insulin gene polymorphism is quite interesting. The risk from the insulin gene is associated with a variable number tandem repeat (VNTR) in the promoter at the 5′ end of the insulin gene rather than the sequence of proinsulin itself. Individuals with a greater number of repeats in the VNTR of their insulin gene are at lower risk of developing diabetes possibly because they express more insulin within their thymus (53). Thus, the leading hypothesis is that the insulin promoter VNTR contributes to diabetes risk by altering thymic insulin expression, since negative selection of T lymphocytes occurs within the thymus and T lymphocytes targeting insulin/proinsulin are likely major factors in islet β-cell destruction. In an analogous manner, the *AIRE* mutation that underlies the APS-1 syndrome (with a 15% risk for type 1A diabetes) also influences thymic insulin expression and presumably negative selection of T lymphocytes (4).

The C1858T polymorphism of the protein tyrosine phosphatase nonreceptor-type 22 (*PTPN22*) gene codes for a tryptophan rather than an arginine at position 620 of the lymphoid protein tyrosine phosphatase (LYP) and is associated with risk for type 1A diabetes (27). Bottini et al. discovered the association of this polymorphism for type 1A diabetes, and shortly thereafter the same polymorphism was associated with rheumatoid arthritis, as well as multiple additional autoimmune diseases (59). The magnitude of the association with the *PTPN22* gene was sufficient enough for rapid confirmation. Though the *PTPN22* C1858T polymorphism interrupts a major pathway for PTPN22 signaling in T lymphocytes, it is not clear whether it is a gain of function rather than loss of function that contributes to diabetes risk.

MULTIPLE AUTOIMMUNE DISORDERS

The genes underlying immune-mediated diabetes both for monogenic disorders (e.g., the IPEX syndrome and APS-1) and more typical type 1A diabetes (polygenic) influence both the development of diabetes and a series of other autoimmune diseases. This has been well documented for the IPEX syndrome where children usually died as neonates due to overwhelming autoimmune enteritis. Bone marrow transplantation appears to reverse the syndrome, as one would expect for a disease dependent on loss of regulatory T lymphocytes. Characteristic autoimmune diseases in patients with

APS-1 are mucocutaneous candidiasis, hypoparathyroidism, Addison's disease, and type 1A diabetes (15% of patients). In general, individuals with type 1A diabetes have a higher risk for other autoimmune disorders, including thyroiditis, Graves' disease, Addison's disease, and celiac disease. The latter three diseases, like type 1A diabetes, are strongly associated with the *HLA-DR3-DQ2* haplotype and both Addison's and celiac diseases are also associated with the *HLA-DR4-DQ8* haplotype. A few non-MHC polymorphisms associated with type 1A diabetes are also associated with multiple autoimmune disorders, and most likely the combination or interaction of MHC and non-MHC polymorphisms determine the observed associations.

CONCLUSION

Type 1A diabetes develops in the setting of genetic susceptibility, and for certain defined MHC genotypes (e.g. DR3-DQ2/DR4-DQ8), high risk can be identified at birth with additional stratification by MHC haplotype sharing (with the high-risk cohort defined as inheriting both MHC haplotypes identical by descent to a proband sibling). Analysis of risk for islet autoimmunity indicates that DR3-DQ2/DR4-DQ8 siblings have as high as 85% risk with sharing of both MHC haplotypes identical by descent with their proband. There is a significantly higher risk in DR3-DQ2/DR4-DQ8 children from the general population if they lack both the *HLA-DPB1*0402* and the *HLA-DRB1*0403* protective alleles. The positive predictive value for anti-islet autoimmunity in children from the general population based on HLA class II alleles (*HLA-DRB1*, *HLA-DQB1*, and *HLA-DPB1*) is 19% versus a 2% risk in DR3-DQ2/DR4-DQ8 children with either the DRB1*0403 or DPB1*0402 protective allele, and a general population risk of approximately 0.4% (43). Thus, an appreciable risk can be identified for the MHC subgroup lacking the *HLA-DPB1*0402* and *HLA-DRB1*0403* protective alleles. The DR3-DQ2/DR4-DQ8 genotype in the DAISY population, however, represents only 38% of children persistently positive for anti-islet autoantibodies and 46% of children diagnosed with diabetes to date. Thus, the requirement of a DR3-DQ2/DR4-DQ8 genotype for selection into a high-risk group is associated with less than 50% sensitivity. We believe that the identification of additional diabetes-associated polymorphisms within the MHC will allow improved prediction of type 1A diabetes. The non-MHC loci, except for the insulin gene, might not contribute materially to prediction given their low reported odds ratios, but likely reveal important pathways of disease pathogenesis. These pathways are related to T-cell signaling and tolerance induction, and potentially influence the development of innate immunity. Type 1A diabetes to date is not influenced by the major type 2 diabetes gene TCF7L2, and the genetic etiology of the diseases are likely distinct (5). Thus, we believe that much can be learned about the pathophysiology of type 1A diabetes with the elucidation of the etiological pathways that are associated with non-MHC loci, and for improving the genetic prediction of type 1A diabetes, further studies of MHC and MHC-linked regions may yield important information.

ACKNOWLEDGMENTS

This work was supported by the National Institutes of Health (DK32083, DK057538), Diabetes Autoimmunity Study in the Young (DAISY, DK32493), Autoimmunity Prevention Center (AI050864), Diabetes Endocrine Research Center

(P30 DK57516), Clinical Research Centers (MO1 RR00069, MO1 RR00051), the Immune Tolerance Network (AI15416), the American Diabetes Association, the Juvenile Diabetes Research Foundation, and the Children's Diabetes Foundation.

REFERENCES

1. Wildin RS, Ramsdell F, Peake J, et al. X-linked neonatal diabetes mellitus, enteropathy and endocrinopathy syndrome is the human equivalent of mouse scurfy. Nat Genet 2001; 27(1):18–20.
2. Aaltonen J, Björses P, Perheentupa J, et al. An autoimmune disease, APECED, caused by mutations in a novel gene featuring two PHD-type zinc-finger domains. Nat Genet 1997; 17(4):399–403.
3. Halonen M, Eskelin P, Myhre AG, et al. AIRE mutations and human leukocyte antigen genotypes as determinants of the autoimmune polyendocrinopathy-candidiasis-ectodermal dystrophy phenotype. J Clin Endocrinol Metab 2002; 87(6):2568–2574.
4. Anderson MS, Venanzi ES, Klein L, et al. Projection of an immunological self shadow within the thymus by the aire protein. Science 2002; 298(5597):1395–1401.
5. Field SF, Howson JM, Smyth DJ, et al. Analysis of the type 2 diabetes gene, TCF7L2, in 13,795 type 1 diabetes cases and control subjects. Diabetologia 2007; 50(1):212–213.
6. Imagawa A, Hanafusa T, Itoh N, et al. Immunological abnormalities in islets at diagnosis paralleled further deterioration of glycaemic control in patients with recent-onset Type I (insulin-dependent) diabetes mellitus. Diabetologia 1999; 42(5):574–578.
7. Hyoty H and Taylor KW. The role of viruses in human diabetes. Diabetologia 2002; 45 (10):1353–1361.
8. Norris JM, Barriga K, Klingensmith G, et al. Timing of cereal exposure in infancy and risk of islet autoimmunity. The Diabetes Autoimmunity Study in the Young (DAISY). JAMA 2003; 290(13):1713–1720.
9. Norris JM. Can the sunshine vitamin shed light on type 1 diabetes?. Lancet 2001; 358 (9292):1476–1478.
10. Zipris D, Lien E, Xie JX, et al. TLR activation synergizes with Kilham rat virus infection to induce diabetes in BBDR rats. J Immunol 2005; 174(1):131–142.
11. Ellerman KE and Like AA. Susceptibility to diabetes is widely distributed in normal class IIu haplotype rats. Diabetologia 2000; 43(7):890–898.
12. Devendra D, Jasinski J, Melanitou E, et al. Interferon-{alpha} as a mediator of poly-inosinic: polycytidylic acid-induced Type 1 diabetes. Diabetes 2005; 54(9):2549–2556.
13. Rubenstein P. The HLA system in congenital rubella patients with and without diabetes. Diabetes 1982; 31:1088–1091.
14. Rabinowe SL, George KL, Loughlin R, et al. Congenital rubella. Monoclonal antibody-defined T cell abnormalities in young adults. Am J Med 1986; 81(5):779–782.
15. Libman I, Songer T, LaPorte R. How many people in the U.S. have IDDM? Diabetes Care 1993; 16(5):841–842.
16. Rewers M. The changing face of the epidemiology of insulin-dependent diabetes mellitus (IDDM): research designs and models of disease causation. Ann Med 1991; 23 (4):419–426.
17. Rewers M, Bugawan TL, Norris JM, et al. Newborn screening for HLA markers associated with IDDM: diabetes autoimmunity study in the young (DAISY). Diabetologia 1996; 39(7):807–812.
18. Liese AD, D'Agostino RB Jr., Hamman RF, et al. The burden of diabetes mellitus among US youth: prevalence estimates from the SEARCH for Diabetes in Youth Study. Pediatrics 2006; 118(4):1510–1518.
19. Onkamo P, Vaananen S, Karvonen M, et al. Worldwide increase in incidence of Type I diabetes—the analysis of the data on published incidence trends. Diabetologia 1999. 42(12):1395–1403.
20. Bach JF. Protective role of infections and vaccinations on autoimmune diseases. J Autoimmun 2001; 16(3):347–353.

21. McKinney PA, Okasha M, Parslow RC, et al. Early social mixing and childhood Type 1 diabetes mellitus: a case-control study in Yorkshire, UK. Diabet Med 2000; 17 (3):236–242.
22. Kwon OJ, Brautbar C, Weintrob N, et al. Immunogenetics of HLA class II in Israeli Ashkenazi Jewish, Israeli non-Ashkenazi Jewish, and in Israeli Arab IDDM patients. Hum Immunol 2001; 62(1):85–91.
23. Redondo MJ, Yu L, Hawa M, et al. Heterogeneity of type I diabetes: analysis of monozygotic twins in Great Britain and the United States. Diabetologia 2001; 44 (3):354–362.
24. Kaprio J, Tuomilehto J, Koskenvuo M, et al. Concordance for type 1 (insulin-dependent) and type 2 (non-insulin-dependent) diabetes mellitus in a population-based cohort of twins in Finland. Diabetologia 1992; 35(11):1060–1067.
25. Kumar D, Gemayel NS, Deapen D, et al. North-American twins with IDDM. Genetic, etiological, and clinical significance of disease concordance according to age, zygosity, and the interval after diagnosis in first twin. Diabetes 1993; 42(9):1351–1363.
26. Metcalfe KA, Hitman GA, Rowe RE, et al. Concordance for type 1 diabetes in identical twins is affected by insulin genotype. Diabetes Care 2001; 24(5):838–842.
27. Concannon P, Erlich HA, Julier C, et al. Type 1 diabetes: evidence for susceptibility loci from four genome-wide linkage scans in 1,435 multiplex families. Diabetes 2005; 54 (10):2995–3001.
28. Lambert AP, Gillespie KM, Thomson G, et al. Absolute risk of childhood-onset type 1 diabetes defined by human leukocyte antigen Class II genotype: a population-based study in the United Kingdom. J Clin Endocrinol Metab 2004; 89(8):4037–4043.
29. Noble JA, Valdes AM, Cook M, et al. The role of HLA class II genes in insulin-dependent diabetes mellitus: molecular analysis of 180 Caucasian, multiplex families. Am J Hum Genet 1996; 59(5):1134–1148.
30. Cucca F, Dudbridge F, Loddo M, et al. The HLA-DPB1–associated component of the IDDM1 and its relationship to the major loci HLA-DQB1, -DQA1, and -DRB1. Diabetes 2001; 50(5):1200–1205.
31. Redondo MJ, Kawasaki E, Mulgrew CL, et al. DR and DQ associated protection from type 1 diabetes: comparison of DRB1*1401 and DQA1*0102-DQB1*0602. J Clin Endocrinol Metab 2000; 85(10):3793–3797.
32. She JX. Susceptibility to type I diabetes: HLA-DQ and DR revisited. Immunol Today 1996; 17(7):323–329.
33. Nepom BS, Schwartz D, Palmer JP, et al. Transcomplementation of HLA genes in IDDM. Diabetes 1987; 36(1):114–117.
34. Rich SS, Concannon P. Challenges and strategies for investigating the genetic complexity of common human diseases. Diabetes 2002; 51(suppl 3):S288–S294.
35. Noble JA, Valdes AM, Bugawan TL, et al. The HLA class I A locus affects susceptibility to type 1 diabetes. Hum Immunol 2002; 63(8):657–664.
36. Ide A, Babu SR, Robles DT, et al. Homozygosity for premature stop codon of the MHC class I chain-related gene A (MIC-A) is associated with early activation of islet autoimmunity of DR3/4-DQ2/8 high risk DAISY relatives. J Clin Immunol 2005; 25(4):303–308.
37. Cruz TD, Valdes AM, Santiago A, et al. DPB1 alleles are associated with type 1 diabetes susceptibility in multiple ethnic groups. Diabetes 2004; 53(8):2158–2163.
38. Valdes AM, Erlich HA, Noble JA. Human leukocyte antigen class I B and C loci contribute to Type 1 Diabetes (T1D) susceptibility and age at T1D onset. Hum Immunol 2005; 66(3):301–313.
39. Johansson S, Lie BA, Todd JA, et al. Evidence of at least two type 1 diabetes susceptibility genes in the HLA complex distinct from HLA-DQB1, -DQA1 and -DRB1. Genes Immun 2003; 4(1):46–53.
40. Risch N. Genetics of IDDM: evidence for complex inheritance with HLA. Genet Epidemiol 1989; 6(1):143–148.
41. Risch N. Assessing the role of HLA-linked and unlinked determinants of disease. Am J Hum Genet 1987; 40(1):1–14.
42. Aly TA, Ide A, Jahromi MM, et al. Extreme genetic risk for Type 1A diabetes. Proc Natl Acad Sci U S A 2006; 103(38):14074–14079.

43. Baschal EE, Aly TA, Babu SR, et al. HLA-DPB1*0402 protects against type 1A diabetic autoimmunity in the highest risk DR3-DQB1*0201/DR4-DQB1*0302 DAISY population. Diabetes 2007; 56(9):2405–2409.
44. Alper CA, Larsen CE, Dubey DP, et al. The haplotype structure of the human major histocompatibility complex. Hum Immunol 2006; 67(1–2):73–84.
45. Awdeh ZL, Raum D, Yunis EJ, et al. Extended HLA/complement allele haplotypes: evidence for T/t-like complex in man. Proc Natl Acad Sci U S A 1983; 80(1):259–263.
46. Ide A, Babu SR, Robles DT, et al. "Extended" A1, B8, DR3 haplotype shows remarkable linkage disequilibrium but is similar to nonextended haplotypes in terms of diabetes risk. Diabetes 2005; 54(6):1879–1883.
47. Valdes AM, Wapelhorst B, Concannon P, et al. Extended DR3-D6S273-HLA-B haplotypes are associated with increased susceptibility to type 1 diabetes in US Caucasians. Tissue Antigens 2005; 65(1):115–119.
48. Price P, Witt C, Allcock R, et al. The genetic basis for the association of the 8.1 ancestral haplotype (A1,B8,DR3) with multiple immunopathological diseases. Immunol Rev 1999; 167(2):257–274.
49. Bilbao JR, Calvo B, Aransay AM, et al. Conserved extended haplotypes discriminate HLA-DR3-homozygous Basque patients with type 1 diabetes mellitus and celiac disease. Genes Immun 2006; 7(7):550–554.
50. Aly TA, Eller E, Ide A, et al. Multi-SNP analysis of MHC region: remarkable conservation of HLA-A1-B8-DR3 haplotype. Diabetes 2006; 55(5):1265–1269.
51. Qu HQ, Montpetit A, Ge B, et al. Toward further mapping of the association between the IL2RA locus and type 1 diabetes. Diabetes 2007; 56(4):1174–1176.
52. Vella A, Cooper JD, Lowe CE, et al. Localization of a type 1 diabetes locus in the IL2RA/CD25 region by use of tag single-nucleotide polymorphisms. Am J Hum Genet 2005; 76(5):773–779.
53. Pugliese A, Zeller M, Fernandez A, et al. The insulin gene is transcribed in the human thymus and transcription levels correlate with allelic variation at the INS VNTR-IDDM2 susceptibility locus for type I diabetes. Nat Genet 1997; 15(3):293–297.
54. Rewers A, Babu S, Wang TB, et al. Ethnic differences in the associations between the HLA-DRB1*04 subtypes and type 1 diabetes. Ann N Y Acad Sci 2003; 1005(11):301–309.
55. Noble JA, Valdes AM, Thomson G, et al. The HLA class II locus DPB1 can influence susceptibility to type 1 diabetes. Diabetes 2000; 49(1):121–125.
56. Roach JC, Deutsch K, Li S, et al. Genetic mapping at 3-kilobase resolution reveals inositol 1,4,5-triphosphate receptor 3 as a risk factor for type 1 diabetes in Sweden. Am J Hum Genet 2006; 79(4):614–627.
57. Alizadeh BZ, Eerligh P, van der Slik AR, et al. MICA marks additional risk factors for Type 1 diabetes on extended HLA haplotypes: an association and meta-analysis. Mol Immunol 2007; 44(11):2806–2812.
58. Donner H, Rau H, Walfish PG, et al. CTLA4 alanine-17 confers genetic susceptibility to Graves' disease and to type 1 diabetes mellitus. J Clin Endocrinol Metab 1997; 82(1):143–146.
59. Bottini N, Muscumeci L, Alonso A, et al. A functional variant of lymphoid tyrosine phosphatase is associated with type I diabetes. Nat Genet 2004; 36(4):337–338.
60. Smyth DJ, Cooper JD, Bailey R, et al. A genome-wide association study of nonsynonymous SNPs identifies a type 1 diabetes locus in the interferon-induced helicase (IFIH1) region. Nat Genet 2006; 38(6):617–619.
61. Qu H, Bharaj B, Liu XQ, et al. Assessing the validity of the association between the SUM04 M55V variant and risk of type 1 diabetes. Nat Genet 2005; 37(2):111–112.

4   Early-Life Diet and Risk of Type 1 Diabetes

Melissa D. Simpson and Jill M. Norris

Department of Preventive Medicine and Biometrics, University of Colorado at Denver and Health Sciences Center, Denver, Colorado, U.S.A.

INTRODUCTION

Early-life diet is important in normal health and development for all children as it can have far-reaching and irreversible health consequences. Those consequences, whether beneficial or detrimental, are the result of a complex interplay between genetic predispositions, dietary content, and the timing of exposure to novel dietary components during infancy and early childhood. Multiple published studies implicate early-life diet as an important factor in the pathogenesis of type 1 diabetes (1). What is not clearly understood is the mechanism through which early-life diet acts to either precipitate or delay the onset of type 1 diabetes. Two main details have been investigated with regard to this relationship: the types of foods in an infant's diet and the timing of introduction to these foods. To further complicate the picture, there is not always agreement between studies about specific findings or their interpretation. In spite of (and sometimes as a result of) the information available, there is no consensus about any overarching mechanisms that might unite current scientific findings into a cohesive picture regarding the contribution that early-life diet makes in the development of type 1 diabetes.

Several theories exist about the manner in which early-life diet can affect the pathogenesis of type 1 diabetes. For the purposes of this chapter they will be somewhat arbitrarily identified as follows: the oral tolerance/antigen theory, the gut permeability theory, and the oxidative stress theory. Each of these theories will be described in detail, early-life diet factors will be explored within their contexts, and finally evidence from the literature will be considered. While each theory will be discussed separately, they are likely not mutually exclusive and a distinct possibility exists that type 1 diabetes pathogenesis is the result of biological interactions between them.

Investigators have employed a variety of study designs to explore the relationships between diet and type 1 diabetes. The initial studies were case-control designs wherein the infant diet exposures of children with type 1 diabetes were compared with those of children without diabetes. As is the case with all designs of this nature, they are subject to data inaccuracies, and recall and selection biases. In the 1990s, birth cohorts in Germany (BABYDIAB), Colorado (DAISY), and Finland (DIPP) were initiated to prospectively follow high-risk children for the development of islet autoimmunity (IA). This outcome is an intermediate that is highly predictive of type 1 diabetes (2,3) and is more feasible to use in a prospective study since it appears at an earlier age than does type 1 diabetes. While all types of studies will be reviewed herein, emphasis will be placed on those that have the most informative data to address the hypotheses.

ORAL TOLERANCE/ANTIGENS THEORY

Oral tolerance is defined as the induction of antigen-specific immunological tolerance brought about by ingesting protein antigens (4). Ingested foods have unique antigenic characteristics that gastrointestinal (GI) mucosal immune tissue recognizes but is programmed to ignore, thereby allowing the body to tolerate the antigens found in food. Because mucosal immune tissue or gut-associated lymphoid tissue (GALT) is the largest and most extensive of the immune system, oral tolerance is a major component of peripheral tolerance. Lack of peripheral tolerance has been implicated in the development of many autoimmune diseases (5,6). The process of oral tolerance is ongoing but there are times during development when the gut immune system is more active with respect to oral tolerance (7). In addition, it is thought that there is a dose-dependent response wherein high oral doses of antigen suppress humoral immunity and low oral doses induce cell-mediated tolerance (4). Regardless of the mechanism, the overriding theme is that repetitive exposure to antigenic proteins in the diet prompts the immune system to tolerate them as harmless.

In order to properly maintain immunological homeostasis, normal oral tolerance is essential. In the case of type 1 diabetes, it is thought that disruption of this system allows the immune system to initiate immune responses against antigens normally tolerated when ingested. When this immune response is initiated, a cycle of exposure and inflammation is induced with the result potentially being IA, which is the first step in the pathway to type 1 diabetes. The early-life dietary factors that may be of special importance in this process include breast-feeding, and exposures to bovine insulin, cow's milk proteins, cereals, omega-3 polyunsaturated fatty acids (n-3 PUFAs), or vitamin D.

Breast milk contains many beneficial components that help ensure normal GI and physiological development during infancy, including immunoglobulins, human insulin, and the appropriate balance of macronutrients essential for human development. These components help establish normal gut environment, nutrient metabolism, and immune function. All three of these factors are important in oral tolerance.

The immunoglobulins contained in breast milk confer passive immunity on an infant who is breast-fed. These molecules train an infant's naïve immune system for normal immune function later in childhood and into adult life. A normally functioning immune system is essential for generation of oral tolerance because of its intrinsic checks and balances intended to differentiate between harmless and harmful foreign antigens and microbes. Because it appears that a great deal of oral tolerance is formed early in life, it also appears intuitive that early-life exposure to the immunoglobulins present in breast milk is imperative in this process.

In addition to immune factors, breast milk also contains human insulin. Exposure to human insulin via breast milk may help in developing tolerance to human insulin, which first occurs in the GALT (4). If lack of tolerance to insulin is a precipitating factor in the development of type 1 diabetes, then exposure to breast milk may have a protective effect on the risk of type 1 diabetes by helping the child to develop tolerance to insulin (6). In support of this hypothesis, a pilot study in children at increased risk for type 1 diabetes showed that children consuming breast milk with higher concentrations of insulin had lower antibody response to insulin from foreign sources than infants consuming breast milk with lower concentrations of insulin (8).

Given the theory of oral tolerance, one might expect that breast-feeding initiation as well as longer duration of breast-feeding may result in a lower risk of type 1 diabetes. However, the epidemiological evidence has been inconsistent. While some studies have found a decreased risk of type 1 diabetes in breast-fed children, others have found equivocal results (1). These studies were case-control design and were accordingly subject to inaccuracies, and recall and selection biases (9). Interestingly, the three prospective studies investigating predictors of IA found no association between either breast-feeding initiation or duration and the appearance of IA in children at increased risk for type 1 diabetes (10–12).

Another mechanism by which breast milk may protect against type 1 diabetes is via decreased exposure to breast-milk substitutes. Infants who are not breast-fed or are not exclusively breast-fed are exposed to breast-milk substitutes, such as infant formulas, which may contain diabetogenic antigens. Therefore, variation in the age at introduction to these substitutes may be a more important variable than overall breast-feeding duration in terms of diabetes risk and may, in part, explain why overall breast-feeding duration is not consistently associated with type 1 diabetes risk in the above studies.

Cow's milk, primarily in the form of cow's milk–based formulas, is a common component of the diet of the infant who receives little or no breast milk. While the association between cow's milk and cow's milk–based infant formulas has been examined extensively, there is still disagreement not only on the nature of this relationship as it pertains to timing of exposure but also on what is present in cow's milk that may be associated with increased risk.

The timing of introduction to foreign antigens is an important factor in the development or disruption of oral tolerance. Many case-control studies have found an inverse association between the age at exposure to cow's milk and type 1 diabetes (13–17). These findings may suggest that infants exposed early in life to cow's milk are more susceptible to disruption in oral tolerance, possibly due to prolonged exposure that results from earlier exposure, a sensitive period effect, or a combination of both. However, like the breast-milk studies, there have been multiple case-control studies that have failed to find an association between the timing of cow's milk introduction and type 1 diabetes (18,19). In addition, all three of the cohort studies discussed above examined age at exposure to cow's milk as well, and found no association between exposure and risk for development of IA (10–12).

Studies have also addressed this question by measuring antibodies in cow's milk proteins, such as bovine serum albumin and β-lactoglobulin, and found that newly diagnosed type 1 diabetic patients had higher antibody levels to bovine serum albumin (20) and β-lactoglobulin (21) than their healthy counterparts. Because associations were seen with different cow's milk proteins, these results indicate that there may be multiple ways in which to disrupt normal oral tolerance, or that disruption in oral tolerance is the result of a constellation of exposures. However, these studies were done in children with existing diabetes, so it is unknown whether these antibodies are elevated prior to the development of clinical diabetes or autoimmunity. This information would inform as to whether elevated antibodies are a marker of the disruption of oral tolerance, which subsequently results in disease, or whether they are simply a marker of the autoimmune process that leads to type 1 diabetes, or perhaps a consequence of the disease itself.

Bovine insulin is another protein in cow's milk that may have a role in oral tolerance disruption. Its molecular structure differs from that of human insulin by three amino acids and it is this feature that researchers believe is the origin of its role in type 1 diabetes (6). Because it is structurally similar to human insulin, it is able to gain access to the GALT while other more dissimilar antigenic proteins will pass through the GI tract without being absorbed. It is hypothesized that once exposed to the GALT, bovine insulin is different enough from human insulin that it may initiate an immune response that lacks the specificity to differentiate between human and bovine insulin, thus generating antibodies that are cross reactive, potentially resulting in type 1 diabetes.

In a study comparing how different infant formulas affect antibody response to bovine insulin and islet autoantibodies, investigators found that infants who were fed a hydrolyzed protein-based infant formula had lower levels of antibodies to bovine insulin at three months of age compared with those who were fed a cow's milk–based infant formula. Moreover, the children receiving the hydrolyzed infant formula had lower levels of islet autoantibodies at 12 months of age than the children receiving cow's milk–based formula (22). While the authors concluded that exposure to bovine insulin at an early stage in the development of the GI tract can predispose children to the formation of islet autoantibodies, further confirmation is needed.

Another observation that may lend support for the theory of oral tolerance as it pertains to bovine insulin is the finding that children born to mothers who have type 1 diabetes have a lower incidence of type 1 diabetes when compared with their counterparts who are born to fathers with the disease (23). Although there are many possible explanations for this relationship, in this case the relevancy lies in the fact that ingestion of amniotic fluid represents the earliest possible dietary exposure for mammals. In the case of a mother who has type 1 diabetes, her fetus is presumably exposed to consistently administered high levels of insulin orally via the amniotic fluid, and therefore may be undergoing early programming for tolerance to orally ingested insulin. In contrast, infants with fathers who have type 1 diabetes carry similar genetic risk but are more likely to develop type 1 diabetes in the absence of high insulin exposure. This hypothesis has not yet been tested.

In addition to breast-milk substitutes, such as infant formulas, the infant is exposed to other dietary antigens in the first year of life that may impact oral tolerance. In the United States, cereals are often the first solid foods to which the infant is exposed, making cereals a potentially important dietary factor to study when defining the role of diet in the development of type 1 diabetes. Like all foods, cereals have antigenic characteristics that could play a role in oral tolerance in infants. Because gluten is the environmental trigger for clinical symptoms of celiac disease, another childhood autoimmune disease, and because it is a component of many cereals, it has been studied in the context of type 1 diabetes as a potentially important environmental exposure as well.

In the biobreeding (BB) diabetes-prone rat, gluten precipitates the onset of IA (24). MacFarlane et al. identified a wheat storage protein called glb1 that may be associated with islet damage, by observing that antibodies to this protein were detectable in patients with diabetes but not in nondiabetic patients (25). Moreover, the timing of introduction of cereals (and/or gluten) during infancy has been examined in all three prospective studies of the development of IA. Both BABYDIAB and DAISY have shown an increased risk for IA associated with exposure to cereals prior to the third month of life when compared with introduction in the fourth to sixth month of life. Norris et al. found that the timing of introduction of any type of cereal was associated with an increased IA risk and also found that there appears to be a U-shaped relationship between risk and age at introduction, the nadir of the curve occurred with introduction in the fourth to sixth months of life (10). In contrast, Ziegler et al. showed the association with gluten specifically and found that a further protective effect was conferred if foods containing gluten were introduced after the sixth month (12). It is important to note that both studies found that the introduction of cereals at less than three months of age resulted in the highest relative risk. These data suggest that there are specific times in infancy wherein exposure is associated with an increased risk of developing IA. The risk associated with early exposure may suggest a mechanism involving an aberrant immune response to cereal antigens in an immature gut immune system among susceptible individuals.

When examining the role of cereals along with the timing of introduction, it is also important to consider whether the increased IA risk is associated with one specific antigen (e.g., gluten), or if it is associated with general antigenic stimulation arising from exposure to an assortment of food antigens. It is interesting that Norris et al. found an effect of timing of cereal introduction in both gluten-containing and non-gluten-containing cereals (10), whereas Ziegler et al. found the association in gluten-containing solid foods but not in non-gluten-containing solid foods (12). Given the difference in the defined dietary variables (the non-gluten-containing food variable in Ziegler et al. contained non-cereal foods), it is difficult to determine whether the two studies actually contradict each other. Interestingly, the Finnish prospective study (DIPP) did not find an association between the timing of introduction to wheat-based foods and the development of IA. However, the finding in the DIPP study that early introduction of fruits and berries was associated with increased risk for IA further supports the idea that general antigenic stimulation is more important than the actual antigen in this disease process (11). Discerning the intricacies of this relationship will be important in future research because it has very practical implications regarding feeding recommendations for infants, particularly those identified as being high risk.

Interestingly, Norris et al. found evidence that a child who is still breast-feeding at the time of introduction to cereals has a reduced risk of IA regardless of the timing of cereal introduction (10). A similar protective relationship between breast-feeding and introduction of gluten has been observed in celiac disease (26). These findings suggest that while not protective independently, breast-feeding may be a protective mediator in the relationship between other dietary factors, including but not limited to cereals, and IA.

The immune system is one of checks and balances between T-helper 1 (Th1) and T-helper 2 (Th2) responses. Lack of oral tolerance may allow a bias towards a Th1 response which is associated with autoimmune pathologies, such as type 1 diabetes (4,27). Dietary factors such as vitamin D and n-3 PUFA's that stimulate a Th2 response may therefore help to protect against the development of IA (7), regardless of, or perhaps specifically in the absence of, oral tolerance.

A case-control study from Norway suggested that children with diabetes were less likely than controls to have been given cod liver oil during infancy (28). This suggests that fish oils may have a role in the process of oral tolerance, perhaps through the immune modulating effects of long-chain PUFAs and/or vitamin D, both of which are present in cod liver oil. Studies in lab animals suggest that both n-3 fatty acids and vitamin D can shift T-cell response to Th2 (29–31), and that n-3 fatty acid supplementation may inhibit the function of antigen-presenting cells (32). Both vitamin D and PUFAs will be discussed in more detail later in the chapter but they are presented here in the context of their potential role in the delay or prevention of disrupted oral tolerance. Because oral tolerance is mediated through a Th2 pathway, it can be seen that shifting the balance toward this more regulatory inflammatory mechanism may help promote its normal development.

GUT PERMEABILITY THEORY

The GI tract is an essential barrier between the body's systems and the outside world. It acts to modulate absorption of nutrients and cull microbes and molecules that could potentially harm the body. There are two barriers in the GI tract intended to prevent ingested foreign antigens, toxins, and macromolecules from gaining access to the systemic circulation. The first barrier is physical and is composed of mucosal cells and their associated tight junctions. This barrier ensures that large molecules will not be allowed into the systemic circulation in the absence of specific receptors on the luminal surface of the mucosal cell's membrane. In the very young, the physical barrier that acts as the interface between the gut and the body may not be as complete as it is later in life. This barrier may confer survival benefits when considering the fact that the infant's primary source of immunologically protective molecules is via ingestion but may also prove detrimental if there is an exposure in this immature environment with which the infant is unable to cope. The second component of the barrier is the GALT and it is the first line of defense for the immune system at the interface between the gut and systemic circulation, as discussed earlier in this chapter. It is here that the immune system is able to defend the body against potentially harmful substances and it is the location for much of the training of the infant's immune system. Because a large proportion of an infant's exposures happen via the GI tract, the GALT is one of the main sites for immune maturation in infants and has been implicated as the major source for food hypersensitivities as well (7).

One theory currently under investigation is that children who are predisposed to type 1 diabetes have increased gut permeability, resulting in increased exposures that may lead to type 1 diabetes. As described above, there is a single layer of cells that protect the internal milieu from the environment in the intestinal lumen. Any compromise of this layer of cells exposes the immunologically reactive submucosa to all of the contents of the intestinal lumen. In addition, it is thought that dietary hypersensitivities or mistimed dietary exposures may exacerbate gut permeability in those at risk (33). Animal studies suggest that gut permeability could result in passage of environmental antigens that trigger the autoimmune response leading to type 1 diabetes (34–38). Investigators have suggested that this increased permeability could be related, in part, to dietary exposures in infancy (35,36). For example, breast-feeding may facilitate gut closure, and other dietary factors, such as gluten, may actually prolong or exacerbate gut permeability.

As discussed above in relation to oral tolerance, breast milk confers important immune factors upon the infant, which in turn may play a role in gut permeability. Because the first couple of months of life are the period when the GI tract is normally the most permeable (39,40), it is important that there are sufficient protective factors in place during this sensitive time. Breast milk is the source of this immune protection for the infant during early life, and in this capacity the immune molecules that are transferred are responsible for guarding against pathogens present in the GI tract. Moreover, there is evidence that breast milk has a direct role in the closure of the gut mucosa and may help to regulate inappropriate gut inflammatory responses, so its presence may have multiple protective factors that act to maintain an optimal level of gut health (41). This phenomenon becomes especially important in children at increased risk for diabetes because the interaction between their genetic susceptibility and the absence of proper or complete cultivation of gut health facilitated by breast milk may precipitate the onset of IA and diabetes.

On the basis of this discussion, one would expect to see evidence in the literature showing that breast-feeding reduces the risk for IA, but as reported earlier in this chapter, this is not the case. The exception is the finding by Norris et al. that breast-feeding at the time of cereal introduction reduces IA risk (10), which may suggest that breast-feeding has a role in either oral tolerance or gut permeability. The discrepancy between theory and results may be attributed to the complexity of the relationship. The following factors may obscure the true relationship between breast-feeding and IA: (1) the difficulty in defining what duration of breast-feeding is optimal for gut closure, (2) the likelihood that there is an interaction between breast-feeding and the presence of pathogens that prolong gut permeability, or (3) the likelihood that there is an interaction between breast-feeding and the presence of specific antigens in the diet.

Another way in which increased gut permeability could lead to diabetes is through increased exposure to the microbial inhabitants of the intestinal tract. Some of the suggested mechanisms by which microbes may play a role in type 1 diabetes etiology include direct cytolysis of islet cells, molecular mimicry, and lymphocyte activation that favors a Th-1 response (42). These processes may be attributed to the microbes themselves or to a microbe-induced increased gut permeability resulting in increased dietary antigen exposure. Furthermore, if initiation of these mechanisms is predicated by colonization of the GI tract, then breast milk may be an important factor in these hypothesized processes by helping to inhibit colonization.

To date, literature about the role of microbes in type 1 diabetes has focused on enteroviruses. Ex vivo studies have demonstrated that some viruses exhibit a tropism for the pancreas (43), which suggests that viruses may induce islet cell cytolysis. Vaarala et al. found that in infants exposed to cow's milk formulas before the age of three months, those who had a T-cell proliferation response to enterovirus antigen at three months of age had higher concentrations of IgG antibodies to bovine insulin at the age of six and nine months than those who did not have the T-cell proliferation response to enterovirus antigen (44). This finding may support either molecular mimicry or the type of T-helper response as a mechanism. Alternatively, it could suggest an enterovirus-induced increase in gut permeability that results in exposure to dietary antigens. Further studies are needed to identify the role (if any) of microbes and to characterize the nature of that role in humans.

One of the mechanistic explanations for the association between the timing of introduction to cereals in the infant diet and the risk of IA may be the effect of gluten on gut permeability (10,12). Zonulin is a newly identified biomarker for intestinal permeability and is a modulator of small intestinal tight junctions (45). Using celiac disease positive cell lines, investigators identified a relationship between gliadin, which is the portion of gluten known to cause damage in celiac disease, and zonulin. They found that zonulin levels increased as a response to exposure to gluten in these cell lines which, in turn, perpetuated the intestinal permeability to macromolecules, including gliadin. Two studies involving BB rats identified higher levels of zonulin in their diabetes-prone colonies compared with wild-type rats (34,46). Finally, in humans, Sapone et al. found that mean serum zonulin was higher in type 1 diabetes patients compared with their first-degree relatives and controls, and that this elevation was correlated with increased gut permeability in these patients (47). The report that gliadin may activate a zonulin-dependent intracellular pathway in the enterocyte may suggest a cycle of gliadin-induced zonulin production and subsequent increased intestinal permeability. If left unchecked, this cycle could lead to escalating exposures to the body as gliadin intake continues. In order to further test this hypothesis, prospective studies are needed to establish temporality as well as the role of diet in the process.

Also of interest is the many ways that gut permeability and oral tolerance are interrelated. Because the physical barrier in the GI tract is meant to prevent chronic exposure and immune stimulation in the GALT, it is possible that in the face of increased permeability there is increased potential for disruption of oral tolerance. For example, if a dietary antigen is introduced that is capable of delaying closure of the gut, it may allow multiple macromolecules gain access to the GALT, which in turn initiates a Th1-mediated response to these molecules that eventually results in the IA that precedes clinical diabetes.

OXIDATIVE STRESS THEORY

Oxidative stress is a general term used to describe the level of oxidative damage in a cell, tissue, or organ, caused by reactive oxygen species (e.g., free radicals). Free radicals are highly reactive chemical species that, at physiological levels, are part of normal homeostasis, but when allowed to proliferate unchecked, cause biological damage. Because the untoward consequences of oxidative damage are most noticeable in rapidly dividing tissues, the GI tract is one of the places where oxidative stress can have the most profound effects. Normally there are multiple defense mechanisms in place that help prevent free radical formation, inactivate free radicals that are formed (via reduction), and repair the damage done by these species. These defenses can be intrinsic or obtained through the diet; both sources are important in everyday functioning.

Immune function and dysfunction are inextricably tied to the reduction/oxidation (redox) balance of an individual and this relationship that may be significant in the pathogenesis of type 1 diabetes. There is evidence to indicate that diabetics have impaired redox balance characterized by decreased antioxidant defenses and increased byproducts of oxidative damage (48). Studies suggest that a similar imbalance exists among healthy first-degree relatives of type 1 diabetes patients, which can be interpreted as evidence that redox imbalance precedes the onset of clinical disease (49). Because children who develop diabetes may have a preexisting impairment of antioxidant capacity, it is especially important that they have ample exogenous sources of antioxidants and free radical scavengers along with limited exposure to dietary oxidants. The most notable early-life dietary factors that may have a protective effect are breast-feeding and dietary intake of fish oils and vitamins D and E, and that may have a diabetogenic effect is exposure to exogenous free radical substrates like nitrates.

Breast milk is high in antioxidant species including enzymatic antioxidants and vitamins C, E, and β-carotene especially when compared with infant formula (50). These antioxidants may help to bolster the antioxidant capabilities in the infant, which in turn, is essential to proper immune function as evidenced by the observation that healthy infants who were exclusively breast-fed had better overall antioxidant capacity than their contemporaries who were fed formula only (51). Given this observation and the proposed hypothesis that increased oxidative stress may result in type 1 diabetes, one might expect to see a protective effect with breast-feeding, particularly longer durations of breast-feeding, on type 1 diabetes and IA. However, the results concerning longer duration of breast-feeding and diabetes or autoimmunity are equivocal. The lack of a clear relationship may suggest that early infancy, the time when breast-feeding is most likely to occur, is not the most important time for exposure to the antioxidants found in breast milk, at least with respect to the etiology of type 1 diabetes. It is also possible that endogenous antioxidants are more important than those acquired through the diet with respect to their role in type 1 diabetes pathogenesis, or that children at increased risk for type 1 diabetes are less able to utilize dietary antioxidants.

Besides breast milk there are multiple early-life diet exposures that affect antioxidant status, including vitamin E, fish oils, and vitamin D. Vitamin E, or α-tocopherol, is a powerful antioxidant that is important in the control of lipid peroxidation, a marker of oxidative stress. Lipids are one of the basic cellular building blocks and are the molecules that maintain normal membrane receptor and transport function as well as normal membrane fluidity. In addition, when lipid peroxidation occurs, abnormalities in the outer lipid membrane can result in death of the cell and a subsequent immune response.

Two Finnish studies examined whether serum α-tocopherol levels were associated with type 1 diabetes. In the first study, investigators identified 19 type 1 diabetic cases developing within a cohort of 7526 men initially examined at age 20 or older. The diabetic cases, with an average age at onset of 28 years, had significantly lower serum α-tocopherol levels at baseline than healthy age-matched controls (52). In the second study, siblings of type 1 diabetic individuals were followed prospectively for the development of type 1 diabetes. The siblings who progressed to type 1 diabetes had lower serum α-tocopherol levels than the siblings who remained autoantibody negative, although these results were only marginally significant (53). These studies suggest that vitamin E may in some way be protective against type 1 diabetes.

Even though fish oil is not an antioxidant itself, it has been shown to increase antioxidant enzyme activity. In a case-control study from Norway, use of cod liver oil supplements in the first year of life was associated with a lower risk of developing type 1 diabetes (28). The same study found no association between maternal use of fish oil supplements during pregnancy and diabetes in their children. Fronczak et al. found similar negative results when they prospectively investigated the association between in utero exposure to dietary n-3 PUFA and the risk of IA (54). These findings suggest that the most pronounced benefits come from direct exposure to the infant.

Vitamin D possesses immune modulating properties that may provide protection against type 1 diabetes. The protective effect may be through the relationship between oxidative reactions and the balance between Th1 and Th2 cellular responses. The redox status of macrophages (e.g., dendritic cells in the intestine) dictates the type of cytokines that are secreted and therefore the type of helper cell response elicited. If a macrophage has decreased antioxidant capacity then the balance of cytokines is shifted preferentially to a Th1 response (55). Since vitamin D has been shown to help shift the balance back toward the regulatory characteristics of the Th2 response, its role in immunological repair may be one of its mechanisms of action (56).

Multiple studies have examined the role of vitamin D in the pathogenesis of type 1 diabetes. The EURODIAB multicenter case-control study found that diabetic children were less likely to have been given vitamin D supplements in infancy than control children (57). This finding is similar to that found in the previously described case-control study form Norway, where diabetic children were less likely to have been given cod liver oil supplements during infancy compared with controls (28), if one were to assume that it is the vitamin D found in cod liver oil rather than the n-3 fatty acids that is responsible. In a large historical prospective study from Finland, Hypponen et al. studied vitamin D supplementation in infants and found an increased risk for type 1 diabetes in those children who received no vitamin D supplementation compared with those who did receive supplements (58). Aside from cod liver oil and vitamin supplements, the primary sources of vitamin D are sunlight, fatty fish, and vitamin D–fortified dairy foods. The aforementioned studies were limited in that they were only able to examine vitamin D from supplements, but not vitamin D exposure from foods. In a small study within DAISY, Fronczak et al. investigated vitamin D intake during pregnancy and found that increased intake of vitamin D from foods was associated with lower risk of IA in the offspring, but no such association was seen for vitamin D intake from supplements (54).

In addition to the aforementioned dietary factors that may help improve antioxidant capacity, there are dietary factors that can cause oxidative damage, including *N*-nitroso compounds. Nitrates and nitrites are common in the diet and are not harmful substrates unto themselves but can be converted in the body to *N*-nitroso compounds, which are reactive oxidative species capable of initiating and propagating damaging oxidative cascades. These cascades may result in direct β-cell destruction or may lead to chronic immune stimulation that may help to precipitate immune-mediated destruction of β cells.

The epidemiological literature concerning nitrates is sparse but includes two ecological studies that found increased risk of diabetes in areas where there were high levels of nitrates in the drinking water (59,60), as well as two case-control studies that found that children with diabetes consumed diets higher in nitrates and nitrites than children without diabetes (61,62). This question has not yet been examined in the prospective studies of predictors of IA in children at increased risk for type 1 diabetes.

CONCLUSION

From this discussion, it is apparent that a great deal of overlap between these theories may exist and it is possible that all of them have a role in the development of IA and type 1 diabetes. For this reason, it is important to consider the components of early-life diet as risk factors or protective factors in their entirety rather than as mutually exclusive entities. Thinking of them in this way increases the complexity of the relationship between infant diet and the development of IA and type 1 diabetes but also potentially holds the key to the environmental component in the interaction between genes, the environment, and type 1 diabetes.

REFERENCES

1. Virtanen SM, Knip M. Nutritional risk predictors of beta cell autoimmunity and type 1 diabetes at a young age. Am J Clin Nutr 2003; 78(6):1053–1067.
2. LaGasse JM, Brantley MS, Leech NJ, et al. Successful prospective prediction of type 1 diabetes in schoolchildren through multiple defined autoantibodies: an 8-year follow-up of the Washington State Diabetes Prediction Study. Diabetes Care 2002; 25(3):505–511.

3. Verge CF, Gianani R, Kawasaki E, et al. Prediction of type I diabetes in first-degree relatives using a combination of insulin, GAD, and ICA512bdc/IA-2 autoantibodies. Diabetes 1996; 45(7):926–933.
4. Faria AM, Weiner HL Oral tolerance. Immunol Rev 2005; 206:232–259.
5. Sherry NA, Kushner JA, Glandt M, et al. Effects of autoimmunity and immune therapy on beta-cell turnover in type 1 diabetes. Diabetes 2006; 55(12):3238–3245.
6. Vaarala O. Is it dietary insulin? Ann N Y Acad Sci 2006; 1079:350–359.
7. Vaarala O. Gut and the induction of immune tolerance in type 1 diabetes. Diabetes Metab Res Rev 1999; 15(5):353–361.
8. Tiittanen M, Paronen J, Savilahti E, et al. Dietary insulin as an immunogen and tolerogen. Pediatr Allergy Immunol 2006; 17(7):538–543.
9. Norris JM, Beaty B, Klingensmith G, et al. Lack of association between early exposure to cow's milk protein and beta-cell autoimmunity. Diabetes Autoimmunity Study in the Young (DAISY). JAMA 1996; 276(8):609–614.
10. Norris JM, Barriga K, Klingensmith G, et al. Timing of initial cereal exposure in infancy and risk of islet autoimmunity. JAMA 2003; 290(13):1713–1720.
11. Virtanen SM, Kenward MG, Erkkola M, et al. Age at introduction of new foods and advanced beta cell autoimmunity in young children with HLA-conferred susceptibility to type 1 diabetes. Diabetologia 2006; 49(7):1512–1521.
12. Ziegler AG, Schmid S, Huber D, et al. Early infant feeding and risk of developing type 1 diabetes-associated autoantibodies. JAMA 2003; 290(13):1721–1728.
13. Hypponen E, Kenward MG, Virtanen SM, et al. Infant feeding, early weight gain, and risk of type 1 diabetes. Childhood Diabetes in Finland (DiMe) Study Group. Diabetes Care 1999; 22(12):1961–1965.
14. Vaarala O, Saukkonen T, Savilahti E, et al. Development of immune response to cow's milk proteins in infants receiving cow's milk or hydrolyzed formula. J Allergy Clin Immunol 1995; 96(6 pt 1):917–923.
15. Kostraba JN, Cruickshanks KJ, Lawler-Heavner J, et al. Early exposure to cow's milk and solid foods in infancy, genetic predisposition, and risk of IDDM. Diabetes 1993; 42(2):288–295.
16. Sipetic S, Vlajinac H, Kocev N, et al. Early infant diet and risk of type 1 diabetes mellitus in Belgrade children. Nutrition 2005; 21(4):474–479.
17. Virtanen SM, Rasanen L, Ylonen K, et al. Early introduction of dairy products associated with increased risk of IDDM in Finnish children. The Childhood in Diabetes in Finland Study Group. Diabetes 1993; 42(12):1786–1790.
18. Fort P, Lanes R, Dahlem S, et al. Breast feeding and insulin-dependent diabetes mellitus in children. J Am Coll Nutr 1986; 5(5):439–441.
19. Samuelsson U, Ludvigsson J. Seasonal variation of birth month and breastfeeding in children with diabetes mellitus. J Pediatr Endocrinol Metab 2001; 14(1):43–46.
20. Perez-Bravo F, Oyarzun A, Carrasco E, et al. Duration of breast feeding and bovine serum albumin antibody levels in type 1 diabetes: a case-control study [see comment]. Pediatr Diabetes 2003; 4(4):157–161.
21. Karlsson MG, Garcia J, Ludvigsson J. Cow's milk proteins cause similar Th1- and Th2-like immune response in diabetic and healthy children. Diabetologia 2001; 44(9): 1140–1147.
22. Akerblom HK, Virtanen SM, Ilonen J, et al. Dietary manipulation of beta cell autoimmunity in infants at increased risk of type 1 diabetes: a pilot study. Diabetologia 2005; 48(5):829–837;[Erratum appears in Diabetologia 2005;48(8):1676. Note: Riikjarv MA [added]; Ormisson A [added]; Ludvigsson J [added]; Dosch HM [added]; Hakulinen T [added]; Knip M [added]].
23. Tuomilehto J, Podar T, Tuomilehto-Wolf E, et al. Evidence for importance of gender and birth cohort for risk of IDDM in offspring of IDDM parents. Diabetologia 1995. 38(8):975–982.
24. Scott FW, Rowsell P, Wang GS, et al. Oral exposure to diabetes-promoting food or immunomodulators in neonates alters gut cytokines and diabetes. Diabetes 2002; 51(1):73–78.

25. MacFarlane AJ, Burghardt KM, Kelly J, et al. A type 1 diabetes-related protein from wheat (*Triticum aestivum*). cDNA clone of a wheat storage globulin, Glb1, linked to islet damage. J Biol Chem 2003; 278(1):54–63.

26. Ivarsson A, Hernell O, Stenlund H, et al. Breast-feeding protects against celiac disease. Am J Clin Nutr 2002; 75(5):914–921.

27. Singh VK, Mehrotra S, Agarwal SS. The paradigm of Th1 and Th2 cytokines: its relevance to autoimmunity and allergy. Review. Immunol Res 1999; 20(2):147–161.

28. Stene LC, Joner G. Norwegian Childhood Diabetes Study Group. Use of cod liver oil during the first year of life is associated with lower risk of childhood-onset type 1 diabetes: a large, population-based, case-control study [see comment]. Am J Clin Nutr 2003; 78(6):1128–1134.

29. Giulietti A, Gysemans C, Stoffels K, et al. Vitamin D deficiency in early life accelerates Type 1 diabetes in non-obese diabetic mice. Diabetologia 2004; 47(3):451–462.

30. Gregori S, Giarratana N, Smiroldo S, et al. A 1alpha,25-dihydroxyvitamin D(3) analog enhances regulatory T-cells and arrests autoimmune diabetes in NOD mice. Diabetes 2002; 51(5):1367–1374.

31. Kleemann R, Scott FW, Worz-Pagenstert U, et al. Impact of dietary fat on Th1/Th2 cytokine gene expression in the pancreas and gut of diabetes-prone BB rats. J Autoimmun 1998; 11(1):97–103.

32. Hughes DA, Pinder AC. n-3 polyunsaturated fatty acids inhibit the antigen-presenting function of human monocytes. Am J Clin Nutr 2000; 71(1 suppl):357S–360S.

33. Liu Z, Li N, Neu J. Tight junctions, leaky intestines, and pediatric diseases. Acta Paediatr 2005; 94(4):386–393.

34. Neu J, Reverte CM, Mackey AD, et al. Changes in intestinal morphology and permeability in the biobreeding rat before the onset of type 1 diabetes. J Pediatr Gastroenterol Nutr 2005; 40(5):589–595.

35. Courtois P, Nsimba G, Jijakli H, et al. Gut permeability and intestinal mucins, invertase, and peroxidase in control and diabetes-prone BB rats fed either a protective or a diabetogenic diet. Dig Dis Sci 2005; 50(2):266–275.

36. Courtois P, Jurysta C, Sener A, et al. Quantitative and qualitative alterations of intestinal mucins in BioBreeding rats. Int J Mol Med 2005; 15(1):105–108.

37. Malaisse WJ, Courtois P, Scott FW. Insulin-dependent diabetes and gut dysfunction: the BB rat model. Review. Horm Metab Res 2004; 36(9):585–594.

38. Secondulfo M, Iafusco D, Carratu R, et al. Ultrastructural mucosal alterations and increased intestinal permeability in non-celiac, type I diabetic patients. Dig Liver Dis 2004; 36(1):35–45.

39. Catassi C, Bonucci A, Coppa GV, et al. Intestinal permeability changes during the first month: effect of natural versus artificial feeding. J Pediatr Gastroenterol Nutr 1995; 21(4):383–386.

40. Kuitunen M, Savilahti E, Sarnesto A. Human alpha-lactalbumin and bovine beta-lactoglobulin absorption in infants. Allergy 1994; 49(5):354–360.

41. Lawrence RM, Pane CA. Human breast milk: current concepts of immunology and infectious diseases. Review. Curr Probl Pediatr Adolesc Health Care 2007; 37(1):7–36.

42. Lammi N, Karvonen M, Tuomilehto J. Do microbes have a causal role in type 1 diabetes? Med Sci Monit 2005; 11(3):RA63–RA69.

43. Ylipaasto P, Klingel K, Lindberg AM, et al. Enterovirus infection in human pancreatic islet cells, islet tropism in vivo and receptor involvement in cultured islet beta cells. Diabetologia 2004; 47(2):225–239.

44. Vaarala O, Klemetti P, Juhela S, et al. Effect of coincident enterovirus infection and cow's milk exposure on immunisation to insulin in early infancy. Diabetologia 2002. 45(4):531–534.

45. Fasano A. Intestinal zonulin: open sesame! Gut 2001; 49(2):159–162.

46. Watts T, Berti I, Sapone A, et al. Role of the intestinal tight junction modulator zonulin in the pathogenesis of type I diabetes in BB diabetic-prone rats. Proc Natl Acad Sci U S A 2005; 102(8):2916–2921.

47. Sapone A, de Magistris L, Pietzak M, et al. Zonulin upregulation is associated with increased gut permeability in subjects with type 1 diabetes and their relatives. Diabetes 2006; 55(5):1443–1449.
48. Martin-Gallan P, Carrascosa A, Gussinye M, et al. Estimation of lipoperoxidative damage and antioxidant status in diabetic children: relationship with individual antioxidants. Free Radic Res 2005; 39(9):933–942.
49. Matteucci E, Giampietro O. Oxidative stress in families of type 1 diabetic patients. Diabetes Care 2000; 23(8):1182–1186.
50. Friel JK, Martin SM, Langdon M, et al. Milk from mothers of both premature and full-term infants provides better antioxidant protection than does infant formula. Pediatr Res 2002; 51(5):612–618.
51. Aycicek A, Erel O, Kocyigit A, et al. Breast milk provides better antioxidant power than does formula. Nutrition 2006; 22(6):616–619.
52. Knekt P, Reunanen A, Marniemi J, et al. Low vitamin E status is a potential risk factor for insulin-dependent diabetes mellitus. J Intern Med 1999; 245(1):99–102.
53. Uusitalo L, Knip M, Kenward MG, et al. Serum alpha-tocopherol concentrations and risk of type 1 diabetes mellitus: a cohort study in siblings of affected children. J Pediatr Endocrinol 2005; 18(12):1409–1416.
54. Fronczak CM, Baron AE, Chase HP, et al. In utero dietary exposures and risk of islet autoimmunity in children. Diabetes Care 2003; 26(12):3237–3242.
55. Murata Y, Amao M, Hamuro J. Sequential conversion of the redox status of macrophages dictates the pathological progression of autoimmune diabetes. Eur J Immunol 2003; 33(4):1001–1011.
56. Mathieu C, Badenhoop K. Vitamin D and type 1 diabetes mellitus: state of the art. Trends Endocrinol Metab 2005; 16(6):261–266.
57. The EURODIAB Substudy 2 Study Group. Vitamin D supplement in early childhood and risk for Type I (insulin-dependent) diabetes mellitus. Diabetologia 1999; 42(1):51–54.
58. Hypponen E, Laara E, Reunanen A, et al. Intake of vitamin D and risk of type 1 diabetes: a birth-cohort study. Lancet 2001; 358(9292):1500–1503.
59. Kostraba JN, Gay EC, Rewers M, et al. Nitrate levels in community drinking waters and risk of IDDM. An ecological analysis. Diabetes Care 1992; 15(11):1505–1508.
60. Parslow RC, McKinney PA, Law GR, et al. Incidence of childhood diabetes mellitus in Yorkshire, northern England, is associated with nitrate in drinking water: an ecological analysis [see comment]. Diabetologia 1997; 40(5):550–556.
61. Virtanen SM, Jaakkola L, Rasanen L, et al. Nitrate and nitrite intake and the risk for type 1 diabetes in Finnish children. Childhood Diabetes in Finland Study Group. Diabet Med 1994; 11(7):656–662.
62. Dahlquist GG, Blom LG, Persson LA, et al. Dietary factors and the risk of developing insulin dependent diabetes in childhood. BMJ 1990; 300(6735):1302–1306.

5 Environmental Determinants: The Role of Viruses and Standard of Hygiene

Mikael Knip
Hospital for Children and Adolescents, University of Helsinki, Helsinki, and Department of Pediatrics, Tampere University Hospital, Tampere, Finland

Heikki Hyöty
Department of Virology, University of Tampere, and Department of Clinical Microbiology, Center for Laboratory Medicine, Tampere University Hospital, Tampere, Finland

INTRODUCTION

Type 1 diabetes is perceived as a chronic immune-mediated disease with a subclinical prodrome of variable duration (1). The preclinical period is characterized by selective loss of insulin-producing β cells in the pancreatic islets in genetically susceptible subjects. The most important genes contributing to disease susceptibility are located in the HLA class II locus on the short arm of chromosome 6 (2). Only a relatively small proportion, i.e., less than 10%, of individuals with HLA-conferred disease susceptibility progress, however, to clinical diabetes. This implies that additional factors are needed to trigger and drive β-cell destruction in genetically predisposed subjects. Environmental factors have been implicated in the pathogenesis of type 1 diabetes both as triggers and potentiators of β-cell destruction (3–5), although a critical role of any individual exogenous factor has not been definitely proven so far. In any case, a series of evidence support a crucial contribution of exogenous factors in the development of type 1 diabetes, such as (1) the fact that less than 10% of those with HLA-conferred diabetes susceptibility do progress to clinical disease, (2) a pair-wise concordance of type 1 diabetes of less than 40% among monozygotic twins, (3) a more than 10-fold difference in the disease incidence among Caucasians living in Europe, (4) a several fold increase in the incidence over the last 50 years in most developed countries, and (5) migration studies indicating that the disease incidence has increased in population groups who have moved from a low-incidence to a high-incidence region. This chapter discusses the role of viruses as potential triggers and potentiators of the diabetic disease process. In addition, we consider the standard of hygiene as a possible factor programming the immune system; a high standard favoring weak immune regulation resulting in either Th1 or Th2 polarization of the CD4+ T cells with autoimmune or allergic manifestations as the outcome.

PATHOGENESIS OF TYPE 1 DIABETES

Clinical type 1 diabetes represents end-stage insulitis, and it has been estimated that at the time of diagnosis only 10–20% of the insulin-producing β cells are still functioning. The clinical disease presentation is preceded by an asymptomatic period of highly variable duration (6). Aggressive β-cell destruction may lead to disease manifestation within a few months in infants and young children, while in other individuals the process may continue for years, in some cases even for more than 10 years, before the eventual presentation of overt disease. The appearance of diabetes-associated autoantibodies is the first detectable sign of emerging β-cell autoimmunity. There are four disease-related autoantibodies that have been shown to predict clinical diabetes (7). These include classical islet cell antibodies (ICA) detected by conventional immunofluorescence, insulin autoantibodies (IAA), and autoantibodies to the 65-kDa isoform of glutamic acid decarboxylase (GADA) and the tyrosine phosphatase-related IA-2 molecule (IA-2A). The latter three auto-antibodies can be measured with specific radiobinding assays.

A variety of studies have shown that β-cell autoimmunity might be induced early in life (8,9). Data from the Finnish Diabetes Prediction and Prevention (DIPP) study show that the first autoantibodies may appear before the age of three months, and that about 9% of these children recruited from the general population based on increased HLA DQB1-conferred genetic risk develop persistent positivity for at least one autoantibody by the age of five years, whereas close to 4% seroconvert to persistent positivity for multiple ($\geq$2) antibodies by that age (10). These figures demonstrate that a higher proportion of the population develops signs of β-cell autoimmunity than that progressing to clinical diabetes. Observations from the DIPP study indicate that the spreading of the humoral autoimmune response from one epitope to another and from one antibody to another occurs in a relatively narrow time window (6,11). If such a spreading does not take place within a year after the appearance of the first autoantibodies, it rarely occurs later. These and other observations imply that positivity for a single autoantibody specificity represents in most cases harmless nonprogressive β-cell autoimmunity, while the presence of two or more autoantibodies reflect a progressive process that rarely reverts (12). Accordingly, positivity for multiple autoantibodies can be used as a surrogate marker of clinical diabetes in prospective studies, in young children in particular, since the overwhelming majority of young children with multiple autoantibodies will eventually present with overt diabetes (13). These new insights into the natural history of type 1 diabetes have opened up new possibilities and strategies for assessing the role of environmental factors in the development of diabetes.

A series of observations suggest that β-cell autoimmunity may be triggered by an environmental culprit at any age, although a majority of the processes appear to start early in childhood (14). We hypothesize that the genetic disease susceptibility allows the initiation of a β-cell destructive process resulting in the presentation of clinical type 1 diabetes in some individuals. However, initiation of the process does not necessarily lead to progression to clinical disease. According to our hypothesis there is a need for a driving exogenous antigen playing the same role as gluten in celiac disease. As a matter of fact there are striking similarities between type 1 diabetes and celiac disease from a pathogenetic point of view (15). Both diseases are characterized by genetic susceptibility determined by both HLA and non-HLA genes. The former explain about half of the familial clustering in both diseases, and accordingly the other half must be due to non-HLA genes and/or shared environment. About 20% of Caucasians carry HLA-conferred genetic susceptibility to celiac disease, the overwhelming majority (>95%) of the population in developed countries are daily exposed to gluten-containing cereals, but in spite of that only maximally 1.3% of the population present with clinical disease (16). Accordingly, some other factor(s) in addition to HLA-conferred predisposition and daily gluten intake are needed for progression to overt celiac disease. It seems unlikely that non-HLA genes should totally account for the missing link, and it is tempting to speculate that one may need a triggering gastrointestinal infection inducing a primary target cell damage and/or a proinflammatory cytokine milieu in the gut epithelium to initiate the disease process subsequently driven by dietary gluten toward clinical celiac disease in genetically predisposed individuals. Previous studies have indicated that adenovirus and rotavirus infections might contribute to the pathogenesis of celiac disease (17–19), but only a few studies have focused on the possible role of viruses and other microbes in this disease.

In parallel to celiac disease, about one-fifth of Caucasians carry HLA-conferred susceptibility to type 1 diabetes, whereas the lifetime cumulative incidence of clinical disease can be estimated to be close to 1%, indicating that only about 5% of those with HLA-conferred predisposition progress to overt diabetes. Our hypothesis holds that progression to clinical diabetes requires the combination of genetic disease susceptibility, a critically timed trigger, and high subsequent exposure to a driving antigen (1). If any of these determinants is missing or any of the exogenous factors is inappropriately timed, the risk of type 1 diabetes would be minimal even in the presence of the other predisposing elements. Such a model could explain why only a small minority of those with HLA-conferred diabetes susceptibility do present with overt disease. In addition to the trigger and the driving antigen there are most likely a series of environmental factors modifying the fate and pace of the β-cell destructive process, some having protective and others predisposing effects.

VIRAL INFECTIONS

Viral infections have been implicated in the etiology of type 1 diabetes for more than 100 years. More recently, a variety of studies have been published showing that certain viruses, such as enteroviruses (EV), are capable of inducing diabetes in experimental animals, and seroepidemiological studies have indicated their role in human type 1 diabetes as well (5,20). Table 1 lists viruses suspected to contribute to the diabetic disease process. Viruses may act by at least two possible mechanisms, either via a direct cytolytic effect or by triggering an auto-immune process leading gradually to β-cell destruction (21). The role of molecular mimicry in diabetes-associated autoimmune responses has been indicated by the observations of structural and functional homology between viral structures and β-cell antigens. Persistent or slow virus infections, like in the congenital rubella syndrome (CRS) and cytomegalovirus (CMV) infections, may also be important in the induction of the autoimmune response. The role of viral infections in the etiopathogenesis of human type 1 diabetes has been elucidated by serological and epidemiological studies and case histories (22). Three key hypotheses for the role of viruses in the development of type 1 diabetes are presented in Figure 1.

TABLE 1   Viruses Implicated in the Pathogenesis of Type 1 Diabetes.

Virus	Family	Size (nm)
Enteroviruses	Picornavirus	30
Mumps	Paramyxovirus	100–600
Rubella	Togavirus	60–70
Cytomegalovirus	Herpesvirus	120–300
Rotavirus	Reovirus	100
Ljungan virus	Picornavirus	30
Retroviruses	Retrovirus	100

1. Virus hypothesis
Beta-cell tropic virus damages beta-cells and triggers beta-cell autoimmunity.
Relevant animal model: Encephalomyocarditis virus in mice.

2. Polio hypothesis
Effect of triggering virus is modulated by child's immune
protection and it's ability to neutralize the virus.

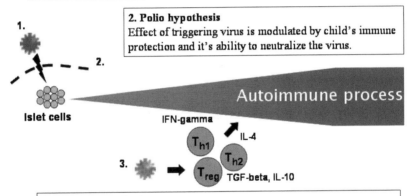

3. Hygiene hypothesis
Virus infections are crucial for the development of immunoregulatory
networks which can downregulate autoimmune process and prevent its
progression to diabetes. Relevant animal model: NOD mouse

FIGURE 1   Three key hypotheses describing various stages of virus-induced diabetes. The *virus hypothesis* is based on an assumption that certain viruses have strong tropism to pancreatic islets. These viruses target to pancreatic islets and trigger the autoimmune process by damaging β cells and activating dendritic cells to present β-cell autoantigens to T cells. The *polio hypothesis* is related to immune protection against these viruses. This protection depends on individual characteristics (e.g., genetic factors) as well as population-dependent factors that are related to the dynamic balance between virus circulation and herd immunity in a given population (maternal antibodies transferred to the infant, in particular). The third hypothesis, the *hygiene hypothesis*, was first proposed to explain the increasing incidence of allergic diseases, and recent observations suggest that it may also be relevant for autoimmune diseases, such as type 1 diabetes. Accordingly, viruses and other microbes are important for the development of immune regulatory networks controlling the autoimmune process. The scarcity of this kind of microbial exposure may lead to inability to downregulate immune responses against self and foreign antigens (allergens).

EV

EV belong to the picornavirus family comprising small, naked icosahedral RNA viruses. The EV genus comprises a series of subgroups that have been formed according to their antigenic properties and, more recently, according to their genetic relationships. Traditional antigenic classification includes the groups of polioviruses, coxsackie B viruses (CBV), coxsackie A viruses (CAV), echoviruses, and new numbered serotypes including altogether more than 100 distinct serotypes. Epidemiological, serological, and biological indications suggest that EV may be involved in the pathogenesis of type 1 diabetes (20,23,24). Infections with different serotypes are common, starting in infancy. The virus frequently causes viremia and spreads to many organs including the pancreas. Most of these infections are mild and subclinical.

The role of EV in the pathogenesis of type 1 diabetes have been strengthened over the last 10 to 20 years, one reason being methodological developments in the diagnosis of EV infections and the other insight that the diabetic disease process starts months and years before the clinical presentation of the disease requiring prospective studies to identify potential triggers and boosters of the process. Gamble and Taylor (25) reported in 1969 parallel changes in the seasonal variation in the incidence of type 1 diabetes and in the frequency of CBV infections. A series of serological case-control studies have shown an increased prevalence of elevated levels of CBV antibodies in patients with newly diagnosed type 1 diabetes (23,24). There are, however, also contradictory results, since some other reports have been unable to find any difference between patients with diabetes and controls (26,27) or even demonstrated decreased levels of CBV antibodies in patients (28).

The first serological studies measured neutralizing EV antibodies that are good markers of infection immunity but poor indicators of a recent infection, if the analyses do not include IgM antibodies. More recent studies have assessed the occurrence of recent or current EV infections by quantifying IgM antibodies with μ-antibody capture methods based on enzyme or radioimmunoassays. With such a methodology patients with newly diagnosed type 1 diabetes were found to have increased IgM class antibodies against EV suggesting an excess of recent infections (29). A Swedish group detected IgM class antibodies to CBV in 40% of children with newly diagnosed type 1 diabetes and in none of the controls (30). The majority of those, who had IgM class antibodies at the diagnosis of diabetes, had experienced previously an EV infection caused by a different serotype, indicated by IgG class antibodies (31). As increased IgM titers reflect an ongoing or recent infection, Fohlman and Friman concluded that these observations suggest that successive infections by different CBV and other EVs increase the risk of manifestation of overt diabetes in genetically susceptible individuals. Such a process fits well into the "Copenhagen model" for the pathogenesis of type 1 diabetes, i.e., the multiple hit hypothesis (32).

The use of polymerase chain reaction (PCR) methodology has enabled the detection of viruses by molecular methods from serum, whole blood, or mononuclear cells with high sensitivity, thus circumventing the indirect approach through antibody-based analyses. An additional advantage is that these methods can be extended to delineate virus nucleotide sequences. Studies from six different countries show an increased frequency of EV detected with PCR from the peripheral circulation in subjects with newly diagnosed type 1 diabetes (Table 2) (33–43). The prevalence of EV mRNA varied from 20% to 64% among the patients

TABLE 2 Enterovirus RNA Detected in Patients with Recently Diagnosed Type 1 Diabetes

Country	Patients		Controls		
	Percentage	N	Percentage	N	Reference
U.K.	64	14	4	45	33
	41	55	31	43	34
	27	110	5	182	36
France	42	12	0	27	35
	38	56	0	37	37
Sweden	50	24	0	24	38
	78	32	8	25	43
Australia	30	206	4	160	39
Japan	38	61	3	58	40
Germany	20–36	50 + 47	2	50	41
Cuba	27	34	3	68	42
Finland	9	58	5	58	unpublished
TOTAL	33	759	5	777	

and from 0% to 31% among the control subjects. The only exception is a Finnish study (Martiskainen et al., unpublished) showing no significant difference between newly diagnosed diabetic children and controls in the frequency of detectable EV RNA in serum samples. Altogether 33% of the patients with newly diagnosed type 1 diabetes had detectable EV mRNA compared with 5% of the controls verifying an increased frequency of EV viremia at the time of clinical presentation of type 1 diabetes.

Finnish prospective studies have repeatedly shown an increased frequency of EV infections among prediabetic subjects compared with unaffected controls and an unequivocal temporal association between EV infections and the appearance of the first diabetes-associated autoantibodies (44–48). The latter observation strongly indicates that EV are capable of triggering β-cell autoimmunity. There are two prospective reports from Germany and Colorado, U.S.A., showing no association between EV infections and β-cell autoimmunity (49,50). Those studies are hampered, however, by limitations due to long sampling intervals and a narrow methodological arsenal. Short sampling intervals (optimally 3 months or less) are critical, when the aim is to assess the temporal association between EV infections and seroconversion to positivity for diabetes-associated autoantibodies.

Two studies from Northern Europe have indicated that maternal enteroviral infections during pregnancy may be associated with later development of type 1 diabetes in the offspring. Dahlquist et al. (51) analyzed maternal sera taken at delivery and observed the closest relation between IgM to CBV3 and type 1 diabetes in the children. A Finnish survey tested sera obtained at the end of the first trimester and showed that the strongest association between CBV5 and type 1 diabetes in offspring under the age of three at diagnosis but not in those older than three years (44). A more recent Finnish study in a larger cohort of pregnant women did not, however, support the earlier observation that EV infections during the first trimester are associated with an increased risk of type 1 diabetes in the offspring (52).

Taken together, most cross-sectional studies in patients with newly diagnosed type 1 diabetes support the hypothesis that EV can precipitate clinical disease in subjects with signs of β-cell autoimmunity. Data from prospective studies

TABLE 3 Summary of Studies Demonstrating EV in Human Pancreatic Tissue

Type of patients	Proportion of patients with virus in pancreas tissue	Methods used for virus detection	Tropism of the virus to islets[a]	Serotype of the virus	Reference
Type 1 diabetes	1/1	IHC	Yes	CBV4	57
	1/1	Virus isolation	ND	CBV4	58
	4/65	IHC	Yes	ND	62
	3/6	IHC, EM, virus isolation	Yes	CBV4[b]	63
Fatal enterovirus infection	1/1	IHC	Yes	CBV3	59
	8/14	IHC	Yes	CBV2, CBV3, CBV4, CBV5	60
	5/9	ISH	Yes	CBV	61
	7/12	ISH	Yes	CBV	62

[a]Enterovirus was detected predominantly or exclusively in pancreatic islets while exocrine pancreas was mostly negative.
[b]Coxsackievirus B4 was isolated from the islets of one patient.
Abbreviations: IHC, immunohistochemistry; ISH, *in situ* hybridization; EM, electron microscopy; ND, not determined; CBV, coxsackie B viruses.

suggest that EV may trigger β-cell autoimmunity and boost existing β-cell autoimmunity. It is also possible that the frequent detection of EV in the blood of patients with type 1 diabetes reflects persistent replication of the virus in the pancreas or some other infectious focus. EV persistence has been described in chronic myocarditis and cardiomyopathies where EV persists in cardiac tissue leading to severe cell damage and failure in organ function. In a recent Finnish study EV was detected in intestinal biopsy samples from 75% of patients with type 1 diabetes compared to 10% of control subjects (53). This new discovery suggests that gut mucosa may be an important infectious focus in type 1 diabetes.

The tropism phenomenon (the characteristics of a virus to infect a particular tissue or cell type), in which the attachment of virus to the viral receptors on cell surface and the interaction of the viral genome with intracellular proteins are central features, is thought to explain why some variants of EV are diabetogenic and others are not (31). It has been proposed that pancreatic β-cell tropic variants of EVs are present in the general population and that they are able to induce β-cell damage in susceptible individuals (54). *In vitro* studies have shown that EV are capable of infecting β cells and inducing functional impairment and cell death (55,56). Such a capacity seems to be shared by a wide range of serotypes, but the extent of the cellular lesions appears to be characteristic of individual virus strains. EV have strong tropism to human islets also in vivo, as EVs have been detected selectively in pancreatic islets but not in exocrine pancreas both in systemic EV infections and in some patients affected by type 1 diabetes (Table 3) (57–63). In a recent study, Dotta et al. detected EV in the pancreases of three out of six patients with recently diagnosed type 1 diabetes and isolated CBV4 virus from one of the pancreases (63). They also found natural killer cell infiltration in the infected islets suggesting activation of the innate immune system. The EV-infected islets showed decreased β-cell function in vitro. These findings raise the possibility that patients with type 1 diabetes may have a persistent (chronic) EV infection in their pancreatic islets. Further studies are needed to define whether tropism to human islets is a specific characteristic of coxsackie B serotypes or a more common feature of several different EV serotypes.

Could a Diabetogenic Enterovirus Infection Qualify as a Trigger of Type 1 Diabetes?

As mentioned earlier, the first signs of β-cell autoimmunity may appear very early in life. The authors have focused their research on defining the characteristics of the trigger(s) of β-cell autoimmunity by observing subjects with increased HLA-conferred diabetes susceptibility prospectively from birth with frequent follow-up visits with an interval of 3 to 6 months up to the age of 2 years and thereafter with an interval of 6 to 12 months (64). These studies have revealed that there is an unequivocal temporal variation in the appearance of the first diabetes-associated autoantibodies reflecting the initiation of the disease process and paralleling the seasonal variation previously observed in the presentation of clinical diabetes (9,65). Most initial autoantibodies appear during the cold period in the fall and winter while rarely in the spring or in the summer. There also seems to be some variation from one year to another in the timing and height of the autoantibody peaks. When studying families with more than one child experiencing seroconversion to auto-antibody positivity, we have noticed that the autoantibodies rarely appear simultaneously in seroconverting siblings (66). The first autoantibodies do emerge, however, more often than expected during the same season among such siblings but infrequently in the same year. On the basis of these observations we conclude that the trigger of β-cell autoimmunity (1) has a seasonal pattern, being more common during the cold season; (2) shows some temporal variation from year to year; and (3) does not necessarily induce β-cell autoimmunity at the same time in all genetically susceptible siblings within the same family.

On the basis of the characteristics listed above, some exogenous factors implicated as potential triggers of β-cell autoimmunity may be excluded. These include exogenous factors with a stable or consistently increasing exposure, such as most dietary components in early childhood. The pattern of autoantibody appearance strongly points to the role of infectious agents with conspicuous seasonal variation as triggers of β-cell autoimmunity. Such variations are typical for viral infections, and the pattern of laboratory confirmed EV infections in Finland fits well into the proposed role of EV infections as triggers of β-cell autoimmunity. In addition to viral infections, one should also consider other environmental variables with seasonal variation. There is definitely seasonal variation in the amount of daylight and sunshine hours, especially in Northern Europe, the region with the highest incidence of type 1 diabetes in the world (67). Without oral substitution, the sun light-dependent synthesis of vitamin D in the skin is the most important source of this immunologically active hormone. Some studies have indicated that the lack of oral vitamin D substitution in infancy increases the subsequent risk of type 1 diabetes (68,69). The following two arguments do, however, speak against the role of vitamin D deficiency as a trigger of β-cell autoimmunity: (1) there is a general recommendation that all young children should be substituted with daily vitamin D drops in Northern Europe, and this recommendation is implemented by more than 95% of the parents at least up to the age of two years; and (2) there are regions with a low incidence of type 1 diabetes in Northern Europe, e.g., Russian Karelia having an annual incidence rate of 7.8 per 100,000 children under the age of 15 years in the time period 1990–1999 compared with that of 42 in Finland (70), while there were no significant differences in the circulating vitamin D concentrations in pregnant women and schoolchildren between Russian Karelia and Finland (71). It has been shown that the mean HbA1c level varies over the year in children with manifest type 1 diabetes, with the highest values in the fall and winter and with lower levels in the spring and summer (72–74). This may reflect improved insulin sensitivity in the spring and summer due to more physical exercise. Improved insulin sensitivity diminishes β-cell stress, as the work load on the β-cells decreases. It is, however, unlikely that there should be substantial seasonal variation in the physical exercise in very young children, the target group in whom the seasonal variation in the appearance of the first diabetes-associated autoantibodies have been observed.

Accordingly we are left with viral infections as the most likely explanation to the seasonal variation in the emergence of the first signs of β-cell autoimmunity. Taking into account the timing and profiles of autoantibody peaks observed in the Finnish DIPP study, EV infections appear to be one of the most probable triggers of β-cell autoimmunity. This is further supported by our previous observations of a strong temporal relationship between EV infections and the appearance of the first diabetes-associated autoantibodies in prospective series of young children with increased genetic susceptibility to type 1 diabetes (44–48). The implicated link between EV infections and β-cell autoimmunity has been questioned, since most of the supportive data have come out of Finnish studies, and two other prospective studies, i.e., BABYDIAB in Germany and the Diabetes Autoimmunity Study in the Young (DAISY) in Denver, Colorado, have failed to demonstrate any association between EV infections and β-cell autoimmunity (49,50). There are, however, at least three critical issues with a decisive impact on the ability of any prospective study to provide meaningful observations in this context. The first one is the size of the study and the number of subjects who develop signs of β-cell autoimmunity; factors clearly related to the statistical power of the study (75). Each prospective study has so far included less than 50 seroconverters, which confers a high risk of missing even major influences of EV infections on β-cell autoimmunity. A second critical consideration is the study design and the sampling interval. Long sampling intervals definitely hamper the possibility to detect EV infections from collected samples. In the BABYDIAB study, coxsackie virus antibodies were measured from serum samples taken at the age of 9 months, 2 years, 5 years, and 8 years, and in DAISY, the samples were obtained at the age of 9 months, 15 months, 2 years, and then annually. In contrast, the DIPP study has a more frequent sampling schedule collecting samples with an interval of 3 to 6 months over the first 2 years of life and subsequently with an interval of 6 to12 months. The third crucial point is related to the type of samples collected and the methodological arsenal used for the detection of EV infections, taking into account that there are more than 100 different serotypes. The DIPP study used the most extensive strategy including detection of EV RNA with PCR from serum and stool samples, and analysis of IgA, IgM, and IgG class EV antibodies using both group- and serotype-specific assays. The impact of these differences are reflected by the substantially lower frequency of infections diagnosed, e.g., in the BABYDIAB cohort compared with the DIPP study (7% vs. 81% of the children had an EV infection by the age of 2 years). It is unlikely that such a difference could be due to a lower frequency of EV infections in Germany, as EV infections actually seem to be more common in the background population in Germany than in Finland (76).

The frequency of EV infections has decreased over the last decades in the background population in developed countries, e.g., in Finland and Sweden (76). These countries have in spite of that a high and increasing incidence of type 1 diabetes among children. This appears to be paradoxical. The paradox can, however, be explained by the so called "poliohypothesis" introduced by Viskari et al. (77). The polioviruses comprise three serotypes among more than 100 EV serotypes. When the frequency of acute poliovirus infections started to decrease at the beginning of the last century among the general population in countries with an increasing standard of hygiene, the incidence of paralytic polio being a complication of the acute infection began to increase. This was obviously the consequence of the concerted action of decreased levels of protective maternal poliovirus antibodies transferred transplacentally and through breast milk to the infant and the delay of infections to the age when the maternal antibodies had already declined, leading to a situation where the risk of the infant to get the first poliovirus infection at the time when no maternal protection was around increased. In the absence of maternal neutralizing antibodies, poliovirus was able to spread from the intestine to the blood and then to the central nervous system where it has strong tropism to motoneurons leading to their damage and subsequent paralysis. Similarly, the decreasing frequency of EV infections in the background population would increase the susceptibility of young children to the diabetogenic effect of EVs. The same phenomenon may also contribute to the marked international variation in the incidence of type 1 diabetes, as EV infections seem to be rare in countries where the rate of type 1 diabetes is high (77).

Other Viruses
Mumps
Gundersen (78), in his classical study in 1927, reported an increase in the number of cases with type 1 diabetes two to four years after a mumps epidemic. Subsequently, there have been numerous case reports describing a temporal relationship between mumps and clinical presentation of diabetes (4). In epidemiological studies, peaks in the incidence of childhood type 1 diabetes have been observed two to four years after mumps epidemics. Serological evidence of an association between mumps infection and type 1 diabetes has been difficult to obtain because of the long interval between the infection and the clinical manifestation of type 1 diabetes. A Finnish study reported decreased IgG class mumps antibody titers in children with newly diagnosed type 1 diabetes compared with those in controls, the finding being interpreted as indicative of an abnormal immunological response to mumps infection (79). Interestingly, in patient series collected earlier, when natural mumps was still common in Finland, IgG class mumps virus antibodies were not decreased, and IgA antibodies were elevated in diabetic children. This decline in mumps antibody levels may reflect the elimination of cases with mumps-induced type 1 diabetes by the triple vaccine comprising mumps, measles, and rubella.

Rubella
Diabetes has been observed in 10–20% of patients with the CRS with a latent period of 5 to 25 years (4). However, a recent study showed that signs of humoral β-cell autoimmunity are extremely rare among patients with the CRS, indicating that CRS-associated diabetes may be caused by other than autoimmune mechanisms (80).

CMV
The human CMV can be transmitted before birth, like the rubella virus, either transplacentally or at conception from an infected parent carrying the CMV genome in his or her genomic DNA. CMV infections may also be transmitted prenatally or postnatally through close contact or breast milk. CMV has been implicated in the development of type 1 diabetes by a case report of an infant with congenital CMV

infection who presented with diabetes at the age of 13 months (81). In a Swedish prospective study, 16,474 newborn infants were screened for congenital CMV infections by virus isolation from the urine, and 76 infants were found to be infected. Only one out of 73 infected individuals (1.4%) manifested type 1 diabetes, when observed up to the age of seven years or more, whereas 38 of 19,483 controls (0.2%) became affected by diabetes (82). This observation suggests that congenital CMV infection is not a major trigger of type 1 diabetes.

Hiltunen et al. found comparable levels of CMV IgG and IgM antibodies in children with newly diagnosed type 1 diabetes and in control children, while the patients had higher IgA antibodies than the controls (83). The latter observation may reflect reactivated or persistent CMV infections in children with recent-onset diabetes. No association was observed between ICA and CMV antibodies. Neither could any differences be seen in the CMV antibodies in early pregnancy between mothers whose offspring later presented with clinical type 1 diabetes and control mothers. During prospective follow-up of unaffected siblings of children with diabetes no seroconversions could be detected in CMV antibodies, and no changes could be seen in CMV antibodies in relation to seroconversion to positivity for ICA or progression to clinical diabetes in the siblings. Accordingly, no evidence was found in favor of the hypothesis that primary CMV infections in utero or in childhood could promote or precipitate type 1 diabetes. If CMV infections play a role in the pathogenesis of this disease, it must be limited to an extremely small proportion of cases.

Rotavirus

Honeyman et al. (84) reported some years ago molecular homology between the VP7 protein of rotavirus and T-cell epitopes in the protein tyrosine phosphatase–related IA-2 molecule and in the 65-kDa isoform of glutamic acid decarboxylase. In a prospective study of infants genetically predisposed to type 1 diabetes, they observed that the appearance of diabetes-associated autoantibodies was associated with significant rises in rotavirus antibodies, indicating that rotavirus infections may induce β-cell autoimmunity in genetically susceptible infants (85). A Finnish prospective study showed that about 16% of infants and young children with HLA-conferred susceptibility to type 1 diabetes experienced a rotavirus infection during the six-month window preceding the detection of the first diabetes-associated autoantibodies, whereas 15% of the control subjects matched for gender, birth date, delivery hospital, and HLA genotype had signs of a rotavirus infection during the corresponding time period (86). That observation does not lend support to the role of rotavirus infections as triggers of β-cell autoimmunity.

Ljungan Virus

A Swedish group has recently reported that the development of autoimmune diabetes in captured wild bank voles is associated with the Ljungan virus, a novel picornavirus isolated from bank voles (87). While this virus can clearly cause a diabetes-like disease in certain circumstances in bank voles, it has not been convincingly shown that it could infect humans or induce type 1 diabetes in man. However, the Swedish group also reported that young children with newly diagnosed type 1 diabetes had increased titers of Ljungan virus antibodies and implicated that bank voles might play a role as a zoonotic reservoir and vector for a potentially diabetogenic virus in man. Further studies are, however, needed to confirm this hypothesis.

Retroviruses

The human genome contains numerous retroviral sequences, a majority of which is noninfectious. Endogenous retroviruses exist as viral DNA integrated into the genome of every cell in the host, and they are transmitted vertically to the next generation via germline DNA. Retroviruses have been associated with autoimmune diabetes in animal models such as the NOD mouse (88). Retroviruses have not been consistently shown to be involved in the development of human type 1 diabetes, although IAA from patients with type 1 diabetes and unaffected first-degree relatives have been observed to cross-react with the retroviral antigen p73 (89), indicating that IAA-positive sera contain antibodies that recognize both insulin and p73. There is also some evidence that T-cell responses to superantigens encoded by human retrovirus K18 may lead to an autoimmune attack against the β cells (90).

THE HYGIENE HYPOTHESIS

The hygiene hypothesis postulates a relationship between the increasing incidence and prevalence of immune-mediated diseases in modern society and a childhood environment characterized by a decreased pathogen exposure. The hypothesis was initially introduced to explain the increasing frequency of atopic eczema and asthma in developed countries (91). Recently, the hygiene hypothesis has been implicated to contribute to the increasing incidence of autoimmune diseases such as type 1 diabetes (92). It is conceivable that a decreased microbial load in early life may have a major impact on the programming of the immune system, and the gut-associated lymphoid tissue (GALT) in particular.

Role of the Standard of Hygiene in the Development of Immune-Mediated Diseases Including Type 1 Diabetes

Type 1 diabetes is the most common autoimmune disease in childhood (93), while allergic disorders, such as asthma and allergic rhinoconjunctivitis, represent the most frequent chronic diseases in that age group (94). Convincing data show that the incidence of type 1 diabetes has increased considerably in most industrialized countries after World War II; e.g., in Finland the incidence rate has increased fivefold over the last 50 years (1). There are also strong indications that the prevalence of allergic diseases has increased substantially in Western countries over the same time period, although improved and more extensive diagnostic strategies most likely explain part of the increase in allergic disorders (95).

The autoimmune attack on the β-cells characteristic of type 1 diabetes is considered to be T-helper 1 (Th1)-mediated (96–98). CD4+ T cells are divided into subsets, such as Th1 and Th2 effector T cells and regulatory T cells according to their functional profile. Th1 cells facilitate cell-mediated immune responses by secreting, e.g., gamma-interferon (INFγ) and interleukin 2 (IL-2), while Th2 cells induce humoral immune responses by secreting, e.g., IL-4 and IL-10 (99). Regulatory T cells can be separated into naturally occurring regulatory T cells, which originate from the thymus, and adaptive regulatory T cells, which are induced in the periphery (100,101). Natural regulatory T cells express characteristically CD4, CD25, CTLA-4, and Foxp3 transcription regulator, which is considered to be a specific marker for CD4+CD25^{high} regulatory T cells (102–104). In humans, it has been shown that Foxp3-expressing CD4+CD25^{high} regulatory T cells can be induced from peripheral CD4+CD25-T cells upon stimulation (105,106). Several viruses and other microbes have been shown to activate regulatory T cells, which may play a role in the development of virus-induced tissue pathology and the eradication of the virus (107).

From an immunological point of view, the mechanisms behind the development of organ-specific autoimmune disorders and allergy represent the antipodes of each other. In organ-specific autoimmune diseases, autoreactive T cells are assumed to attack and destroy the target tissue, while allergic disorders are characterized by a strong humoral immune response including IgE antibodies against environmental antigens, i.e., allergens. Accordingly, organ-specific autoimmune disorders are perceived as a Th1-polarized process, and allergic diseases as a Th2-biased condition. Although this is likely an oversimplification of biologically multifaceted disease processes, where regulatory T cells are strongly involved, there are observations indicating that allergic diseases are less frequent in patients with an organ-specific autoimmune disease than in unaffected subjects (108,109). Hence, it is intriguing that both autoimmune disorders and allergic diseases have become more and more common in parallel over the last half of the 20th century in populations with increasing prosperity and improving standard of hygiene.

A series of evidence suggest that the maturation of the immune system over the first few years of life is an important determinant of autoimmune and allergic diseases. The first signs of β-cell autoimmunity preceding the progression to clinical type 1 diabetes emerge already in infancy (8,9), and similarly, infants are affected by allergic diseases such as food allergy presenting with gastrointestinal, respiratory, and/or cutaneous symptoms. Microbial infections are thought to be important in this maturation process and certain degree of exposure to microbial agents may be needed for the development of a proper balance and regulation of the Th1- and Th2-type immune responses. Several studies have implicated that early childhood infections may be linked to decreased risk of allergic diseases (110,111). In the United States, serologic evidence of acquisition of certain infections, mainly food-borne and orofecal infections, is associated with a reduced likelihood of presenting with hay fever and asthma later in life (112).

The effect of microbes might be very complex. Certain viral infections may predispose to these diseases, e.g., respiratory syncytial virus and rhinoviruses may increase the risk of asthma or precipitate its symptom, while other viruses may protect from the same diseases, as hepatitis A virus seem to protect from asthma. Thus, the evaluation of the role of microbes, their mutual interactions, and interactions with host susceptibility genes and other host-related factors in the pathogenesis of these diseases is complicated. A series of genes regulate the individual susceptibility to type 1 diabetes and allergy, and many of them are known to be involved in the resistance to microbial infections and to play a role in the infectious process. The commensal microflora may also contribute to the maturation of the immune system in infants and young children (113).

Recent Data in Favor of the Hygiene Hypothesis

The Karelian Republic of the Russian Federation is an area immediately east of Finland with a total population of approximately 720,000 inhabitants. One of the steepest gradients in standard of living worldwide is present at the border between Russian Karelia and Finland with a sevenfold difference in the gross national product. Accordingly, these two populations comprise a "living laboratory" providing a unique possibility to test the hygiene hypothesis and gene-environment interactions in the development of immune-mediated diseases.

Recent studies have shown that there are substantial differences in the frequency of allergy between Russian Karelia and Finland both among schoolchildren and adults. Skin prick tests (SPT) among seven- to nine-year-old schoolchildren revealed that SPT positivity to birch and cat was about three times more frequent in Finland (114). In a population based study of two generations von Herzen et al. showed that SPT positivity to airborne and food allergens were less common both among schoolchildren and their mothers in Russian Karelia compared with their counterparts in Finland (115). In our own studies we have observed that the incidence rate of type 1 diabetes among children under the age of 15 years was almost six times lower in Russian Karelia than in Finland (7.4 vs. 41.4/100,000 children) over a 10-year time period (1990–1999) (Fig. 2A) (70). There was no significant difference in the frequency of HLA DQ genotypes conferring type 1 diabetes susceptibility or protection between Finland and Russian Karelia strongly suggesting that lifestyle and/or environmental factors must be major contributors to the steep difference in the incidence rate of type 1 diabetes between these two areas. In another study we analyzed the frequency of diabetes-associated autoantibodies, i.e., ICA, IAA, GADA, and IA-2A. There was no difference in the frequency of ICA, IAA, or GADA between the two populations, but Finnish schoolchildren often tested about four times more positive for IA-2A, which usually appears as the last autoantibody reactivity during the preclinical disease process. The data suggest that signs of β-cell autoimmunity are induced as frequently in children in Russian Karelia as in Finland. However, the Karelian children seem to be characterized by a less frequent and/or retarded progression in their prediabetic disease process (116). These findings indicate that the Russian Karelian environment and/or lifestyle are less diabetogenic than that in Finland.

In the same series we observed that Finnish schoolchildren tested positive for celiac disease-associated tissue transglutaminase autoantibodies 2.5 times more frequently than Karelian children (Fig. 2B) (117). This implies that celiac disease-associated autoimmunity is more than two times more frequent in Finland than in Russian Karelia. This difference was confirmed by small bowel biopsies carried out from subjects positive for transglutaminase antibodies in both countries. The prevalence of biopsy-proven celiac disease was one in 496 children in Karelia compared with one in 107 children in Finland. Autoantibodies to the thyroid gland were also about six times less frequent among schoolchildren in Russian Karelia compared with their Finnish peers. The fact that the studied populations share partly the same ancestry and that the frequency of HLA genes predisposing to autoimmune diseases is quite similar suggests that environmental and life-style associated factors play a major role in the development of thyroid autoimmunity (118).

Total and allergen-specific IgE were measured in 350 children in Finland and in 350 children of Finnish-Karelian ancestry in Russian Karelia. Karelian schoolchildren had significantly higher concentrations of total IgE than their Finnish counterparts, which may reflect an increased exposure to parasite infections in Russian Karelia. In contrast the Finnish schoolchildren had significantly higher levels of birch and cat-specific IgE suggesting increased allergic sensitization to these common allergens in Finland. Altogether allergic sensitization to these allergens was detected in 22% of the children in Finland compared with 6 % of the children in Russian Karelia (Fig. 2C; $p < 0.001$) (119). In the same study we compared the frequency of signs of several microbial infections in 7- to 14-year-old children in Russian Karelia and in Finland. EV antibodies were analyzed as an

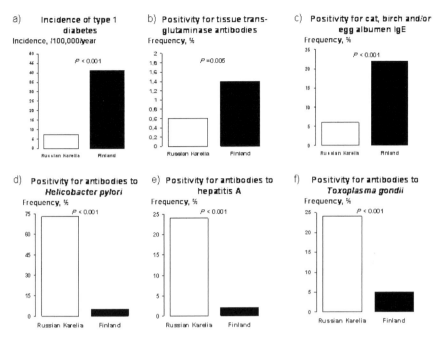

FIGURE 2 The mirror image of autoimmunity/allergy and infectious diseases among schoolchildren in Russian Karelia and in Finland. The Russian Karelian children had a sixfold lower incidence of type 1 diabetes over the time period 1990–1999 **(A)** (70), a 2.5-fold lower prevalence of tissue transglutaminase antibodies **(B)** (117), and an almost fourfold lower frequency of allergen-specific IgE to cat, birch, and/or egg albumen **(C)** (119) than their Finnish peers, whereas they had a 15-fold higher prevalence of *Helicobacter pylori* antibodies, **(D)**, a 12-fold higher prevalence of hepatitis A antibodies **(E)**, and a fivefold higher prevalence of *Toxoplasma gondii* antibodies **(F)** than the Finnish schoolchildren (119).

indicator of exposure to one plausible trigger of β-cell autoimmunity. In addition, *Helicobacter pylori*, hepatitis A virus, and *Toxoplasma gondii* antibodies were measured as indicators of the microbial load. All these microbial infections were significantly more frequent in Russian Karelia than in Finland (Fig. 2D–F) (119). In addition, some of the microbes, EV in particular, were associated with decreased risk of IgE-mediated allergic sensitization. These findings are in line with the hygiene hypothesis and suggest that the conspicuous difference in microbial exposures between the two countries may partly explain the higher incidence of type 1 diabetes and allergy in Finland. This is also consistent with our observations in other countries suggesting that a clean environment and a low frequency of EV infections may increase the risk of type 1 diabetes by reducing the levels of protective maternal antibodies and thereby making the infants more susceptible for such infections (120).

How to Test the Hygiene Hypothesis in Type 1 Diabetes?

All the studies referred to in the section above have been performed either in schoolchildren or young adults. Accordingly, they are not able to address early events in the disease process, which in type 1 diabetes and most other immune-mediated diseases start months and years before the emergence of clinical signs. It would be essential to study the maturation of the immune system in young children living in contrasting socioeconomic conditions and with different standards of hygiene. The optimal design would be a prospective birth cohort study monitoring the participants closely over the first years of life. One aim of such a study would be to identify which factors protect the children living in an environment with low standard of hygiene against type 1 diabetes and other immune-mediated diseases. Another aim would be to define the mechanisms and molecular pathways which mediate this effect. The overall goal should be to design effective preventive treatments for type 1 diabetes and other immune-mediated diseases based on the observations made in such a prospective birth cohort study. By using modern methods of functional genomics it will be possible to identify potential differences in the expression profile of immunologically active molecules in young children taking part in the prospective birth cohort study.

A prospective birth cohort study will render it possible to define the timing of the appearance of the first signs of β-cell autoimmunity. This approach will facilitate the search for environmental triggers of β-cell autoimmunity. Such a study will also enable the identification of both genetic and environmental determinants of the progression rate from seroconversion to autoantibody positivity to the manifestation of clinical type 1 diabetes. The size of the study cohort should be large enough to provide an opportunity to assess gene-environment interactions affecting the appearance and progression of β-cell autoimmunity and allergy. The study will make it possible to explore the role of microbes and parasites in the gastrointestinal tract in the emergence of signs of autoimmunity and allergy, since there would be considerable differences in the microbial load between the young children from the populations to be studied. The study setting should also be designed in order to open up new opportunities to analyze the interplay between early infant nutrition, gastrointestinal microflora, and gut immunity in the development of type 1 diabetes and other immune-mediated diseases.

PERSPECTIVES FOR THE FUTURE

The identification of exogenous factors triggering and driving β-cell destruction offers potential means for intervention aimed at the prevention of type 1 diabetes. Therefore, it is important to pursue studies on the role of environmental factors in the pathogenesis of this disease. Environmental modification is likely to offer the most powerful strategy for effective disease prevention, since such an approach can target the whole population or at least that proportion of the population carrying increased genetic disease susceptibility and would therefore prevent both sporadic and familial type 1 diabetes, if successful. This consideration is crucial, since the sporadic cases comprise 83–98% of all children with newly diagnosed diabetes according to a comparative European survey (121). Previous success stories in other diseases such as the elimination of dietary gluten in celiac disease and the use of antibiotics for the treatment of *H. pylori* infection in patients with gastritis or gastric ulcers clearly show the huge therapeutic potential of such a strategy.

It is important to keep in mind that there are gene-environment interactions operating in all phases of the disease process of type 1 diabetes, not only in the induction phase of β-cell autoimmunity. The delineation of such interactions is challenging and requires both new methodological tools and study cohorts large enough for the analyses of interactions. So far there are only a few examples of gene-environment interactions implicated in the development of type 1 diabetes.

HLA risk alleles for type 1 diabetes have been linked to the appearance of auto-antibodies subsequent to EV infections (39) and to increased immune responsiveness to EV antigens (122). The recent identification of a diabetes-associated genetic polymorphism in the gene on chromosome 2 encoding the interferon-induced helicase protein raises the interesting possibility of an interaction between that genetic polymorphism and EV infections, as the encoded protein functions as an intracellular receptor for EV RNA (123). It recognizes viral dsRNA, which is synthesized during EV replication leading to type 1 interferon production and activation of the innate immune system. Another consideration that has to be taken into account is that there may be interactions between two or more environmental factors. One needs, however, extensive study cohorts to be able to identify such interactions. A recent Finnish study implied that two environmental risk factors for type 1 diabetes, i.e., an early EV infection and early exposure to cow's milk can, when present concomitantly, boost the immune response to bovine insulin in infants with increased HLA-defined disease predisposition (124).

The scientific challenges in the near future are to define the most likely environmental culprit(s) and booster(s) of β-cell autoimmunity and to delineate how exogenous factors affect the natural history of type 1 diabetes. A new consortium comprising six prospective birth cohort studies, the German BABYDIAB Study, the American DAISY, and the Finnish DIPP Study among others, and observing risk individuals from birth through signs of β-cell autoimmunity to clinical disease provide an optimal setting for successful explorative work (125). The Environmental Determinants in Diabetes of the Young (TEDDY) consortium has been funded by the National Institute of Diabetes, Digestive and Kidney Diseases (NIDDK) and has started to recruit participating families in the fall of 2004. We also have to keep our eyes and minds open for potential protective environmental factors, since family studies have shown that all high-risk individuals do not progress to clinical diabetes within a foreseeable period of time (126,127).

ACKNOWLEDGMENTS

This research was supported by the Juvenile Diabetes Research Foundation International, Type 1 Diabetes Targeted Program co-funded by the Research Council for Health, Academy of Finland, the Juvenile Diabetes Foundation International and the Sigrid Jusélius Foundation, the Foundation for Diabetes Research in Finland, Finska Läkaresällskapet, the Päivikki and Sakari Sohlberg Foundation, Tampere Tuberculosis Foundation, and the Novo Nordisk Foundation.

REFERENCES

1. Knip M, Veijola R, Virtanen SM, et al. Environmental triggers and determinants of β-cell autoimmunity and type 1 diabetes. Diabetes 2005; 54(suppl 2):S125–S136.
2. Ilonen J, Sjöroos M, Knip M, et al. Estimation of genetic risk for type 1 diabetes. Am J Med Genet 2002; 115:30–36.
3. Dahlquist G. Environmental risk factors in human Type 1 diabetes: an epidemiological perspective. Diabetes Metab Rev 1995; 11:37–46.
4. Åkerblom HK, Knip M. Putative environmental factors in type 1 diabetes. Diabetes Metab Rev 1998; 14:31–67.
5. Åkerblom HK, Vaarala O, Hyöty H, et al. Environmental factors in the etiology of type 1 diabetes. Am J Med Genet 2002; 115:18–29.
6. Knip M. Natural course of preclinical type 1 diabetes. Horm Res 2002; 57(suppl 1):6–11.

7. Knip M. Can we predict type 1 diabetes in the general population? Diabetes Care 2002; 25:623–625.
8. Ziegler AG, Hummel M, Schenker M, et al. Autoantibody appearance and risk for development of childhood diabetes in offspring of parents with type 1 diabetes: the 2-year analysis of the German BABYDIAB Study. Diabetes 1999; 48:460–468.
9. Kimpimäki T, Kupila A, Hämäläinen AM, et al. The first signs of ß-cell autoimmunity appear in infancy in genetically susceptible children from the general population: the Finnish Type 1 diabetes prediction and prevention study. J Clin Endocrinol Metab 2001; 86:4782–4788.
10. Kukko M, Kimpimäki T, Korhonen S, et al. Dynamics of diabetes-associated autoantibodies in young children with HLA-conferred risk of type 1 diabetes recruited from the general population. J Clin Endocrinol Metab 2005; 90:2712–2717.
11. Kupila A, Muona P, Ronkainen M, et al. Genetic risk determines the emergence of diabetes-associated autoantibodies in young children. Diabetes 2002; 51:646–651.
12. Mrena S, Virtanen S, Laippala P, et al. Models for predicting type 1 diabetes in siblings of affected children. Diabetes Care 2006; 29:662–667.
13. Kimpimäki T, Kulmala P, Savola K, et al. Disease-associated autoantibodies as surrogate markers of type 1 diabetes in young children at increased genetic risk. J Clin Endocrinol Metab 2000; 85:1126–1130.
14. Leslie RD, Delli Castelli M. Age-dependent influences on the origins of autoimmune diabetes: evidence and implications. Diabetes 2004; 53:3033–3040.
15. Alaedini A, Green PH. Narrative review: celiac disease: understanding a complex autoimmune disorder. Ann Intern Med 2005; 142:289–298.
16. Mäki M, Mustalahti K, Kokkonen J, et al. Prevalence of celiac disease in children in Finland. N Engl J Med 2003; 348:2517–2524.
17. Kagnoff MF, Paterson YJ, Kumar PJ, et al. Evidence for the role of human intestinal adenovirus in the pathogenesis of celiac disease. Gut 1987; 28:995–1001.
18. Lähdeaho ML, Parkkonen P, Reunala T, et al. Antibodies to the E1bprotein-derived peptides of enteric adenovirus type 40 are associated with celiac disease and dermatitis herpetiformis. Clin Immunol Immunopathol 1993; 69:300–305.
19. Stene LC, Honeyman MC, Hoffenberg EJ, et al. Rotavirus infection frequency and risk of celiac disease autoimmunity in early childhood: a longitudinal study. Am J Gastroenterol 2006; 101:2333–2334.
20. Hyoty H, Taylor KW. The role of viruses in human diabetes. Diabetologia 2002; 45:1353–1361.
21. Yoon JW. Role of viruses in the pathogenesis of IDDM. Ann Med 1991; 23:437–445.
22. Szopa TM, Titchener PA, Portwood ND, et al. Diabetes mellitus due to viruses—some recent developments. Diabetologia 1993; 36:687–695.
23. Barrett-Connor E. Is insulin-dependent diabetes mellitus caused by Coxsackie B infection? A review of the epidemiologic evidence. Rev Infect Dis 1985; 7:207–215.
24. Banatvala JE. Insulin-dependent (juvenile-onset, type 1) diabetes mellitus. Coxsackie B viruses revisited. Prog Med Virol 1987; 34:33–54.
25. Gamble DR, Taylor KW. Seasonal incidence of diabetes mellitus. Br Med J 1969; 3: 631–633.
26. Orchard TJ, Atchison RW, Becker D, et al. Coxsackie infection and diabetes. Lancet 1983; 2:631.
27. Mertens T, Grüneklee D, Eggers HJ. Neutralizing antibodies against Coxsackie B viruses in patients with recent onset of type 1 diabetes. Eur J Pediatr 1983; 140:293–294.
28. Palmer JP, Cooney MK, Ward RH, et al. Reduced Coxsackie antibody titres in Type 1 (insulin-dependent) diabetic patients presenting during an outbreak of Coxsackie B3 and B4 infection. Diabetologia 1982; 22:426–429.
29. Graves PM, Norris JM, Pallansch MA, et al. The role of enteroviral infections in the development of IDDM: limitations of current approaches. Diabetes 1997; 46:161–168.
30. Frisk G, Fohlman J, Kobbah M, et al. High frequency of Coxsackie-B-virus-specific IgM in children developing type 1 diabetes during a period of high diabetes morbidity. J Med Virol 1985; 17:219–227.
31. Fohlman J, Friman G. Is juvenile diabetes a viral disease? Ann Med 1993; 25:569–574.
32. Nerup J, Mandrup-Poulsen T, Mølvig J, et al. Mechanisms of pancreatic beta-cell destruction in Type 1 diabetes. Diabetes Care 1988; 11(suppl 1):16–23.

33. Clements GB, Galbraith DN, Taylor KW. Coxsackie B virus infection and onset of childhood diabetes. Lancet 1995; 346:221–223.
34. Foy CA, Quirke P, Lewis FA, et al. Detection of common viruses using the polymerase chain reaction to assess levels of viral presence in type 1 (insulin-dependent) diabetic patients. Diabet Med 1995; 12:1002–1008.
35. Andreoletti L, Hober D, Hober-Vandenberghe C, et al. Detection of coxsackie B virus RNA sequences in whole blood samples from adult patients at the onset of type I diabetes mellitus. J Med Virol 1997; 52:121–127.
36. Nairn C, Galbraith DN, Taylor KW, et al. Enterovirus variants in the serum of children at the onset of Type 1 diabetes mellitus. Diabet Med 1999; 16:509–513.
37. Chehadeh W, Weill J, Vantyghem MC, et al. Increased level of interferon-alpha in blood of patients with insulin-dependent diabetes mellitus: relationship with coxsackievirus B infection. J Infect Dis 2000; 181:1929–1939.
38. Yin H, Berg AK, Tuvemo T, et al. Enterovirus RNA is found in peripheral blood mononuclear cells in a majority of type 1 diabetic children at onset. Diabetes 2002; 51:1964–1971.
39. Craig ME, Howard NJ, Silink M, et al. Reduced frequency of HLA DRB1*03-DQB1*02 in children with type 1 diabetes associated with enterovirus RNA. J Infect Dis 2003; 187:1562–1570.
40. Kawashima H, Ihara T, Ioi H, et al. Enterovirus-related type 1 diabetes mellitus and antibodies to glutamic acid decarboxylase in Japan. J Infect 2004; 49:147–151.
41. Moya-Suri V, Schlosser M, Zimmermann K, et al. Enterovirus RNA sequences in sera of schoolchildren in the general population and their association with type 1-diabetes-associated autoantibodies. J Med Microbiol 2005; 54:879–883.
42. Sarmiento L, Cabrera-Rode E, Lekuleni L, et al. Occurrence of enterovirus RNA in serum of children with newly diagnosed type 1 diabetes and islet cell autoantibody-positive subjects in a population with a low incidence of type 1 diabetes. Autoimmunity 2007; 40:540–545.
43. Elfaitouri A, Berg AK, Frisk G, et al. Recent enterovirus infection in type 1 diabetes: evidence with a novel IgM method. J Med Virol 2007; 79:1861–1867.
44. Hyöty H, Hiltunen M, Knip M, et al. A prospective study of the role of Coxsackie B and other enterovirus infections in the pathogenesis of IDDM. Diabetes 1995; 44:652–657.
45. Hiltunen M, Hyöty H, Knip M, et al. ICA seroconversion in children is temporally associated with enterovirus infections. J Infect Dis 1997; 175:554–560.
46. Lönnrot M, Salminen K, Knip M, et al. Enterovirus RNA in serum is a risk factor for beta-cell autoimmunity and clinical type 1 diabetes: a prospective study. J Med Virol 2000; 61:214–220.
47. Lönnrot M, Korpela K, Knip M, et al. Enterovirus infection as a risk factor for ß-cell autoimmunity in a prospectively observed birth cohort—the Finnish Diabetes Prediction and Prevention (DIPP) study. Diabetes 2000; 49:1314–1318.
48. Salminen K, Sadeharju K, Lönnrot M, et al. Enterovirus infections are associated with the induction of beta-cell autoimmunity in a prospective birth cohort study. J Med Virol 2003; 69:91–98.
49. Fuchtenbusch M, Irnstetter A, Jager G, et al. No evidence for an association of coxsackie virus infections during pregnancy and early childhood with development of islet autoantibodies in offspring of mothers or fathers with type 1 diabetes. J Autoimmun 2001; 17:333–340.
50. Graves PM, Rotbart HA, Nix WA, et al. Prospective study of enteroviral infections and development of beta-cell autoimmunity. Diabetes autoimmunity study in the young (DAISY). Diabetes Res Clin Pract 2003; 59:51–61.
51. Dahlquist CG, Ivarsson S, Lindberg B, et al. Maternal enteroviral infection during pregnancy. Diabetes 1995; 44:408–413.
52. Viskari HR, Roivainen M, Reunanen A, et al. Maternal first-trimester enterovirus infection and future risk of type 1 diabetes in the exposed fetus. Diabetes 2002; 51: 2568–2571.
53. Oikarinen M, Tauriainen S, Honkanen T, et al. Detection of enteroviruses in the intestine of type 1 diabetic patients. Clin Exp Immunol 2007; DOI: 10.1111/j.1365–2249.2007.03529.x.
54. Szopa TM, Ward T, Dronfield DM, et al. Coxsackie B4 viruses with the potential to damage beta cells of the islets are present in clinical isolates. Diabetologia 1990; 33: 325–328.

55. Roivainen M, Rasilainen S, Ylipaasto P, et al. Mechanisms of coxsackievirus-induced damage to human pancreatic beta-cells. J Clin Endocrinol Metab 2000; 85:432–440.

56. Roivainen M, Ylipaasto P, Savolainen C, et al. Functional impairment and killing of human beta cells by enteroviruses: the capacity is shared by a wide range of serotypes, but the extent is a characteristic of individual virus strains. Diabetologia 2002; 45: 693–702.

57. Gladisch R, Hofmann W, Waldherr R. Myocarditis and insulitis following coxsackie virus infection. Z Kardiol 1976; 65:837–849.

58. Yoon JW, Austin M, Onodera T, et al. Isolation of a virus from the pancreas of a child with diabetic ketoacidosis. N Engl J Med 1979; 300:1173–1179.

59. Iwasaki T, Monma N, Satodate R, et al. An immunofluorescent study of generalized Coxsackie virus B3 infection in a newborn infant. Acta Pathol Jpn 1985; 35:741–748.

60. Foulis AK, Farquharson MA, Cameron SO, et al. A search for the presence of the enteroviral capsid protein VP1 in pancreases of patients with type 1 (insulin-dependent) diabetes and pancreases and hearts of infants who died of coxsackie viral myocarditis. Diabetologia 1990; 33:290–298.

61. Foulis AK, McGill M, Farquharson MA, et al. A search for evidence of viral infection in pancreases of newly diagnosed patients with IDDM. Diabetologia 1997; 40:53–61.

62. Ylipaasto P, Klingel K, Lindberg AM, et al. Enterovirus infection in human pancreatic islet cells, islet tropism in vivo and receptor involvement in cultured islet beta cells. Diabetologia 2004; 47:225–239.

63. Dotta F, Censini A, van Halteren A, et al. Coxsackie B4 virus infection of beta cells and natural killer cell insulitis in recent-onset type 1 diabetic patients. Proc Natl Acad Sci U S A 2007; 104:5115–5120.

64. Kupila A, Muona P, Simell T, et al. Feasibility of genetic and immunological prediction of type 1 diabetes in a population-based birth cohort. Diabetologia 2001; 44:290–297.

65. Laron Z. Lessons from recent epidemiological studies in type 1 childhood diabetes. J Pediatr Endocrinol Metab 1999; 12(suppl 3):733–736.

66. Kukko M, Toivonen A, Kupila A, et al. Familial clustering of beta-cell autoimmunity in initially non-diabetic children. Diabetes Metab Res Rev 2006; 22:53–58.

67. Karvonen M, Viik-Kajander M, Moltchanova E, et al. Incidence of childhood type 1 diabetes worldwide. Diabetes Care 2000; 23:1516–1526.

68. The EURODIAB Substudy 2 Study Group: vitamin D supplement in early childhood and risk of Type I (insulin-dependent) diabetes mellitus. Diabetologia 1999; 42:51–54.

69. Hyppönen E, Läärä E, Järvelin MR, et al. Intake of vitamin D and risk of type 1 diabetes: a birth cohort study. Lancet 2001; 358:1500–1504.

70. Kondrashova A, Reunanen A, Romanov A, et al. A sixfold gradient in the incidence of type 1 diabetes at the eastern border of Finland—evidence for the role of environmental factors in the disease pathogenesis. Ann Med 2005; 37:67–72.

71. Viskari H, Kondrashova A, Koskela P, et al. Circulating vitamin D concentrations in two neighboring populations with markedly different incidence of type 1 diabetes. Diabetes Care 2006; 49:1458–1459.

72. Käär ML, Åkerblom HK, Huttunen NP, et al. Metabolic control of children and adolescents with insulin-dependent diabetes mellitus. Acta Paediatr Scand 1984; 73:102–108.

73. Hinde FR, Standen PJ, Mann NP, et al. Seasonal variation of haemoglobin A1 in children with insulin-dependent diabetes mellitus. Eur J Pediatr 1989; 148:146–147.

74. Nordfeldt S, Ludvigsson J. Seasonal variation of HbA1c in intensive treatment of children with type 1 diabetes. J Pediatr Endocrinol Metab 2000; 13:529–535.

75. Dahlquist G. Environmental factors and type 1 diabetes. Diabetes Care 2001; 24:80–182.

76. Viskari H, Ludvigsson J, Uibo R, et al. Relationship between the incidence of type 1 diabetes and maternal enterovirus antibodies—time trends and geographical variation. Diabetologia 2005; 48:1280–1287.

77. Viskari HR, Koskela P, Lönnrot M, et al. Can enterovirus infections explain the increasing incidence of type 1 diabetes? Diabetes Care 2000; 23:414–416.

78. Gundersen E. Is diabetes of infectious origin? J Infect Dis 1927; 41:197–202.

79. Hyöty H, Hiltunen M, Reunanen A, et al. Decline of mumps antibodies in Type 1 (insulin-dependent) diabetic children and a plateau in the rising incidence of Type 1

diabetes after introduction of the mumps-measles-rubella vaccine in Finland. Diabetologia 1993; 36:1303–1308.
80. Viskari H, Paronen J, Keskinen P, et al. Humoral beta-cell autoimmunity is rare in patients with the congenital rubella syndrome. Clin Exp Immunol 2003; 133:378–383.
81. Ward KP, Galloway WH, Auchterlonie IA. Congenital cytomegalovirus infection and diabetes. Lancet 1979; 1:497.
82. Ivarsson SA, Lindberg B, Nilsson KO, et al. The prevalence of type 1 diabetes mellitus at follow-up of Swedish infants congenitally infected with cytomegalovirus. Diabetic Med 1993; 10:521–523.
83. Hiltunen M, Hyöty H, Karjalainen J, et al. Serological evaluation of the role of cytomegalovirus in the pathogenesis of IDDM—a prospective study. Diabetologia 1995; 38:705–710.
84. Honeyman MC, Stone NL, Harrison LC. T-cell epitopes in type 1 diabetes autoantigen tyrosine phosphatase IA-2: potential for mimicry with rotavirus and other environmental agents. Mol Med 1998; 4:231–239.
85. Honeyman MC, Coulson BS, Stone NL, et al. Association between rotavirus infection and pancreatic islet autoimmunity in children at risk of developing type 1 diabetes. Diabetes 2000; 49:1319–1324.
86. Blomquist M, Juhela S, Erkkilä S, et al. Rotavirus infections and development of diabetes-associated autoantibodies during the first 2 years of life. Clin Exp Immunol 2002; 128:511–515.
87. Niklasson B, Heller KE, Schonecker B, et al. Development of type 1 diabetes in wild bank voles associated with islet autoantibodies and the novel ljungan virus. Int J Exp Diabesity Res 2003; 4:35–44.
88. Suenaga K, Yoon JW. Association of beta-cell specific expression of endogenous retrovirus with the development of insulitis and diabetes in NOD mice. Diabetes 1988; 37:1722–1726.
89. Hao W, Serreze DV, McCulloch DK, et al. Insulin (auto) antibodies from human IDDM cross-react with retroviral antigen p73. J Autoimmun 1993; 6:787–798.
90. Conrad B, Weissmahr RN, Böni J, et al. A human endogenous retroviral superantigen as candidate autoimmune gene in type 1 diabetes. Cell 1997; 90:303–313.
91. Strachan DP. Hay fever, hygiene and houshold size. Br Med J 1989; 299:1259–1260.
92. Bach JF. The effect of infections on susceptibility to autoimmune and allergic diseases. New Engl J Med 2002; 347:911–920.
93. Gale EAM. The risk of childhood type 1 diabetes in the 20th century. Diabetes 2002; 51:3353–3361.
94. ISAAC Steering Committee. Worldwide variation in the prevalence of asthma, allergic rhino-conjunctivitis and atopic eczema: IAAC. Lancet 1998; 351:1225–1232.
95. Burney PG, Chinn S, Rona RJ. Has the prevalence of asthma increased in children? Evidence from the national study of health and growth 1973–86. Br Med J 1990; 300:1652–1653.
96. Liblau RS, Singer SM, McDevitt HO. Th1 and Th2 CD4+ T cells in the pathogenesis of organ-specific autoimmune diseases. Immunol Today 1995; 16:34–38.
97. Berman MA, Sandborg CI, Wang Z, et al. Decreased IL-4 production in new onset type I insulin-dependent diabetes mellitus. J Immunol 1996; 157:4690–4696.
98. Kallman BA, Huther M, Tubes M, et al. Systemic bias of cytokine production toward cell-mediated immune regulation in IDDM and toward humoral immunity in Graves' disease. Diabetes 1997; 46:237–243.
99. Lowdell M, Bottazzo GF. Autoimmunity and insulin-dependent diabetes. Lancet 1993; 341:1378–1379.
100. Fontenot JD, Rudensky AY. A well adapted regulatory contrivance: regulatory T cell development and the forkhead family transcription factor Foxp3. Nat Immunol 2005; 6:331–337.
101. Sakaguchi S. Naturally arising Foxp3-expressing CD25+CD4+ regulatory T cells in immunological tolerance to self and non-self. Nat Immunol 2005; 6:345–352.
102. Fontenot JD, Gavin MA, Rudensky AY. Foxp3 programs the development and function of CD4+CD25+ regulatory T cells. Nat Immunol 2003; 4:330–336.
103. Khattri R, Cox T, Yasayko SA, et al. An essential role for Scurfin in CD4+CD25+ T regulatory cells. Nat Immunol 2003; 4:337–342.

104. Yagi H, Nomura T, Nakamura K, et al. Crucial role of FOXP3 in the development and function of human CD25+CD4+ regulatory T cells. Int Immunol 2004; 16:1643–1656.
105. Walker MR, Kasprowicz DJ, Gersuk VH, et al. Induction of FoxP3 and acquisition of T regulatory activity by stimulated human CD4+CD25– T cells. J Clin Invest 2003; 112:1437–1443.
106. Rao PE, Petrone AL, Ponath PD. Differentiation and expansion of T cells with regulatory function from human peripheral lymphocytes by stimulation in the presence of TGF-{beta}. J Immunol 2005; 174:1446–1455.
107. Belkaid Y, Rouse BT. Natural regulatory T cells in infectious diseases. Nat Immunol 2005; 6:353–360.
108. EURODIAB Substudy 2 Group. Decreased prevalence of atopic diseases in children with diabetes. J Pediatr 2000; 137:470–474.
109. Olesen AB, Juul S, Birkebaek N, et al. Association between atopic dermatitis and insulin-dependent diabetes mellitus: a case-control study. Lancet 2001; 357:1749–1752.
110. von Hertzen LC. Puzzling associations between childhood infections and the later occurrence of asthma and atopy. Ann Med 2000; 32:397–400.
111. McKeever TM, Lewis SA, Smith C, et al. Early exposure to infections and antibiotics and the incidence of allergic disease: a birth cohort study with the West Midlands General Practice Research Database. J Allergy Clin Immunol 2002; 109:43–50.
112. Matricardi PM, Rosmini F, Panetta V, et al. Hay fever and asthma in relation to markers of infection in the United States. J Allergy Clin Immunol 2002; 110:381–387.
113. Rakoff-Nahoum S, Medzhitov R. Role of the innate immune system and host-commensal mutualism. Curr Top Microbiol Immunol 2006; 308:1–18.
114. Klemola T, Masyuk V, von Hertzen L, et al. Occurrence of atopy among Russian and Finnish schoolchildren. Allergy 2004; 59:465–466.
115. von Hertzen L, Mäkelä MJ, Petäys T, et al. Growing disparities in atopy between the Finns and the Russians: a comparison of two generations. J Allergy Clin Immunol 2006; 117:151–157.
116. Kondrashova A, Viskari H, Romanov A, et al. Signs of β-cell autoimmunity in non–diabetic schoolchildren: a comparison between Russian Karelia with a low incidence of type 1 diabetes and Finland with a high incidence rate. Diabetes Care 2007; 30:95–100.
117. Kondrashova A, Mustalahti K, Kaukinen K, et al. Lower economic status and inferior hygienic environment protect against celiac disease. Ann Med 2007; 39:DO1: 10.1080/07853890701678689.
118. Kondrashova A, Haapala AM, Viskari H, et al. Serological evidence of thyroid auto-immunity among schoolchildren in two different socioeconomic environments. J Clin Endocrinol Metab 2007; 92:in press.
119. Seiskari T, Kondrashova A, Viskari H, et al. Atopic sensitisation and microbial load - a comparison between Finland and Russian Karelia. Clin Exp Immunol 2007; 148:47–52.
120. Viskari H, Salur L, Uibo R, et al. Correlations between the incidence of type 1 diabetes and enterovirus infections in Europe. J Med Virol 2004; 72:610–617.
121. The EURODIAB ACE Study Group and The EURODIAB ACE Substudy 2 Study Group. Familial risk of type I diabetes in European children. Diabetologia 1998; 41:1151–1156.
122. Sadeharju K, Knip M, Hiltunen P, et al. The HLA-DR phenotype modulates the humoral immune response to enterovirus antigens. Diabetologia 2003; 46:1100–1105.
123. Smyth DJ, Cooper JD, Bailey R, et al. A genome-wide association study of non-synonymous SNPs identifies a type 1 diabetes locus in the interferon-induced helicase (IFIH1) region. Nat Genet 2006; 38:617–619.
124. Vaarala O, Klemetti P, Juhela S, et al. Effect of coincident enterovirus infection and cow's milk exposure on immunisation to insulin in early infancy. Diabetologia 2002; 45:531–534.
125. Hagopian W, Lernmark Å, Rewers MJ, et al. TEDDY—the environmental determinants of diabetes in the young – an observational clinical trial. Ann N Y Acad Sci 2006; 1079: 320–326.
126. Bingley PJ, Christie MR, Bonifacio E, et al. Combined analysis of autoantibodies improves prediction of IDDM in islet cell antibody-positive relatives. Diabetes 1994; 43:1304–1310.
127. Kulmala P, Petersen JS, Vähäsalo P, et al. Prediction of insulin-dependent diabetes mellitus in siblings of diabetic children—a population-based study. J Clin Invest 1998; 101: 327–336.

Tempo and Type 1 Diabetes: The Accelerator Hypothesis

Terence J. Wilkin

Department of Endocrinology and Metabolism, Peninsula Medical School, Plymouth Campus, U.K.

HISTORICAL SETTING

Until 40 or so years ago, diabetes was regarded as a single disorder. Himsworth had commented in the 1930s on the insulin-resistant individual who required larger doses of insulin, but the designations of adult onset and juvenile onset were descriptive and unrelated to any perceived differences in mechanism. In the mid-1960s, the Belgian histopathologist, Willy Gepts, first described infiltration of lymphocytes in the islets of children who died within a few days of developing diabetes (1). He noted similarities to *struma lymphomatosa* of the thyroid, first described by Hashimoto in 1912, but regarded by the late 1950s as "autoimmune" because of the thyroid antibodies found in the serum of such patients. In 1974, Jorn Nerup described an association between childhood diabetes and the immune response or HLA genes on the short arm of chromosome 6 (2) and in the same year Franco Bottazzo and Deborah Doniach famously reported the presence of antibodies to the islet cells in blood samples from people with insulin-dependent diabetes (3).

Together, lymphocytic infiltration of the islets, immunogenetic linkage, and autoantibodies specific to the islets prompted a radical revision in the understanding of diabetes. The prevailing model of diabetes as a single disorder that could present either in childhood (juvenile onset) or later in life (adult onset) was replaced by a classification that clearly distinguished type 1 diabetes from type 2 diabetes (then almost exclusively a disorder of later adulthood). Type 1 became known as autoimmune diabetes, caused by a dysregulated immune system that attacked, and ultimately destroyed, the β cells. Type 2 was a metabolic disorder driven by the demands of insulin resistance.

The past four decades have seen a progressive rise in the incidence of diabetes. While the focus has been on type 2 because of its greater numbers and clinical impact, the pattern has been identical for type 1 (4,5). Whereas type 2 diabetes is widely understood to be linked to obesity and the insulin resistance it causes (6), the rise in type 1 has not been satisfactorily explained though a wide variety of possible triggers has been proposed.

THE ISSUE

Diabetes is of two types. Type 1 is an autoimmune disorder of childhood, characterized by acute onset, ketoacidosis, and insulin dependency. Type 2 is a metabolic disorder of middle life, slow in onset and non-insulin dependent.

These definitions are the basis on which a generation or more has understood diabetes, but they need urgent revision. More than half of patients with type 1 diabetes present in adulthood (7), when their onset is slow and many neither develop acidosis nor require insulin for many years. Type 2 diabetes occurs in teenagers (8), sometimes with ketoacidosis (9), and insulin dependency frequently ensues given time. Clinically, there is little other than tempo to distinguish the two.

Accurate classification depends on a proper understanding of mechanisms, and is important because it guides both treatment and prevention. Commentators have recently begun to question the existing classification of diabetes, because it seems poorly adapted to the changing characteristics of the disease (10,11). As a recent editorial explained, a classification may come to embody outworn concepts that prevent us from seeking or applying new information (10). Established classification may perversely serve to discourage new thinking, and when a classification is questioned, so too must be the mechanisms on which it is based.

The aim of this chapter is to explore the mechanisms on which the current classification, and with it the current understanding of diabetes, is based and to suggest an alternative that may better explain its changing character. It focuses on a single theme—tempo—that may reunify diabetes into a single disorder.

TEMPO: THE CENTRAL CONCEPT

Diabetes develops only when the β cells are unable to produce sufficient insulin for the body's needs. The deficiency might be supply led, as in the monogenic disorders HNF-1α or Kir-6, where there is a primary deficiency in insulin supply (12,13), or demand led, as in insulin resistance. Both may contribute, and probably do in most instances. A measure of β-cell mass, adjusted for insulin sensitivity, describes the functional reserve of the β cells. Reserve falls progressively over time through natural apoptosis though, for most, the decline is probably slow and unimportant because a lifetime is too short for the loss to become critical. In others, the tempo is quicker, and the loss of β cells relative to demand results in first glucose intolerance, and then diabetes (Fig. 1). Crucially, the age at which diabetes develops is linked not so much to the cause of β-cell loss, as to the tempo. Whether slow (no diabetes), moderate (diabetes in adulthood), or rapid (diabetes in childhood), the concept is the same. Age at onset, incidence and, ultimately, prevalence are determined by tempo.

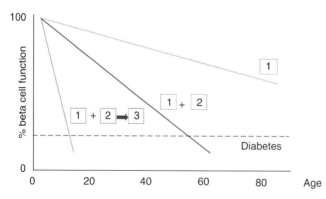

FIGURE 1 The concept of tempo in diabetes and the accelerators that influence it. The first accelerator represents the constitutional variation in β-cell mass at birth and rate of loss during a lifetime. It is seldom, if ever, sufficient to cause diabetes. The second is insulin resistance, which upregulates the β cell both metabolically and antigenically. The third is the immune response, modulated by immune response genes but dependent on insulin resistance for antigenic upregulation of the β cells.

THE HYPOTHESIS

The accelerator hypothesis argues that type 1 and type 2 diabetes are the same disorder of insulin resistance, set against different genetic backgrounds (14). It identifies three accelerators that quicken the tempo of β-cell insufficiency relative to demand. The first accelerator—a constitutionally (intrinsically) variable rate of β-cell apoptosis during life (15)—may be necessary for diabetes to develop, but is seldom in itself sufficient to cause it. It reflects natural differences of β-cell reserve within the population, which may be genetic or programmed during early life. The recently described TCF7L2 gene may be an example (16).

Insulin resistance, the second accelerator, is acquired largely from excess weight gain and physical inactivity. It further increases the rate of β-cell apoptosis through glucotoxicity and lipotoxicity (17,18), and accounts for what has traditionally been termed type 2 diabetes. However, as the environmental pressure from insulin resistance has grown, so the tempo of β-cell loss has quickened, and the age at presentation correspondingly fallen. What was diabetes in adulthood has become diabetes in childhood. People with type 2 diabetes are a subset of the whole population, but a growing subset as obesity—and with it insulin resistance—rises.

For conceptual purposes, people with type 1 and type 2 diabetes have often been viewed as members of separate populations, allowing a degree of overlap between them to account for the type 2 patient who progresses to insulin dependency ["type 1.5" diabetes (19)]. Those who develop type 1 diabetes, however, are in reality as much members of the general population as those who develop type 2, exposed to the same obesogenic environment and demands on the β cell. People with type 1 diabetes merely represent a further subset of the population, subject not only to insulin resistance but also to a third accelerator, genes that encode an immune response to the metabolically upregulated islets. The immune response is conventionally interpreted as autoimmune, but is viewed by the accelerator hypothesis as a physiological and predictable response in immunoreactive individuals. The hypothesis views "autoimmunity" as a response to insulin resistance rather than the cause of the diabetes—an inflammatory response within the β cells whose intensity is associated with significant collateral damage and which further accelerates the tempo. It may be speculated in this context that the glucagon-secreting α cells are spared because they are metabolically downregulated in hyperglycemia.

Immune tolerance is conventionally regarded as absolute, and autoimmunity an abrogation of it. Tolerance clearly raises an issue where the immune response in diabetes is seen by the accelerator hypothesis as a physiological response rather than pathological cause. The author has argued (20), on the basis of others' work before him (21), that the immune system evolved originally as a "housekeeper," programmed to phagocytose the detritus of natural cell death. It retains that primordial function. From this perspective, "autoimmunity" will be antigen driven and specific, its intensity responsive to the rate of apoptosis (antigenic load) and modulated by genetic influences. Self-tolerance and its abrogation are not at issue where clones expand appropriately to remove apoptotic bodies. Antibodies in this context are classic immunological adaptors. They link the specific subparticulate molecules to be cleared to nonspecific Fc receptors of phagocytic neutrophils, which in turn engulf the complex and dispose of it through the reticuloendothelial system (22). At its most intense, the reaction recruits T cells, which are proinflammatory and directly destructive. It has long been recognized that islet cells are both metabolically and immunogenically upregulated when functionally stressed by a rising blood sugar

(23,24). At whatever age it emerges, insulin resistance could be expected to increase β-cell stress and to intensify an immune response in those who are genetically predisposed. The phenomenon of insulin resistance which, as the response to progressively rising body weight, has been largely responsible for reducing the age at presentation of type 2 diabetes over recent time, might be doing just the same for type 1 diabetes by promoting the immunological accelerants of β-cell death in a progressively younger age group. If there is little clinically to distinguish two types of diabetes nowadays, there is little fundamentally either.

Insulin dependency is the end stage toward which all diabetes moves, and the notions of type 1 and type 2 insulin and non-insulin dependency may be artificial. The development of diabetes is just a matter of time, and the hypothesis views tempo as the only feature that distinguishes one "type" from another. Of the three accelerators, the first is intrinsic and the second largely acquired. Except for the rare monogenic forms, genes do not cause diabetes, but fix the level of response to environmental risk. The third accelerator is confined to a small subset of the population and is active only when driven by insulin resistance. Without insulin resistance, "autoimmune" diabetes would not occur, and backward regression of the gradient that describes the rise in type 1 diabetes over recent years bottoms out in the 1950s (25)—a point in time after World War II when the environmental changes associated with the rise in diabetes arguably began. Insulin resistance is associated with visceral fat mass and is widely believed to explain the epidemic rise of type 2 diabetes in the industrially developed world (26). The accelerator hypothesis argues that visceral weight gain is also central to type 1 diabetes, as much responsible for its rising incidence as for that of type 2, and the environmental factor in type 1 diabetes that has eluded epidemiology for so long.

The concept of an etiological link between the two types of diabetes is not new and has been suggested before by the author (27), but the evidence is now stronger. The hypothesis envisages infinite variation in the relative contributions made to β-cell loss by the degree of β-cell upregulation and the intensity of the immune response to it. Little insulin resistance is likely to be needed to accelerate β-cell loss in those carrying the most responsive immunogenotype (type 1 diabetes in childhood), whereas high levels of insulin resistance would be needed to achieve the same tempo of loss in those with protective genotypes (type 2 diabetes in childhood). Indeed, because insulin resistance and genetic susceptibility to it are independent continuums, the hypothesis would view diabetes itself as a continuum of tempos in two dimensions—the combination of highest insulin resistance and greatest immunoreactivity to it at one extreme (youngest onset), and that of the lowest insulin resistance and least reactivity at the other (onset in old age or never), with every shade of tempo in between. Type 1 diabetes is the same as type 2 except for one essential variable: intensity of the immune response to metabolically upregulated islets.

THE EPIDEMIOLOGY OF DIABETES

Over the past 20 years, the incidence of type 2 diabetes in the western world has increased dramatically, a pattern that parallels closely the rising incidence of obesity and (by implication) that of insulin resistance (28). Furthermore, age at presentation has been falling, such that the incidence of type 2 diabetes in American adolescents has increased tenfold and in Japanese school children 36-fold within a generation (29).

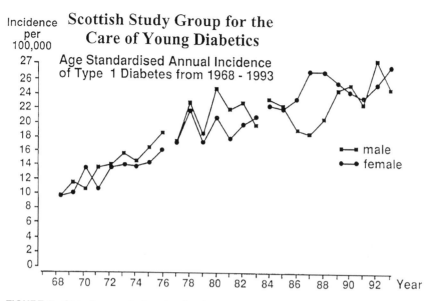

FIGURE 2 One of many studies showing the progressive rise in incidence of type 1 diabetes over the past generation.

Rather strikingly, the same pattern of increasing incidence and younger age at presentation has occurred for type 1 diabetes over the same time period (Fig. 2). Several studies in Europe show a doubling in incidence of type 1 diabetes over the last generation, with a clear shift of presentation to younger age groups (4,5), although the data are largely restricted to children and adolescents. The incidence of type 1 diabetes has been highest around puberty in all populations studied (30). The earlier peak in girls is consistent with their earlier maturation (31). The association between type 1 diabetes and puberty has never been satisfactorily explained, but may once again be an expression of insulin resistance. The hormonal changes of puberty (particularly the rise in growth hormone) places demands on insulin production that already damaged islets may be unable to meet. Again, body mass index (BMI) rises rapidly during puberty, and with it insulin resistance (32).

If the latter were the correct explanation, the accelerator hypothesis would predict a correspondingly earlier presentation of diabetes, as the BMI previously associated with puberty is reached at a progressively younger age. Tuomilehto et al. have reported how, over recent years, the age-at-onset curve for diabetes has risen to include most of early childhood, all but losing its peripubertal peak (33). Others have shown independently that weight gain early in childhood is associated with a higher risk of early type 1 diabetes (34,35), and the same appears to be true for type 2 (8). Most recently, the Childhood Diabetes in Finland Study Group has reported that a relative weight in childhood of >120% is associated with a more than twofold greater risk of developing type 1 diabetes (36). While the image of the emaciated child presenting with type 1 diabetes will undoubtedly persist into the 21st century, reality suggests something different. Audit of a single cohort of British children presenting with type 1 diabetes between 1980 and 2000 suggests that the mean BMI standard deviation score (BMI SDS) at presentation began to exceed that of the control population in the mid-1990s (37).

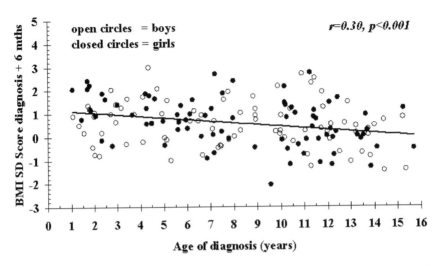

FIGURE 3 Example of the inverse relationship between body mass and age at onset of type 1 diabetes shown repeatedly in populations of children with type 1 diabetes. *Source*: From Ref. 37.

These observations provide important support for the hypothesis. They point to a central role for body mass, and by implication for insulin resistance in the development of type 1 as well as type 2 diabetes. More importantly still, there are now five full-length reports to indicate that, within a population with type 1 diabetes, the heaviest children develop type 1 diabetes and the youngest, true acceleration (37–41) (Fig. 3).

INSULIN RESISTANCE

Many theories have sought to account for insulin resistance. The Thrifty Genotype Hypothesis argues for gene selection against muscle proteolysis during an evolutionary history of recurring famine (42,43). In contrast, the Thrifty Phenotype Hypothesis (44), which first described an association between low birth weight and insulin resistance, explains the link as a gestational programming of the fetus in response to poor maternal nutrition. More recently, the Fetal Insulin Hypothesis has cited observations in families with monogenic glucokinase deficiency to illustrate the dependence of fetal growth on the genetics of fetal and maternal insulin secretion (45). It predicts that a gene or combination of genes responsible for insulin resistance will be found, which leads both to low weight at birth through insulin resistance and to glucose intolerance later in life.

There is a common theme to all three hypotheses: insulin resistance, which might arguably have favored survival in times of famine, leaves many in today's "coke and burger" culture unable to control their blood sugar. None of the theories, however, estimates how much of today's diabetes (the attributable proportion) can be accounted for by insulin resistance already present at birth, nor explains the rising incidence of type 2 diabetes, which, according to the logic of all three hypotheses, should by now be stable or falling as nutrition in pregnancy improves and gene selection operates to deselect the less fit. Insulin resistance acquired through lifestyle change is more likely than genes or gestational experience to underlie the recent rise in diabetes and its ever-younger presentation.

Importantly for the accelerator hypothesis, glucose clamp studies conducted 20 years ago showed that non-insulinized adults with autoimmune diabetes were as insulin resistant as those of comparable glucose tolerance with type 2 diabetes (46). More recently, Fourlanos et al., in a prospective study of children at risk, have shown how those who were more insulin resistant at the outset were more likely to convert to type 1 diabetes during the period of observation (47). Conversion rate is an expression of tempo and a measure of incidence. Seropositive type 2 diabetic adults become insulin dependent more rapidly than those who are seronegative (48), and the rise in proinsulin/insulin ratio that has long been the hallmark of insulin resistance in pre-type 2 diabetes also characterizes pre-type 1 diabetes (49). These observations together provide robust support for the "overlay" and "accelerator" concepts. The slower tempo of progression in adults has provided the means of demonstrating that all diabetics are associated with insulin resistance (the second accelerator) and that a subgroup advances more rapidly to insulin dependency as a result of an immune response (the third accelerator).

PATHOPHYSIOLOGY OF DIABETES

Type 1 diabetes is associated with autoantibodies and activated lymphocytes that are reactive with β-cell antigens (50). Its course is characterized by a symptomless prediabetic phase whose presence may be inferred from immune markers. Pre-type 1 diabetes is a period of accelerated β-cell loss, whose tempo varies from acute in those who present young to subacute or chronic in those who present later in life (51). The differences in tempo are assumed to be under genetic control, since those who develop type 1 diabetes in childhood tend to carry more intensely responsive HLA genes from those who develop it later in life (52,53). β-Cell "autoimmunity" appears to start early in life, insofar as immune markers predictive of future diabetes can be present as early as nine months of age (54). Analysis of the prediabetic phase among people recruited to large type 1 diabetes prevention studies, such as DPT-1, suggests that disturbances of glucose control are present months or years before clinical onset (55).

To be successful, a unifying hypothesis should be able to address all circumstances, and until recently, the development of neonatal type 1 diabetes within the first few weeks of life was difficult to reconcile with β-cell loss driven by insulin resistance. However, newly described mutations in the Kir-6 gene, which encodes insulin release, appear able to account for the majority of such cases under the age of six months, and possibly more (13). This is a monogenic disorder of insulin release but, if common variants of the gene were found in the population at large, polymorphisms that reduced rather than prevented the release of insulin, insulin resistance may once again be implicated in a type 1 (insulin requiring) diabetes that differed from type 2 only in genetic background. Common variants have been described of the glucokinase gene responsible for MODY2, but in contrast to disturbed insulin release, β cells subject to glucokinase deficiency are glucose insensitive and protected against upregulation by hyperglycemia (56).

Type 2 diabetes results from a combination of insulin resistance and defective insulin response (57). Blood insulin concentrations are raised, at least initially, but are never sufficient to meet the resistance that entrains them. Like type 2, type 1 diabetes also presents after a variable period of prediabetes, whose presence may be revealed not just by autoantibodies, but by high fasting insulin/glucose ratios and later by glycosuria or hyperglycemia in circumstances that temporarily increase insulin resistance—typically pregnancy, thyrotoxicosis, or a course of anti-inflammatory steroids. Between 17–63% of women whose glycosuria during pregnancy is attributable to glucose intolerance will subsequently become diabetic, depending on the series quoted (58). Of these, a proportion [around 20% according to one study (59)] will develop type 1 diabetes, underscoring the principle to be established here that the prediabetes of type 1 and type 2 differ only in tempo, not in outcome. Both represent a period of accelerated β-cell loss.

PROGRESSION FROM PREDIABETES TO DIABETES

If the tempo of progression can be slowed, the incidence of disease will fall, so that understanding the process of progression is likely to prove important to the prevention of diabetes. The construct proposed earlier proposed supply-led and demand-led hyperglycemia to denote a lack of insulin supply and a failure of its action, respectively, and Figure 4 illustrates the kinetics of insulin and glucose that might be expected in exclusively supply-led diabetes such as the monogenic HNF-1α mutation (MODY 3) (12). Insulin release falls progressively throughout life, and glucose levels rise as a consequence. The lower body weight of people with the HNF-1α mutation reflects their relative lack of insulin, which is a strongly anabolic hormone.

Type 1 diabetes is also regarded conventionally as a supply-led disorder, where autoimmune destruction of the β cells is deemed responsible for the fall in insulin that leads to both hyperglycemia and loss of weight that commonly precede its onset. Two observations, however, cast doubt on the supply-led nature of type 1 diabetes—the higher BMI that has repeatedly been observed during the early years of children who go on to develop type 1 diabetes (36,60–62) and their higher levels of insulin and insulin resistance (46,47,63). Such observations, and the fact that the first evidence of insulin dependency in those with type 2 diabetes, as with type 1, is usually weight loss suggest that there may be parallels in progression of the two disorders that merit scrutiny.

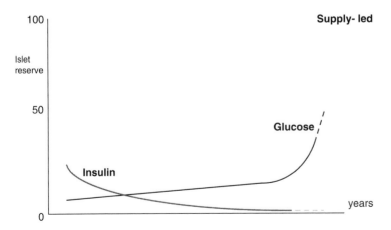

FIGURE 4 The excursions in insulin and glucose that might be expected over time when hyperglycemia is exclusively supply led—the result of β-cell dysfunction.

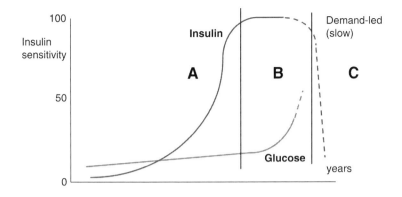

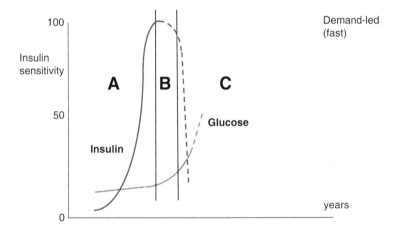

FIGURE 5 (*Upper and lower panel*) The kinetics of insulin release and glucose control in demand-led diabetes without the third accelerator (HLA gene—slow tempo) and with the third accelerator (fast tempo), as envisaged by the accelerator hypothesis.

Again, for the sake of simplicity, the natural history of diabetes can be divided into three phases—prediabetes (phase A), insulin-independent diabetes (phase B), and insulin-dependent diabetes (phase C) (Fig. 5). What follows is the (speculative) case for a single process of progression in both types of diabetes, where only the tempo differs. Both type 1 and type 2 diabetes, it is argued, are demand led, the rate of β-cell loss in response to the demand being the determinant of the age at onset.

In type 2 diabetes (Fig. 5, upper panel), where the gradient of progression to insulin dependency is gentle, there is a protracted window of time (phase B) during which the production of insulin is failing slowly but sufficient to sustain reasonable health. The diagnosis is invariably made in this phase, by chance or as a result of nonspecific symptoms. Indeed, many patients have been diabetic for years by the time the diagnosis is made. So slow is the progression that medication is often used to treat the blood glucose level more than the

Without the 3rd accelerator

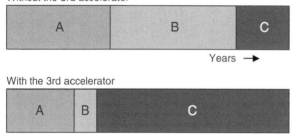

Years ➡

With the 3rd accelerator

FIGURE 6 The relative durations of the prediabetic (**A**), insulin-independent (**B**), and insulin-dependent (**C**) phases of diabetes in people with (type 1 diabetes) or without (type 2 diabetes) the third accelerator, as envisaged by the accelerator hypothesis.

symptoms. By contrast, it is proposed that the presence in type 1 diabetes of the third (immunogenetic) accelerator may propel a child through phase B so rapidly that it is often (usually) missed clinically (Fig. 5, lower panel). The fact that a phase B exists in type 1 diabetes is nevertheless clear from the honeymoon period, and the fact that people with less-reactive immunogenotypes spend more time in the insulin-independent state [type 1.5 diabetes (19)]. Latent autoimmune diabetes of adulthood (LADA) is similarly interpreted to be an expression of demand-led β-cell insufficiency in which the HLA genotype does not accelerate the patient into insulin dependency over days or weeks, but over months or years.

What in type 2 diabetes progresses slowly from mounting hyperinsulinemia through decompensation (saturation of β-cell reserve) to hypoinsulinemia and insulin dependency (Fig. 6), progresses rapidly in type 1 diabetes. The tempo is accelerated, but the same phases apply, suggesting that the same process—the same disorder—may be present.

SUSCEPTIBILITY AND RISK

Type 2 diabetes is prevalent in industrially developed societies. It affects up to 30% of some populations (64), suggesting that susceptibility to diabetes is common, though not universal, insofar as some of those apparently at greatest risk—the pathologically obese—never develop the disease.

The probability of developing a multifactorial disorder such as diabetes is made up of two components—genetic susceptibility and environmental risk. Each contributes to the probability of disease as a proportion so that, if one rises, the other inevitably falls. Concordance among monozygotic twin pairs is used to calculate the genetic contribution, and is said to lie at around 75% in type 2 diabetes (rising to 95% if those with glucose intolerance alone are included) (65), but only 20% in type 1 (66). However, it will be clear that heritability is not fixed, for any rise in the contribution from environmental risk will reduce the contribution from genetic susceptibility. If the Accelerator Hypothesis is correct in ascribing the increased incidence of type 1 diabetes to rising body mass on the basis of tempo, it should be able to show a rising BMI at onset over time and a falling need for the high-susceptibility alleles associated with the HLADR3/DR4 serotype.

Evidence for obesity as the risk responsible for the rising incidence of type 1 diabetes comes from both the United Kingdom and the United States. A study in the south of England shows a progressive rise in BMI at diagnosis among children over the past 20 years (41) (Fig. 7). These data are important because they show

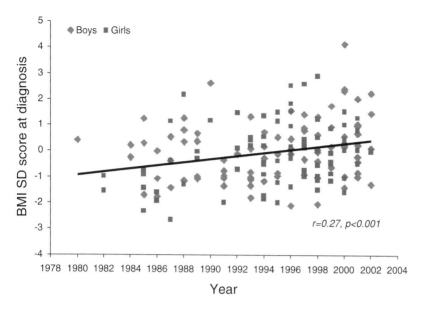

FIGURE 7 Evidence of the secular rise in body mass of children at the onset of type 1 diabetes. *Source*: From Ref. 37.

not simply a rise in obesity among diabetic children over a 20-year period, but a progressively increasing BMI at the time of onset. Corresponding data from Pittsburgh showed a threefold rise in the frequency of overweight (BMI > 85th percentile) at onset of type 1 diabetes among children from the early 1980s to the late 1990s (67).

VARIANTS ON THE HYPOTHESIS

All commentators agree that the rise in incidence of type 1 diabetes over recent decades has been the result of environmental rather than genetic change. The gene pool cannot have altered significantly in such a brief period, and the falling contribution of HLA genes to the probability of disease is witness to rising environmental risk. However, variants of the accelerator hypothesis have interpreted the change in environmental pressure in different ways.

The concept of double diabetes retains discrete mechanisms for type 1 and type 2 diabetes, and sees them operating together in parallel rather than in sequence (68). It explains the rise in childhood diabetes as a rise in the metabolic component alongside, and independent of, the autoimmune component. The concept of coexistence of the two mechanisms in the one child is entirely valid, but has different implications for prevention. Reduction in insulin resistance, whether achieved through lifestyle change or medication, will target the one mechanism, but not the other. According to the double diabetes concept, autoimmune insulitis would not respond to insulin sensitization nor insulin resistance to immunoregulation, so that two independent interventions would arguably be needed to address two independent pathologies.

The "Overload Hypothesis" lists a wide variety of factors, environmental and constitutional, that could overload the islets and hasten β-cell loss (69). Whether puberty, growth velocity, stress or physical inactivity, they all have insulin resistance in common and in this respect do not differ from the accelerator principle. However, the overload hypothesis does seek to make a clear distinction between factors that initiate type 1 diabetes (triggers) and factors that determine its rate of progression thereafter. It argues that the environmental factors that are causing an increase in childhood-onset diabetes and a shift to a younger age at onset must be operating after the initiation of autoimmunity because the factors deemed to trigger the disease (enteroviral infection and early weaning are cited as examples) are decreasing.

It nevertheless remains possible that type 1 diabetes is unrelated to viral infection (evidence has proved elusive) and that early weaning merely means less weight gain early on, a factor later deemed favorable in progression of the disease. The overload hypothesis continues to view the immunological reaction in type 1 diabetes as the primary event (autoimmunity) rather than a genetically modulated response, and in this respect differs fundamentally from the accelerator hypothesis.

LIMITATIONS AND CHALLENGES

The accelerator hypothesis may be criticized for failing to address the wealth of animal evidence cited in support of autoimmunity—but it does not do so dismissively. The BB rat, NOD mouse, and other models suggest that the immune system can spontaneously cause β-cell disease and diabetes. The pathways involved have been teased apart meticulously, and the immunological processes described in detail. However, the issue for the hypothesis is not so much whether a dysregulated immune system can destroy the β-cell mass (which clearly it can), but whether the process described in inbred rodents under pathogen-free conditions necessarily relates to outbred man. The mutated animal models may merely undergo a process spontaneously that in man needs environmental pressure. If this were the case, the immune response in man could arguably be interpreted as secondary, and the process in rodents one of normal immunology in unnatural circumstances.

Three studies have emerged since the hypothesis was first published that challenge it wholly or in part. The first, from Birmingham, United Kingdom, was unable to confirm the key prediction of an inverse correlation between BMI and age at onset population in a cohort of type 1 diabetic children (70). Five other studies, all of them larger, have nevertheless been able to show this correlation (37–41). The earlier study may have suffered the imprecision of small numbers, of racial mix (South-Asian children have a higher risk of type 1 diabetes for a given BMI) and of variable weight loss prior to onset (other studies have recorded weight after rehydration and refeeding). It is also important that the groups tested represent whole rather than selected populations, although most, if not all, children with diabetes will be referred to a specialist department where registration is usual.

A study by Dabelea et al. reported an inverse relationship after appropriate adjustments for age-at-diagnosis and BMI (the acceleration predicted) among those whose fasting C-peptide (FCP) levels lay below the median, but none among those whose FCP lay above it (41). The difference was interpreted to mean that any relationship to insulin resistance applied only to a subset of type 1 diabetic children with low β-cell reserve. The one adjustment that was not made, however, may be the crucial one—the HLA genotype. Those children who obeyed the prediction were younger than those who did not. The younger the diabetic child at diagnosis, the more likely is he/she to carry high-susceptibility HLA genes (71), and so it is possible, even probable, that the proportion of children carrying high-susceptibility HLA genes was greater in the younger group than in the older group. The only difference in behavior between the two groups may have been one of tempo, and while the age range studied was sufficient to demonstrate the predicted inverse relationship in the younger group carrying more intensely reactive HLA genes, it may not have been wide enough to demonstrate the corresponding relationship for the older group carrying less reactive genes. Indeed, as HLA genes are the third accelerator of β-cell loss, presenting the data in this way may have served to support the hypothesis for the entire group rather than qualify it according to FCP.

The recently discovered TCF7L2 gene, mentioned earlier, is associated with an odds ratio of 1.36 for type 2 diabetes among adults (72). On the basis that if the accelerator hypothesis were correct, the gene should appear with a similar frequency in type 1 as in type 2 diabetes, Field et al. recently genotyped 6200 children with type 1 diabetes and 7600 controls under the age of 17 years (73). The odds ratio in the children with type 1 diabetes was not significantly different from 1.0, from which the authors concluded that type 1 and type 2 diabetes were not the same disorders. However, the argument appears to be flawed (74). The accelerator hypothesis proposes that "type 1 and type 2 diabetes are the same disorder of insulin resistance *set against different genetic backgrounds*" (17). An environmental pressure that converts susceptibility into disease will select the most susceptible first. The hypothesis is based on tempo, and as HLA genes and TCF7L2 segregate independently, only the most susceptible (HLA) would be expected to succumb in childhood. As the incidence of type 2 diabetes in childhood increases because the environmental pressure continues to rise, so will the frequency of TCF7L2 in childhood diabetes, as the hypothesis predicts.

BODY MASS: THE ELUSIVE "TRIGGER" OF TYPE 1 DIABETES

If the rising incidence and earlier presentation of diabetes were to be explained by an ever-heavier population at all ages, weight gain would have as much a role in the changing demography of type 1 diabetes as it has in that of type 2. Ascribing the rising incidence of type 1 diabetes to metabolic rather than to immunological factors has novel and important implications. Clinical research over the past 30 years has focused almost exclusively on exogenous factors (viruses, toxins, allergens) deemed able to initiate, facilitate, or intensify autoimmune damage to the β cell. Although many have been proposed (75), none has been confirmed, and apart from body mass, none shows correlations within type 1 diabetic populations to suggest the dose-responsiveness needed for cause and effect. The prevalence of obesity has trebled over the past generation. Insulin resistance, resulting from a combination of obesity and physical inactivity, is a serious candidate for the "elusive" environmental factor responsible for the rising incidence of type 1 diabetes, and as such, a true accelerator.

The rise in incidence of diabetes in "westernized" countries over recent time has occurred over a period too brief for changes in the gene pool to exert an influence. Similarly, there is no evidence of falling birth weight over the same period to suggest a deterioration in fetal quality and attendant risk of insulin resistance, as the fetal origins hypothesis proposes—indeed, birth weights have risen. More likely, it is the progressive increase in body weight after birth, with the rising prevalence of obesity at all ages over the past 30 or more years, which is responsible.

The accelerator hypothesis at its simplest can be reduced to the unfavorable interplay between two variables: insulin resistance and β-cell apoptosis. Apoptosis occurs naturally throughout life at a variable rate, but may be intrinsically higher in those who are susceptible to diabetes. Insulin resistance—whether present at birth or acquired through the accumulation of visceral fat during life—accelerates β-cell loss and makes demands on insulin secretion that in some cannot be met.

Immune damage of the β cells is the third accelerator, restricted by genotype to a small and independent minority of the population. At its most aggressive, the immune response might be sufficient to cause diabetes by itself, though an accelerator different from insulin resistance would be needed to account for the increase in apoptosis, which provokes it. The hypothesis predicts that in older patients, where β-cell autoreactivity is less aggressive, those with islet-cell auto-immunity and most likely to develop diabetes will already have the diabetic phenotype—a low β-cell mass and high insulin resistance. Those who do not might be expected to remain seropositive but healthy, to succumb only when the intrinsic β-cell mass wanes and/or insulin resistance rises with the corpulence of advancing age.

Tempo, and tempo alone it is argued, distinguishes what in the past have been described as two separate types of diabetes. The three phases in the pro-gression to overt diabetes—prediabetes, insulin-independent diabetes, and insulin-dependent diabetes can all be identified in both types, differing only (though sometimes substantially) in their relative duration. Not to take account of these phases and their differences in tempo will make it conceptually difficult to regard as two equivalent diabetic states where insulin is needed from the outset in one, but only (if ever) after a long period of clinical diabetes in the other. The requirement for insulin in both cases is nevertheless reached at exactly corre-sponding points in the progression of prediabetes. All people with diabetes move toward this point of insulin dependence—some reach it very quickly, others perhaps not in a lifetime.

A hypothesis postulating body mass as a primary risk factor in the etiology of type 1, as well as type 2, diabetes is novel, but eminently testable. Ultimately, it will be necessary to establish whether strategies to reduce the second accelerator (insulin resistance) in those at risk from type 1 diabetes, through weight loss, metformin, or one of the thiazolidinediones (76), is paralleled by a deceleration in the third—immune damage to the β cells—and by the slowing of conversion from risk to disease. The notion that type 1 could represent merely the accelerated development of type 2 diabetes is important if it implies that strategies currently on trial to suppress the immunological accelerator of type 1 diabetes [e.g., anti-CD3 (77,78)] leave unchanged the insulin resistance that provoked it. Of course, inter-vention that prevents the immune response may be expected to reduce the tempo of type 1 diabetes, as was the case with cyclosporine, but the control of weight gain further upstream, and with it insulin resistance, could be a more fundamental means of avoiding diabetes, safer and cheaper (80).

CONCLUSION

Diabetes used to be straightforward. There was a childhood type that required insulin and an adult type that did not. Adult-onset diabetes seldom presented before the age of 50, and most died with it rather than of it. Childhood diabetes presented acutely, and was sometimes life threatening. The adult diabetic was overweight, and the child underweight. This tableau of contrasts has changed dramatically over the course of a single generation. Diabetes is now more common, it presents at an earlier age, many adults require insulin and many children do not. Such has been the convergence in phenotype of the young diabetic that the current system of classification finds it difficult to distinguish the childhood diabetic as type 1 or type 2. Classifications are important in formulating appropriate treatment and in directing prevention. The current classification of diabetes may need changing, and the accelerator hypothesis, if confirmed, offers a structure on which such a change might be based.

REFERENCES

1. Gepts W. Pathologic anatomy of the pancreas in juvenile diabetes mellitus. Diabetes 1965; 14:619–633.
2. Nerup J, Platz P, Anderssen OO. HLA antigens and diabetes mellitus. Lancet 1974; 2:864–866.
3. Bottazzo GF, Florin-Christensen A, Doniach D. Islet-cell antibodies in diabetes mellitus with autoimmune polyendocrine deficiencies. Lancet 1974; 2:1279–1283.
4. Onkamo P, Vaananen S, Karvonen M, et al. Worldwide increase of type 1 diabetes—analysis of the data on published incidence trends. Diabetologia 1999; 42:1395–1403.
5. Gale EAM The rise of childhood type 1 diabetes in the 20th century. Diabetes 2002; 51:3353–3361.
6. Shuldiner AR, Yang R, Gong DW. Resistin, obesity and insulin resistance—the emerging role of the adipocyte as an endocrine organ. N Engl J Med 2001 Nov 1; 345 (18):1345–1346.
7. Molbak AG, Christau B, Marner B, et al. Incidence of insulin-dependent diabetes in age groups over 30 years in Denmark. Diabet Med 1994; 11:650–655.
8. Rosenbloom AL, Joe JR, Young RS, et al. Emerging epidemic of type 2 diabetes in youth. Diabetes Care 1999; 22:345–354.
9. Aizawa T, Funase Y, Katakura M, et al. Ketosis-onset diabetes in young adults with subsequent non-insulin-dependency, a link between IDDM and NIDDM? Diabet Med 1997; 14:989–991.
10. Gale EA. Declassifying diabetes. Diabetologia 2006; 49:1989–1995.
11. Wilkin TJ. Changing perspectives in diabetes: their impact on its classification. Diabetologia 2007 (in press).
12. Velho C, Froguel P. Maturity-onset diabetes of the young (MODY), MODY genes and non-insulin-dependent diabetes mellitus. Diabetes Metab 1997; 23(suppl 2):34–37.
13. Pearson ER, Flechtner I, Njolstad PR, et al. Switching from insulin to oral sulfonylureas in patients with diabetes due to Kir6.2 mutations. N Engl J Med 2006; 355:467–477.
14. Wilkin TJ. The accelerator hypothesis: weight gain as the missing link between Type I and Type II diabetes. Diabetologia 2001; 44:914–922.
15. Mauricio D, Mandrup-Poulsen T. Apoptosis and the pathogenesis of IDDM: a question of life and death. Diabetes 1998; 47:537–543.
16. Saxena R, Gianniny L, Burtt NP, et al. Common single nucleotide polymorphisms in TCF7L2 are reproducibly associated with type 2 diabetes and reduce the insulin response to glucose in nondiabetic individuals. Diabetes 2006; 55:2890–2895.
17. Maedler K, Donath MY. Beta-cells in type 2 diabetes: a loss of function and mass. Horm Res 2004; 62(suppl 3):67–73.
18. Robertson RP, Harmon J, Tran PO, et al. Beta-cell glucose toxicity, lipotoxicity, and chronic oxidative stress in type 2 diabetes. Diabetes 2004; 53(suppl 1): S119–S124.
19. Juneja R, Palmer JP. Type 1½ diabetes: myth or reality? Autoimmunity 1999; 29:65–83.
20. Wilkin TJ. Autoimmunity: attack or defence? Autoimmunity 1989; 3:57–73.
21. Grabar P. Autoantibodies and the physiological role of immunoglobulins. Immunol Today 1983; 4:337–340.
22. Roitt I, Brostoff J, Male D. Immunology. London: Churchill Livingstone, 1995:1.5–1.6.

23. Bjork E, Kampe O, Karlsson FA, et al. Glucose regulation of the autoantigen GAD65 in human pancreatic islets. J Clin Endocrinol Metab 1992; 75:574–576.

24. Judkowski V, Krakowski M, Rodriguez E, et al. Increased islet antigen presentation leads to type-1 diabetes in mice with autoimmune susceptibility. Eur J Immunol 2004; 34:1031–1040.

25. Gale EA. The rise of childhood type 1 diabetes in the 20th century. Diabetes 2002; 51:3353–3361.

26. Zimmet P. Globalization, coca-colonization and the chronic disease epidemic: can the Doomsday scenario be averted? J Intern Med 2000; 247:301–310.

27. Wilkin TJ. Early nutrition and diabetes mellitus (Editorial). Br Med J 1993; 306:283–284.

28. National Task Force on the Prevention and Treatment of Obesity. Overweight, obesity, and health risk. Arch Intern Med 2000; 160:898–904.

29. Kitagawa T, Owada M, Urakami T, et al. Increased incidence of non-insulin dependent diabetes mellitus among Japanese schoolchildren correlates with an increased intake of animal protein and fat. Clin Pediatr (Phila) 1998; 37:111–115.

30. Akerblom HK, Reunanen A. The epidemiology of insulin-dependent diabetes mellitus (IDDM) in Finland and in northern Europe. Diabetes Care 1985; 8(suppl 1):10–16.

31. Staines A, Bodansky HJ, Lilley HE, et al. The epidemiology of diabetes mellitus in the United Kingdom: the Yorkshire Regional Childhood Diabetes Register. Diabetologia 1993; 36:1282–1287.

32. Moran A, Jacobs DR Jr., Steinberger J, et al. Insulin resistance during puberty: results from clamp studies in 357 children. Diabetes 1999; 48:2039–2044.

33. Tuomilehto J, Virtala E, Karvonen M, et al. Increase in incidence of insulin-dependent diabetes mellitus among children in Finland. J Epidemiol 1995; 24:984–992.

34. Johansson C, Samuelsson U, Ludvigsson J. A high weight gain in early life is associated with an increased risk of type 1 (insulin-dependent) diabetes mellitus. Diabetologia 1994; 37:91–94.

35. Hypponen E, Kenward MG, Virtanen SM, et al. Infant feeding, early weight gain and risk of type 1 diabetes. Childhood diabetes in Finland (DiME) Study Group. Diabetes Care 1999; 22:1961–1965.

36. Hypponen E, Virtanen SM, Kenward MG, et al. Obesity, increased linear growth, and risk of type 1 diabetes in children. Childhood Diabetes in Finland Study Group. Diabetes Care 2000; 23:1755–1760.

37. Betts P, Mulligan J, Ward P, et al. Increasing body weight predicts the earlier onset of insulin-dependant diabetes in childhood: testing the "accelerator hypothesis" (2). Diabet Med 2005; 22:144–151.

38. Kibirige M, Metcalf B, Renuka R, et al. Testing the accelerator hypothesis: the relationship between body mass and age at diagnosis of type 1 diabetes. Diabetes Care 2003; 26:2865–2870.

39. Knerr I, Wolf J, Reinehr T, et al. The "accelerator hypothesis": relationship between weight, height, body mass index and age at diagnosis in a large cohort of 9,248 German and Austrian children with type 1 diabetes mellitus. Diabetologia. 2005; 48:2501–2504.

40. Kordonouri O, Hartmann R: Higher body weight is associated with earlier onset of type 1 diabetes: confirming the accelerator hypothesis. Diabetic Med 2005; 22:1783–1784.

41. Dabelea D, D'Agostino RB Jr., Mayer-Davis EJ, et al. Testing the accelerator hypothesis: Body size, beta-cell function, and age at onset of type 1 (autoimmune) diabetes. Diabetes Care 2006; 29:290–294.

42. Neel JV. Diabetes mellitus: a 'thrifty' genotype rendered detrimental by 'progress'? Am J Hum Genet 1962; 14:353–362.

43. Reaven GM. Hypothesis: muscle insulin resistance is the ('not so') thrifty genotype. Diabetologia 1998; 41:482–484.

44. Hales CN, Barker DJP. Type 2 (non insulin-dependent) diabetes: the thrifty phenotype hypothesis. Diabetologia 1992; 35:595–601.

45. Hattersley AT, Tooke JE. The fetal insulin hypothesis: an alternative explanation of the association of low birth weight with diabetes and vascular disease. Lancet 1999; 353:1789–1792.

46. Gray RS, Borsey DQ, Irvine WJ, et al. Non-insulin-treated ICA positive diabetics are equally insulin-resistant. Diabetes Metab 1983; 9:292–296.
47. Fourlanos S, Narendran P, Byrnes GB, et al. Insulin resistance is a risk factor for progression to type 1 diabetes. Diabetologia 2004; 47:1661–1667.
48. Turner R, Stratton I, Horton V, et al. UKPDS 25: autoantibodies to islet-cell cytoplasm and glutamic acid carboxylase for prediction of insulin requirement in type 2 diabetes. UK prospective diabetes Study Group. Lancet 1997; 350:1288–1293.
49. Rodrigue-Villar C, Conget I, Casamitjana R, et al. High proinsulin levels in late pre-IDDM stage. Diabetes Res Clin Pract 1997; 37:145–148.
50. Atkinson MA, Maclaren NK. The pathogenesis of insulin-dependent diabetes mellitus. N Engl J Med 1994; 331:1428–1436.
51. Eisenbarth GS, Gianani R, Yu L, et al. Dual-parameter model for prediction of type I diabetes mellitus. Proc Assoc Am Physicians 1998; 110:126–135.
52. Demaine AG, Hibberd ML, Mangles D, et al. A new marker in the HLA class I region is associated with the age at onset of IDDM. Diabetologia 1995; 38:623–628.
53. Cailla-Zucman S, Garchon HJ, Timsit J, et al. Age-dependent HLA genetic heterogeneity of type 1 insulin-dependent diabetes mellitus. J Clin Invest 1992; 90:2242–2250.
54. Ziegler AG, Hummel M, Schenker M, et al. Autoantibody appearance and risk for development of childhood diabetes in offspring of parents with type 1 diabetes: the 2-year analysis of the German BABYDIAB Study. Diabetes 1999; 48:460–468.
55. Barker JM, McFann K, Harrison LC, et al. Pre-type 1 diabetes dysmetabolism: maximal sensitivity achieved with both oral and intravenous glucose tolerance testing. J Pediatr 2007; 150:31.e6–36.e6.
56. Weedon MN, Frayling TM, Shields B, et al. Genetic regulation of birth weight and fasting glucose by a common polymorphism in the islet cell promoter of the glucokinase gene. Diabetes 2005; 54:576–581.
57. Turner RC, Holman RR, Matthews DR, et al. Relative contributions of insulin deficiency and insulin resistance in maturity-onset diabetes. Lancet 1982; 1: 596–598.
58. Kjos SL, Buchanan TA. Gestational diabetes mellitus. New Engl J Med 1999; 341:1749–1756.
59. Damm P, Kuhl C, Buschard K, et al. Prevalence and predictive value of islet cell antibodies and insulin autoantibodies in women with gestational diabetes. Diabet Med 1994; 11:558–563.
60. Baum JD, Ounsted M, Smith MA. Weight gain in infancy and subsequent development of diabetes mellitus in childhood. Lancet 1975; 2:866.
61. Johansson C, Samuelsson U, Ludvigsson J. A high weight gain in early life is associated with an increased risk of type 1 (insulin-dependent) diabetes. Diabetologia 1994; 37:91–94.
62. Bruining GJ. Association between infant growth before onset of juvenile type-1 diabetes and autoantibodies to IA-2. Netherlands Kolibrie study group of childhood diabetes. Lancet 2000; 356:655–656.
63. Hawa Ml, Bonfanti R, Valeri C, et al. No evidence for genetically determined alteration in insulin secretion or sensitivity predisposing to type 1 diabetes: a study of identical twins. Diabetes Care. 2005; 28:1415–1418.
64. Zimmet PZ, McCarty DJ, de Courten MP. The global epidemiology of non-insulin-dependent diabetes mellitus and the metabolic syndrome. J Diabetes Complications 1997; 11:60–68.
65. Medici F, Hawa M, Ianari A, et al. Concordance rate for type 2 diabetes mellitus in monozygotic twins: an actuarial analysis. Diabetologia 1999; 42:146–150.
66. Kaprio J, Tuomilehto J, Koskenvuo M, et al. Concordance for type 1 (insulin-dependent) and type 2 (non-insulin-dependent) diabetes mellitus in a population-based cohort of twins in Finland. Diabetologia 1992; 35:1060–1067.
67. Libman IM, Pietropaolo M, Arslanian SA, et al. Changing prevalence of overweight children and adolescents at onset of insulin-treated diabetes. Diabetes Care 2003; 26:2871–2875.
68. Libman IM, Becker DJ. Coexistence of type 1 and type 2 diabetes mellitus: "double" diabetes? Pediatr Diabetes 2003; 4:110–113.

69. Dahlquist G. Can we slow the rising incidence of childhood-onset autoimmune diabetes? The overload hypothesis. Diabetologia 2006; 49:20–24.
70. Porter JR, Barrett TJ. Braking the accelerator hypothesis? Diabetologia 2004; 47:352–3563.
71. Tait BD, Harrison LC, Drummond BP, et al. HLA antigens and age at diagnosis of insulin-dependent diabetes mellitus. Hum Immunol 1995; 42:116–122.
72. Florez JC, Jablonski KA, Balley N, et al. TCF7L2 polymorphisms and progression to diabetes in the Diabetes Prevention Program. N Engl J Med 2006; 355:241–250.
73. Field SF, Howson JMM, Smyth DJ, et al. Analysis of the type 2 diabetes gene TCF7L2 in 13,795 type 1 diabetes cases and control subjects. Diabetologia 2007; 50:212–213.
74. Wilkin TJ. The accelerator hypothesis cannot be tested using the type 2 diabetes gene, TCF7L2. Diabetologia 2007 (in press).
75. Dahlquist G. The aetiology of type 1 diabetes: an epidemiological perspective. Acta Paediatr Suppl 1998; 425:5–10.
76. Day C. Thiazolidinediones: a new class of antidiabetic drugs. Diabet Med 1999; 16:179–192.
77. Harlan DM, von Herrath M. Immune intervention with anti-CD3 in diabetes. Nat Med 2005; 11:716–718.
78. Herold KC, Gitelman SE, Masharani U, et al. A single course of anti-CD3 monoclonal antibody hOKT3gamma1(Ala–Ala) results in improvement in C-peptide responses and clinical parameters for at least 2 years after onset of type 1 diabetes. Diabetes 2005; 54:1763–1769.
79. Dupre J, Stiller CR, Gent M, et al. Clinical trials of cyclosporin in IDDM. Diabetes Care 1988; 11(suppl 1):37–44.
80. Wilkin T, Ludvigsson J, Greenbaum C, et al. Future intervention trials in type 1 diabetes. Diabetes Care 2004; 27:996–997.

7 Epidemiology of Type 2 Diabetes in Children and Adolescents

Kristen Nadeau
Department of Pediatrics, University of Colorado at Denver and The Children's Hospital, Denver, Colorado, U.S.A.

Dana Dabelea
Department of Preventive Medicine and Biometrics, University of Colorado at Denver, Denver, Colorado, U.S.A.

INTRODUCTION

Historically, diabetes in youth was believed to be almost entirely Type 1 (autoimmune and insulin dependent) diabetes. In contrast, those over 30 years at the time of onset were considered to have type 2 diabetes (T2DM), defined as diabetes resulting from insulin resistance (IR), with a concomitant insulin secretory defect (1). Although T2DM has been traditionally viewed as an adult disease, as risk increases with advancing age, the question of whether T2DM is a pediatric disease is now being answered in the affirmative. An increasing proportion of youth with apparent T2DM is reported, especially in minority populations (2–4).

The epidemiology of T2DM in youth is yet unclear because of its relative rarity, the infrequency of comprehensive registries, and the small number of appropriate, population-based studies. Most available data come from reviews of diabetes clinics, not population-based studies. Therefore, the true magnitude of T2DM in youth may be underestimated. Since the classification of diabetes based on etiopathogenesis is new (1), there is potential for misclassification of different types of diabetes in youth. There is, therefore, a need for large population-based studies using standardized case definitions to define the magnitude of the problem of childhood T2DM. This chapter summarizes data on the global epidemiology of T2DM in youth.

PREVALENCE

Population-Based Studies
Population-based studies, where all individuals within a geographical area undergo diabetes screening, are ideal to determine prevalence, as they capture even undiagnosed cases. However, among the limited number of available population-based studies of T2DM in youth, few test oral glucose tolerance [the gold standard for diabetes mellitus (DM) diagnosis] and many lack key data essential to differentiate T2DM from T1DM. Studies lacking screening for undiagnosed diabetes may underreport T2DM, as the disease is sometimes asymptomatic. Table 1 and 2 summarize the most important epidemiologic studies of prevalence and incidence of T2DM in youth.

TABLE 1 Studies of Prevalence of Type 2 Diabetes in Youth

Study/location	Race/ethnicity	Age-group	Prevalence (per 1000)	Period	Reference
NHANES III/U.S.A.	Multiethnic	12–19	1.3	1988–1994	5
NHANES/U.S.A.	Multiethnic	12–19	3.0	1999–2002	6
Manitoba/Canada	Oji-Cree Indians	4–19	11.1	1996–1997	12
Indian Health Service	American Indians & Alaska natives	15–19	5.4	1998	14
Arizona/U.S.A.	Pima Indians	10–14	22.3	1992–1996	4
		15–19	50.9		
SEARCH/U.S.A.	Native-Americans	10–19	1.74	2001	15
	African-Americans		1.05		
	Asian/Pacific Islander		0.54		
	Hispanics		0.48		
	Non-Hispanic whites		0.19		
Taiwan	Taiwanese	6–18	0.09 males	1993–1999	16
			0.15 females		
Israel	Israeli	17	0.36 males	2005	17
			0.1 females		
Saudi Arabia	Arabian	<14	1.2	2000	19
		14–29	7.9		

Abbreviation: NHANES, National Health and Nutrition Examination Survey.

TABLE 2 Studies of Incidence of Type 2 Diabetes in Youth

Study/location	Race/ethnicity	Age-group	Incidence (per 100,000/year)	Period	Reference
Arizona/U.S.A.	Pima Indians	5–14	331.9	1991–1903	196
SEARCH/U.S.A.	Native-Americans	15–19	49.4	2002–2003	21
	Asian/Pacific Islander		22.7		
	African-Americans		19.4		
	Hispanics		17.0		
	Non-Hispanic whites		5.6		
Chicago/U.S.A.	African-American	0–17	15.2	1985–1994	25
	Latino		10.7		
Cincinnati/U.S.A.	Hispanic & African-American	10–19	7.2	1994	26
Japan	Japanese	Primary & junior high school	1.73	1974–1980	23
			2.76	1981–2002	
Japan	Japanese	Primary high school	2	1991–1995	24
			13.9		
U.K.	Blacks	0–17	2.9	2004–2005	31
	South Asians		1.25		
	Whites		0.35		
Australia	Indigenous	0–17	16.0	1990–2002	33
	Non-indigenous		1.0		

In the United States, the National Health and Nutrition Examination Survey (NHANES) III provided data on a sample of 2867 patients aged 12 to 19 years, collected between 1988 and 1994 (5). Thirteen of these adolescents had diabetes, of whom four were classified as T2DM, implying a T2DM prevalence of 0.13%. All four with presumed T2DM were of non-Hispanic black or Mexican-American origin. An additional 22 adolescents had HbA1c $> 6\%$, but did not meet the formal criteria for diabetes. The differentiation between T1DM and T2DM was based only on the use of insulin, likely underestimating the T2DM prevalence, as many youth with T2DM are also treated with insulin.

More recent U.S. data are available from NHANES 1999–2002, using the same definitions of diabetes (6). The prevalence of diabetes was 0.5%, among over 4000 adolescents completing self-report information; 44% of these cases were classified as T2DM, implying a prevalence of 0.2%; 0.11% required both insulin and oral medications, hence probably having T2DM and, thus, increasing the prevalence to 0.3%. While the NHANES-based prevalence appears to be rising, a heightened awareness of T2DM could also increase the identification of undiagnosed cases. Among over 1400 NHANES subjects with fasting glucose measures, the prevalence of impaired fasting glucose (IFG) was 11% (using a cutoff of 5.6 mmol/L), or 1.5% (using a cutoff of 6.1 mmol/L), unchanged from NHANES III. Unfortunately, no data were provided on undiagnosed diabetes. In addition, the use of self-report has obvious limitations as does the poor differentiation between T1DM and T2DM.

The U.S. National Survey of Children's Health (NSCH) (7) was a population-based cross-sectional parental telephone survey of random households completed from January 2003 through July 2004, including 102,353 children < 18 years of age. This analysis provided a nationally representative prevalence estimate of 3.2 cases per 1000 children. Unfortunately, there was no differentiation as to diabetes type.

A study of fourth grader Mexican Americans found a T2DM prevalence of 0.3%, and a prevalence of 0.14% of each of impaired glucose tolerance (IGT) and IFG (8). A study of eighth graders from 12 U.S. middle schools, selected for high-risk ethnicity (56% Hispanic, mean age 13.6 years), reported that 6.2% had IFG (fasting plasma glucose (FPG) ≥ 6.1 mmol/L), 2.3% had IGT, and 0.4% had undiagnosed diabetes (FPG ≥ 7.0 mmol/L) (9).

T2DM appears to be strikingly common among Native North American youth. Thirty years of data collected among the Pima Indians of Arizona have shown increasing rates of antibody negative diabetes among children, as well as a female preponderance (4). From 1967–1976 to 1987–1996, the T2DM prevalence in Pima youth increased from 2.4% to 3.8% in males and from 2.7% to 5.3% in females, the highest rates reported in youth to date. In the 1991–1992 Navajo Health and Nutrition Survey, the prevalence of diabetes (type unknown) among Navajo youth aged 12 to 19 years was 1.4% and one of every two identified cases was diagnosed by screening (10). Among Canadian First Nation youth aged 6 to 17 years, T2DM prevalence was also very high, and reportedly increasing (11). For example, screening studies of the Oji-Cree First Nation in Sandy Lake (12) and Therese Point (13) report a prevalence of T2DM of 3.6% and 4%, respectively, in girls aged 10 to 19 years. A study of American Indian and Alaskan Native adolescents also reported increasing prevalence of T2DM among 15- to 19-year-olds (0.32% in 1990 to 0.54% in 1998) (14).

SEARCH for Diabetes in Youth is a U.S. large, multicenter, multiethnic collaborative study of physician-diagnosed primary diabetes in youth less than 20 years of age. SEARCH identified 6379 youth with diabetes prevalent in 2001, in a population of approximately 3.5 million youth (15). A total of 769 had T2DM, as assessed by the health care provider. Prevalence of T2DM was estimated at 0.22 per 1000, being much lower in youth aged 0 to 9 years (0.01/1000) than in those aged 10 to 19 years (0.42/1000). Among the 1349 DM cases in children aged 0 to 9 years, only 11 had T2DM, making T1DM the most prevalent diabetes type. Among the

6030 cases in youth aged 10 to 19 years, the highest prevalence of T2DM was observed among Native Americans (1.74/1000), followed by African-Americans (1.05/1000), Asian/Pacific Islanders (0.54/1000), Hispanics (0.48/1000), and non-Hispanic whites (0.19/1000). In this age group, T2DM accounted for about 6% of diabetes diagnosed in non-Hispanic whites, 22% in Hispanics, 33% in African-Americans, 40% in Asian/Pacific Islanders, and 76% in Native American youth.

A screening program for glycosuria was carried out in 3 million 6- to 18-year-old Taiwanese students (16), with fasting blood glucose measured if glycosuria persisted. The prevalence of undiagnosed diabetes was 9 and 15 per 100,000 boys and girls, respectively. A three-year follow-up of those with diabetes found that 54% still carried a diagnosis of T2DM, 10% T1DM, 9% secondary diabetes, 20% nondiabetic, and 8% with no definite diagnosis, clearly implicating T2DM as the leading cause of childhood diabetes in Taiwan. Another large study evaluated over 70,000 17-year-old Israeli military conscripts (17). T2DM (defined as diagnostic fasting, two hour or random blood glucose, but not requiring insulin treatment) was found in 0.036% of males, and 0.01% of females. A screening study of 1647 Turkish adolescents identified 1.96% with IFG, but no cases of T2DM (18). Data from a Saudi Arabian screening study (19) found T2DM in 0.12% and IGT in 0.25% of children below 14 years. In those aged 14 to 29 years, the prevalence of T2DM was 0.79%, while IGT was 0.21%. Of note, the pediatric Saudi data, consistent with adult data from this population, indicate a very high prevalence of T2DM in the Middle-East, rivaled only by Asian/Pacific Islanders, and indigenous peoples from North America and Australasia (20).

INCIDENCE

Population-Based Studies

SEARCH for Diabetes in Youth is the first population-based U.S. study to provide comprehensive estimates of T2DM incidence in youth according to race and ethnicity. In 2002 and 2003, a total of 2435 youth with newly diagnosed diabetes were ascertained covering over 10 million person-years (21). Among children aged < 10 years, most had T1DM, regardless of race and ethnicity, with only 19 children having T2DM. Overall, T2DM was relatively infrequent, except among 10- to 14-year-old and 15- to 19-year-old minority groups. The rates of T2DM were the highest among Native Americans (25.3/100,000 per year and 49.4/100,000 per year for ages 10 to 14 and 15 to 19 years, respectively), followed by African-Americans (22.3 and 19.4), Asian/Pacific Islanders (11.8 and 22.7), and Hispanic youth (8.9 and 17.0), and were low (3.0 and 5.6) among non-Hispanic whites. Consistent with previous reports (4,22), SEARCH demonstrates that T2DM contributes considerably to the overall diabetes incidence among minority youth age ≥ 10 years, and rates are ~60% higher in females than in males. SEARCH estimates that the annual number of newly diagnosed youth with T2DM in the United States is approximately 3700.

A large survey of pediatric T2DM has been undertaken in Japan, where urine dipstick screening programs for renal disease have been used to screen for DM by follow-up of those with glycosuria. Significant methodological limitations exist, as glycosuria is an insensitive screening tool for diabetes. In the most recent Japanese report, involving almost 9 million children screened between 1974 and 2002 (23), the overall annual incidence of T2DM was 2.63/100,00 per year. The annual incidence after 1981 was significantly higher than that before 1980 (2.75 vs. 1.73/100,000 per year, $p < 0.0001$). However, there were no further changes in the incidence of T2DM from 1981 to 2002. The annual incidence was significantly higher for junior high school versus primary school students (6.43 vs. 0.78/100,00 per year, $p < 0.0001$). Over 80% of those with T2DM were obese, and almost 60% had a positive family history of diabetes in first or second degree relatives. Similarly, Kitagawa et al. (3) screened Tokyo schoolchildren for glycosuria yearly from 1974 to 1981. Using glucose—and tolbutamide—tolerance tests in combination with other data, they estimated that the yearly incidence of T2DM among elementary and junior high school students was 3.2/100,000 per year. In an extension of this study through 1995, T2DM incidence reportedly increased from 1991 to 1995, particularly among older children, to 2/100,000 per year for elementary and 13.9/100,000 per year for junior high school students (24).

Trends in incidence rates over time need to be interpreted cautiously for several reasons. First, recent recognition that insulin requirement and diabetic ketoacidosis are not exclusive to T1DM may result in classification of T2DM in a patient who previously would have been labeled as having T1DM. Second, with increasing awareness of and surveillance for T2DM, undiagnosed cases of T2DM are more likely to be uncovered at earlier ages than in the past. The effect of these factors cannot always be determined, but is likely to contribute to the reported rises in incidence.

Clinic-Based Studies

Many publications rely on data collected from diabetes clinics. A strength of such studies is that pediatrician assignment of DM type is likely to be more accurate (though not always uniform) than in population-based studies. However, a particular clinic population may not accurately represent the general population.

Several clinic-based studies report an increased incidence of T2DM. For example, T2DM incidence rates rose by 9% per year from 1985 to 1994, on the basis of medical records of 735 African-American and Latino children with insulin-treated diabetes in Chicago (25). The incidence was higher in African-Americans than in Latinos (15.2 vs. 10.7/100,000 per year), with a female predominance. Presentation of T2DM was typically around puberty. Similarly, among 1027 consecutive patients attending a Cincinnati diabetes clinic (26), T2DM incidence increased by 10-fold, from 0.7/100,000 per year in 1982 to 7.2/100,00 per year in 1994. Onset was typically around puberty, the majority were African-Americans, and the female:male ratio was 1.7:1. Among 569 children and adolescents presenting to a Florida diabetes clinic between 1994 and 1998 (27), the proportion of new cases with T2DM rose from 9.4% to 20%. Significant predictors of T2DM were Hispanic or African-American race or ethnicity and female gender. In Arkansas, new-onset non-Type 1 DM increased fivefold in youth aged 8 to 21 years between 1990 and 1995 (22), and predictors included African-American race, female gender, and older age at diagnosis. An analysis of the U.S. Indian Health Service outpatient database revealed a 68% increase in the prevalence of diabetes between 1990 and 1998 among adolescents aged 15 to 19, from 3.2 per 1000 to 5.4 per 1000 (28). During this period, the rate for those <15 years remained stable and relatively low at 1.2 per 1000.

Similarly, a study in Thailand (29) reported a rise in the proportion with T2DM referred to a diabetes clinic from 5% to 17% during 1997 to 1999. A Hungarian study (30) from 1989 to 2001 also reported rising incidence rates over time, with 57% of T2DM cases and 77% of IGT cases being diagnosed in the last six years of the study (30). Finally, a study of 0- to 16-year-olds from United Kingdom identified 67 cases of T2DM (defined as DM with elevated insulin or C-peptide levels and/or the absence of DM-associated antibodies) during the period 2004–2005 (31). The U.K. T2DM incidence was 0.53/100,000 per year and was higher in blacks (3.9/100,000 per year) and South Asians (1.25/100,000 per year) compared with whites (0.35/100,000 per year). The 2004–2005 incidence was 2.5 times higher than the 2003 U.K. prevalence data. However, the overall incidence of T2DM in this study compared with the U.K. incidence of T1DM (15–20/100,000 per year) (32) indicates that T2DM is still relatively infrequent in the United Kingdom.

A detailed study from the only pediatric diabetes clinic serving approximately two million Australians, documented a rise in the incidence of T2DM among youth aged 0 to 17 years (33). Between 1990 and 2002, average annual rises in the incidence of pediatric T2DM were 23% in the indigenous and 31% in the nonindigenous population. By study completion, the estimated annual incidences were approximately 16/100,000 per year in the indigenous population and 1/100,000 per year in the nonindigenous population. Similarly, in an analysis of 14- to 20-year-olds attending a New Zealand diabetes clinic, the prevalence of T2DM rose from 1.8% in 1996 to 11.0% in 2002 (34). T2DM rose from 12.5% of new diabetes cases in 1997 to 1999 to 35.7% in 2000–2001. In contrast to other studies, only 50% with T2DM were female, perhaps reflecting the fact that unlike other studies, most of the subjects developed diabetes after puberty (mean age of onset being 15 years). Indeed, Taiwanese data reveal that the female predominance decreases with increasing age, and within the 16- to 18-year-old group, the incidence of diabetes was equal for males and females (16).

While much evidence supports an increasing incidence and prevalence of T2DM among youth, it is possible that this rise is predominantly a feature of high-risk ethnic groups. Well-designed studies of youth in Germany, Austria, France, and the United Kingdom (35–37), all indicate that T2DM remains a rarity in these populations, accounting for only 1–2% of all diabetes cases. A survey of all children (aged 0–16 years) with diabetes from 177 U.K. pediatric diabetes centers found that <1% of all cases were due to T2DM, with a predominance of females and South Asians (36). A single center in France (38) reported that only 2% of 382 children (aged 1–16 years) with diabetes had T2DM. Using an Austrian national register, Rami et al. (39) found that T2DM represented only 1.5% of all newly diagnosed cases of diabetes under the age of 15 years from 1999 to 2001, giving an incidence of 0.25/100,000 per year. In contrast, while the U.S. SEARCH data support the notion that T2DM in youth is predominantly occurring in high-risk ethnic groups, T2DM accounts for 14.9% of all diabetes cases among NHW adolescents aged 10 years and older. Although differences in obesity rates between U.S. and European youth are likely contributors, the full explanation for these discrepancies remains uncertain.

EPIDEMIOLOGY OF RISK FACTORS FOR T2DM IN YOUTH

The literature regarding risk factors of T2DM in children and adolescents is less robust than in adults. However, available data confirm similar risk factors in youth and adults. Some of the more important factors are discussed below.

Race and Ethnicity
Race/ethnicity is recognized as an important risk factor in the development of T2DM in adults. The influence of race and ethnicity appears to be even stronger for

youth-onset T2DM. Indeed, in multiple studies, the only pediatric cases of T2DM are of non-European backgrounds. Higher prevalences have been seen in Asians, Hispanics, indigenous peoples (U.S.A., Canada, Australia), and African-Americans, with the highest rates in the world being observed in Pima Indians (22,28,40).

Obesity, Diet, and Physical Activity

The rise in T2DM rates mirrors growth in urbanization and economic development, and the associated increase in overweight and obesity. The risk of T2DM increases with increasing weight (41–43), weight gain (44,45), body mass index (BMI) (46–48), waist-to-hip ratio (49,50), and central fat deposition (51,52). The temporal trends in the prevalence of overweight and obesity in the United States (53,54) through the year 2000 have paralleled steady increases in adult T2DM prevalence (55,56). As in adults, there is a strong relationship between obesity and the prevalence of T2DM in youth (32). Data reported in 2005 from a single U.S. school district (57) indicates that obese children are over twofold more likely to have diabetes than normal weight children. Japanese studies demonstrate a rise in pediatric T2DM incidence, paralleling rises in obesity from 1975 to 1995 (24). A Turkish study of 196 obese 7 to 18 year olds, found that 35 (18%) had IGT and six (3%) had T2DM (58). Currently 85% of children with T2DM are overweight or obese at diagnosis (59), and mean BMI in children with T2DM has been reported to be as high as 35 to 38 kg/m^2 (22,26). A lifestyle predisposing to obesity also seems to characterize families of adolescents with T2DM (60).

The prevalence of obesity in youth is increasing globally. For example, among Japanese children, obesity increased from 5% to 8% from 1976 to 1992 (61). Trend analyses indicate increased adiposity among U.S. youth since 1960 (62–64), with an increase of at least 50% since 1976 (65). The U.S. National Longitudinal Survey of Youth, a prospective cohort study, found that the prevalence of overweight increased annually from 1986 to 1998 by 3.2% in non-Hispanic white youth, by 5.8% in African-Americans, and by 4.3% in Hispanics. Thus by 1998, 21.5% of African-Americans, 21.8% of Hispanics, and 12.3% of non-Hispanic white youth were overweight (66). During 1999–2000, 15% of 6- to 19-year olds were overweight compared with 11% in 1994–1998, with the greatest increases in African-American and Mexican American adolescents (67). In 2003–2004, 17.1% of U.S. children and adolescents were overweight (68). In addition, the heaviest children are much heavier than previously, with the greatest increases taking place in the top decile (69). In Australia, the prevalence of obesity in youth aged 7 to 15 years increased two- to fourfold from 1985 to 1997 (70).

The problem of obesity also extends to developing nations, particularly in relatively affluent urban areas. In India, a recent study reported that 18% of 13- to 18-year-olds were overweight (71), with the prevalence correlating positively with age and socioeconomic status and negatively with physical activity. Obesity is also increasingly observed in indigenous populations, such as the Ojibwa-Cree community in Canada, where 48–51% of children aged 4 to 19 years are overweight (>90%) (72). Mean weight (adjusted for age, sex, and height) of all Pima Indian boys and girls has also increased over time ($p < 0.0001$), especially among the heavier children (4). Changes in traditional lifestyles among indigenous communities such as a reduction in hunting and gathering and resulting adoption of a more sedentary life and westernized diet are thought to contribute to the rising obesity levels (63).

Obesity is likely linked to recent changes in children's diets (73,74). Fast food and high-fat and/or high-sugar convenience item consumption has increased, while time for family meals has decreased in many societies. Japanese data show that rises in T2DM and obesity parallel increases in fat and animal protein intake (75). Dietary changes are not confined only to the home environment. A survey of Californian public schools found that 85% sold fast food, which in turn accounted for 70% of all food sales (76). Increases in snacking (with increased nutrient density of snacks, including soft drinks) were observed in nationally representative data from over 20,000 U.S. 2- to 18-year-olds during 1973–1994 (77,78). Similar to patterns among adults, overall percent calories from total and saturated fat has decreased among adolescents over the last two decades but remains above national recommendations (78,79).

While diet composition may contribute to obesity, it is likely that the most important aspect in the development of insulin resistance (IR) and T2DM in youth is excess caloric intake relative to caloric expenditure. In youth, physical inactivity has been identified as an important predictor of excess weight gain (80). Concurrent with increases in overweight and obesity, physical activity has decreased among children and adolescents (81). Currently, only a small percentage of U.S. youth report regular strenuous physical activity more than three times per week (82). A national survey of U.S. adolescents demonstrated large ethnic and gender differences in reported inactivity (102), with African-American and Asian/Pacific Islander girls being the least active (83) and non-Hispanic whites of either gender being the most active (84). During middle and high school years, marked declines in physical activity have been observed, particularly among girls, regardless of race (84–86), with 56% of African-American and 31% of non-Hispanic white girls aged 16 to 17 years having no habitual leisure-time physical activity (86). One reason for the decline in physical activity may be the reduction of physical education in schools, with participation rates down from 41.6% in 1991 to 24.5% in 1995 (87). In the developed world, increasing use of computers and television also markedly decrease children's activity level (74).

While many children get little to no physical activity, even those who meet current recommended activity guidelines may still not be exercising sufficiently. A recent detailed study of 1732 children of 9 and 15 years related a composite metabolic score (including IR, lipids, blood pressure, obesity, and fitness) to physical activity assessed objectively by accelerometry (88). The risk of having an elevated metabolic score only began to fall when more than 60 min/day of moderate activity was accumulated, suggesting that the current targets of 30 min/day may be inadequate.

Insulin Resistance

T2DM in youth typically occurs during puberty and is thought to coincide with a physiologic rise (as high as 50%) in IR (2,89,90). Healthy adolescents are able to compensate for the peripubertal rise in IR with an increase in insulin secretion. However, some adolescents' pancreatic β cells cannot overcome this rise in IR, and therefore a relative insulin deficiency develops, eventually leading to T2DM (58,91). In addition, as in adults, both overall obesity (92–94) and central obesity (95,96) have been associated with hyperinsulinemia and dyslipidemia among children and adolescents. In obese adolescents, the additive effects of obesity-related and pubertal IR create additional stress on the pancreas, and may tip the balance over to T2DM (97). Since puberty occurs on average a year earlier in females than males, pubertal IR also begins earlier in females (98). This may partly explain the female predominance in adolescent T2DM, and the earlier age of onset in females (32).

Even when controlling for body weight, there appear to be ethnic differences in insulin sensitivity, with African-American youth having more hyperinsulinemia and IR than those of European ancestry (94,99). Arslanian et al. suggested an explanation for these differences. Using hyperinsulinemic-euglycemic clamps, they found that African-American youth have both lower insulin clearance and higher insulin secretion when compared with youth of European ancestry (100). Using frequently sampled intravenous glucose tolerance tests, other authors demonstrated that both African-American and Hispanic children have more IR than those of European ancestry (101,102).

In adults, physical inactivity is associated with reduced insulin sensitivity, independent of obesity (103), and with an approximately 1.3- to 2-fold increased risk for T2DM among both men (104) and women (105,106). Among youth, physical inactivity has been associated with obesity (81,107) and increased insulin levels, at least among males (108). IR may be improved by simple means such as weight loss (109) or increasing activity levels (110). This improvement has been demonstrated in obese children (111) and in nondiabetic, normal weight children (112), where the more active children had lower fasting insulin and greater insulin sensitivity.

Family History

Many studies show a strong family history among affected youth, with 45–80% having at least one parent with DM and 74–100% having a first- or second-degree relative with T2DM (32,58,113). Children with T2DM are also more likely to have a family history of cardiovascular disease (114). The Bogalusa Heart Study (115) found that children of individuals with T2DM were more likely to be obese and have higher blood pressures, fasting insulin, glucose, and triglycerides. In the Pima Indians, the cumulative incidence of T2DM is highest in offspring if both parents had DM (116). Therefore, genetic factors are likely to play an important role in the risk for T2DM in youth. However, family history does not always imply a genetic cause, as factors such as similar environmental influences within families and the effects of obesity or DM during pregnancy on the offspring also demand consideration.

Psychosocial Factors

Many youth with T2DM are obese, and obesity may play a role in the development of depression (117–119). In addition, negative body image and weight concerns have been associated with subsequent depression in girls in several studies (120,121). Adults with diabetes have twice the odds of depression compared with nondiabetic controls (122). The association between depression and T2DM may be bidirectional, that is, prior history of depression may increase the risk of diabetes onset, and diabetes may increase the risk of subsequent depression (123,124). However, depression has been associated prospectively with IR in nondiabetic subjects (125) and, therefore, it may contribute to the development of T2DM. A link between neurotransmitter and neuroendocrine changes that occur in both depression and diabetes has been suggested (126), and others have pointed to abnormal functioning of the hypothalamic-pituitary axis in both disorders (124).

In the SEARCH study, 2672 youth (aged 10–21 years) who had diabetes for a mean duration of five years had their mood measured using the Center for Epidemiologic Studies Depression Scale (CES-D) (127). As many as 14% had mildly depressed mood (CES-D scores between 16 and 23) while 8.6% had moderately or severely depressed mood (CES-D scores ≥ 24). Females had a higher mean CES-D score than males. After adjusting for demographic factors and duration of diabetes, the prevalence of depressed mood was higher among males with T2DM than those with T1DM and higher among females with comorbidities than those without comorbidities. Higher mean HbA1c and frequency of emergency room visits were associated with depressed mood.

Family functioning has also been reported as an important moderator of the diabetes-depression association in children (128), although data are limited to studies in T1DM. Conflict in the home has been related to poorer adherence to the medical regimen, poorer metabolic control, and diabetic ketoacidosis (129–132). Parental socioeconomic status (SES) is associated inversely with childhood obesity among whites, but higher SES does not seem to protect African-American and Hispanic children against obesity (133). However, neighborhood deprivation has been associated with higher prevalence of T2DM and other cardiovascular disease (CVD) risk factors, independent of individual SES in multiple racial/ethnic groups (134).

RISK FACTORS OPERATING EARLY IN LIFE

Several risk factors for T2DM operating during the fetal or neonatal period have been described. They all appear to act through increasing the risk of obesity at early ages. There is conclusive evidence that the likelihood of persistence of adolescent obesity into adulthood increases with earlier obesity onset (135).

Birth Weight

The intrauterine environment is increasingly recognized as an important contributor to diabetes both in childhood and in adult life. Being either small for gestational age (SGA) or large for gestational age (LGA) was associated with the development of T2DM later in life (136–142). Both genetic and environmental factors are likely to be involved in mediating these relationships. The hypothesis linking low birth weight to T2DM has been termed the thrifty phenotype (143), and suggests that the fetal response to intrauterine malnutrition leads to IR and impaired β-cell development, increasing the risk of DM later in life. Alternatively, the link may lie in the effect of the genes causing both low birth weight and later abnormalities of insulin secretion or sensitivity (144,145). Studies of monozygotic and dizygotic twins have shown that the lower birth weight twin has a greater risk of DM in adulthood, suggesting the importance of environmental and intrauterine factors (146,147).

In four-year-old Asian Indian children, birth weight was negatively associated with 30-minute postload glucose (148). Children born SGA were also more likely to develop later hypertension and dyslipidemia. In comparison to non-Hispanic white babies, Asian Indian babies weigh less (102), have more subcutaneous fat (149), and higher cord insulin and leptin levels (150). The propensity to fat deposition extends to Asian Indian children born in the United Kingdom, who appear to have a greater tendency to central adiposity compared with their Caucasian counterparts (151). A study examining 152 South African 7-year-olds found an inverse correlation between birth weight and insulin secretion following an oral glucose tolerance test (152). In a British study of 7-year-old subjects, ponderal index at birth was inversely related to 30-minute postload glucose concentrations (153). Data in healthy Pima Indian children and young adults show that birth weight was inversely associated with measures of IR, when adjusted for current weight and height (137). Similarly, in a study of young healthy Danes, the insulin sensitivity index (estimated from the frequently sampled intravenous glucose tolerance test) was inversely correlated with birth weight, but no association between birth weight and β-cell function (estimated from the response to intravenous glucose) was noted (154). In case-control studies including French subjects selected from a population-based registry of births (155,156), individuals born SGA demonstrated hyperinsulinemia and IR as early as the age of 20 years when compared with controls born with normal size. In a recent German study, lower birth weight was associated with higher HbA1c among healthy nondiabetic youth (157,158).

Low birth weight followed by rapid catch-up growth in childhood appears to carry a particularly high risk of subsequent T2DM, in both animal models (136) and human observational studies (159–161). A recent prospective, population based survey from India found that subjects with IGT or T2DM as adults tended to have low birth weights but accelerated increases in BMI from 2 to 12 years of age (162). The British prospective Avon Longitudinal Study of Parents and Children (ALSPAC) found that infants who showed catch-up growth during the first two years of life were smaller and thinner at birth and had more maternal indicators of intrauterine growth restraint (smoking), but were larger and fatter than other children at five years.

The association between low birth weight and T2DM could also result from pleiotropic effects of genes influencing both fetal growth and susceptibility to diabetes (163). Fetuses that carry the heterozygous mutation in the glucokinase gene responsible maturity onset diabetes of youth (MODY2) are also approximately half a kilogram lighter at birth than their unaffected sibs (144). These individuals are of low birth weight only when they inherit the mutation from their father. A similar association between paternal T2DM, low birth weight, and T2DM in offspring was reported in Pima Indians (164). Children born to a father with T2DM weighed an average of 186 g less than children from nondiabetic parents, unrelated to birth order, father's height, or social class. No significant differences were seen in birth weight of offspring between diabetic and nondiabetic mothers. Using family-based association methods in parent-offspring trios with T2DM, Huxtable et al. (165) reported a relationship between the insulin gene and T2DM that was mediated exclusively through paternally transmitted class III variable number tandem repeat (VNTR) alleles. These data support the thrifty genotype hypothesis and, moreover, implicate imprinting of genes in the pathogenesis of T2DM.

Exposure to Maternal Diabetes In Utero

Several reports have convincingly shown that exposure to maternal DM in utero is a significant risk factor for obesity, IGT, and T2DM in youth (166). The offspring of women with DM during pregnancy are more obese during childhood and adolescence, as demonstrated by the longitudinal follow-up of offspring of diabetic Pima Indian women (167–170). The offspring of diabetic women were large at birth, and, at every age before age 20 years, they were heavier for height than were the offspring of prediabetic or nondiabetic women. Consequently, at every age before 20 years, offspring of Pima Indian diabetic women had more T2DM than those of prediabetic and nondiabetic women (171). The higher prevalence of T2DM was only partially mediated by the earlier development of obesity in these offspring (172). Similarly, Silverman et al. (173) followed a cohort of offspring of diabetic mothers and found that, although macrosomia disappears after the first year of life, by age eight years, almost half of the offspring have a weight >90th percentile. At 12.3 years of age, these offspring of diabetic mothers had a significantly higher prevalence of IGT than an age- and sex-matched control group (19.3% vs. 2.5%) and two offspring had already developed T2DM. A direct correlation was found between amniotic fluid insulin concentration at weeks 32 to 34 of pregnancy and obesity at ages six and eight years, suggesting a possible mechanism of this excessive weight gain (174).

While intrauterine exposure is often difficult to separate from genetic factors, there is evidence suggesting that obesity and T2DM in offspring of diabetic mothers is not solely due to genetics. To determine the role of exposure to the diabetic intrauterine environment while controlling for genetic susceptibility, the prevalence of T2DM was compared in Pima Indian siblings born before and after their mother developed DM (175). BMI was significantly higher ($+2.6 \text{ kg/m}^2$) in the 62 siblings born after their mothers were diagnosed with T2DM (exposed to the diabetic intrauterine environment) than in the 121 siblings born before. Similarly, within the same Pima Indian family, siblings born after mother's diagnosis of DM had over a threefold higher risk of developing diabetes at an early age than siblings born before the diagnosis of diabetes in the mother (odds ratio, OR = 3.0, $p < 0.01$). Since these differences were not seen in the families of diabetic fathers, it is unlikely that these findings are due to cohort or birth order effects. Among Pima Indian youth, exposure to maternal diabetes and obesity in pregnancy could account for most of the dramatic increase in T2DM prevalence over the last 30 years (4). The extent to which exposure to maternal diabetes and obesity in utero account for the development of T2DM in other populations, however, is unknown.

The mechanisms by which exposure to DM in utero increase the risk of IGT and T2DM are also uncertain. Both fetal IR (and compensatory hyperinsulinemia) (176), and impaired insulin secretion (177–179) have been proposed. Studies in rats injected with streptozotocin or infused with glucose demonstrate that maternal hyperglycemia during gestation leads to decreased insulin sensitivity and secretion in the adult offspring, resulting in IGT (180–182). Among 104 Pima Indian adults with normal glucose tolerance, the acute insulin response was approximately 40% lower in individuals whose mothers had diabetes during pregnancy than in those whose mothers developed diabetes at an early age but after the birth of the subject (177).

Breastfeeding

In population-based studies, breastfeeding is protective against later development of obesity and T2DM (183–186). Even as infants, bottle-fed babies have significantly higher plasma insulin levels and a prolonged insulin response to glucose (187). A longer duration of exclusive breastfeeding also appears highly protective in a dose-dependent manner against overweight and obesity in children of various age groups (188–190). Both behavioral and metabolic explanations for the apparent benefit of breastfeeding have been proposed. Breast-milk composition changes during each feeding, which may be an important satiety signal (191). In contrast, in bottle-fed infants, consumption is regulated mainly via volume, which could result in overfeeding.

In Pima Indians, exclusive breastfeeding for the first two months of life protects against the development of T2DM in adolescence and young adulthood (OR = 0.64, 95% CI = 0.4–0.9) (192,193). Recently, the SEARCH case-control study reported similar results in a group of youth of diverse racial and ethnic backgrounds (194). Prevalence (%) of breast feeding (any duration) was lower among youth with T2DM than among controls (19.5 vs. 27.1 for African-Americans; 50.0 vs. 83.8 for Hispanics; 39.1 vs. 77.6 for non-Hispanic whites, respectively). The overall crude OR for the association of breast feeding and T2DM was 0.26 (95% CI = 0.15–0.46). When current BMI z-score was added to the model, the OR was attenuated (OR = 0.44; 95% CI = 0.14, 1.38), suggesting possible mediation through childhood weight status. These data strongly suggest that breast feeding may be protective against development of T2DM in youth regardless of race and ethnicity, an effect that may be mediated in part by attained weight status in childhood.

CONCLUSIONS

While still developing, emerging evidence regarding the epidemiology of T2DM in youth is consistent with the increasing prevalence and incidence of T2DM in adults, and with the rapidly increasing prevalence of obesity in all age groups. Overall, T2DM is still a relatively infrequent condition in youth; however, particularly high rates and increasing trends are observed among minority racial and ethnic groups, especially indigenous populations experiencing rapid transitions to westernized lifestyles. In addition to accurately describing these trends, several other challenges lay ahead. These include improving the ability to distinguish T2DM from T1DM in adolescents, choosing the appropriate therapies to prevent morbidity and mortality, and implementing interventions that will succeed in making the necessary lifestyle changes in obese adolescents with T2DM. The problem is that, at the population level, obesity and T2DM rates are quite resistant to efforts aimed at modification of an individual's lifestyle. As a WHO World Health Report noted "...obesity is a side-effect of our and our ancestors' continuous struggle to reach a state of complete food security ... and to reduce hard physical labor" (195). Therefore, effective strategies will have to trade off how much of this achievement such populations are willing to give up in return for better health.

REFERENCES

1. American Diabetes Association: report of the expert committee on the diagnosis and classification of diabetes mellitus. Diabetes Care 1997; 20:1183–1197.
2. Dabelea D, Pettitt DJ, Jones KL, et al. Type 2 diabetes mellitus in minority children and adolescents. An emerging problem. Endocrinol Metab Clin North Am 1999; 28:709–729.
3. Kitagawa T, Mano T, Fujita H. The epidemiology of childhood diabetes mellitus in Tokyo metropolitan area. Tohoku J exp Med 1983; 141:171–179.
4. Dabelea D, Hanson RL, Bennett PH, et al. Increasing prevalence of Type II diabetes in American Indian children. Diabetologia 1998; 41:904–910.
5. Fagot-Campagna A, Saaddine JB, Flegal KM, et al. Diabetes, impaired fasting glucose, and elevated HbA1c in U.S. adolescents: the Third National Health and Nutrition Examination Survey. Diabetes Care 2001; 24:834–837.
6. Duncan GE. Prevalence of diabetes and impaired fasting glucose levels among US adolescents: National Health and Nutrition Examination Survey, 1999–2002. Arch Pediatr Adolesc Med 2006; 160:523–528.
7. Lee JM, Herman WH, McPheeters ML, et al. An epidemiologic profile of children with diabetes in the U.S. Diabetes Care 2006; 29:420–421.

8. Hale DE, Danney MM, Caballero M, et al. Prevalence of type 2 diabetes mellitus in urban, Mexican American 4th graders. Diabetes 2002; 51(suppl 2):A25.

9. Baranowski T, Cooper DM, Harrell J, et al. Presence of diabetes risk factors in a large U.S. eighth-grade cohort. Diabetes Care 2006; 29:212–217.

10. Freedman DS, Serdula MK, Percy CA, et al. Obesity, levels of lipids and glucose, and smoking among Navajo adolescents. J Nutr 1997; 127:2120S.

11. Dean H. Incidence and prevalence of type 2 diabetes in youth in Manitoba, Canada. Diabetes 1999; 48:168.

12. Dean HJ, Young TK, Flett B, et al. Screening for type-2 diabetes in aboriginal children in northern Canada. Lancet 1998; 352:1523–1524.

13. Harris SB, Caulfield LE, Sugamori ME, et al. The epidemiology of diabetes in pregnant Native Canadians. A risk profile. Diabetes Care 1997; 20:1422–1425.

14. Acton KJ, Burrows NR, Moore K, et al. Trends in diabetes prevalence among American Indian and Alaska native children, adolescents, and young adults. Am J Public Health 2002; 92:1485–1490.

15. The SEARCH for Diabetes in Youth Study Group. The burden of diabetes among U.S. youth: prevalence estimates from the SEARCH for Diabetes in Youth Study. Pediatrics 2006; 118:1510–1518.

16. Wei JN, Sung FC, Lin CC, et al. National surveillance for type 2 diabetes mellitus in Taiwanese children. JAMA 2003; 290:1345–1350.

17. Bar Dayan Y, Elishkevits K, Grotto I, et al. The prevalence of obesity and associated morbidity among 17-year-old Israeli conscripts. Public Health 2005; 119:385–389.

18. Uckun-Kitapci A, Tezic T, Firat S, et al. Obesity and type 2 diabetes mellitus a population-based study of adolescents. J Pediatr Endocrinol Metab 2004; 17:1633–1640.

19. el-Hazmi MA, Warsy AS. Prevalence of overweight and obesity in diabetic and non-diabetic Saudis. East Mediterr Health J 2000; 6:276–282.

20. Sicree R, Shaw J, Zimmet P. The Global Burden of Diabetes. In: Gan D, ed. Diabetes Atlas. 2nd ed. Brussels: International Diabetes Federation, 2003:15–71.

21. Dabelea D, Bell RA, D'Agostino RB, et al. Incidence of diabetes in youth in the United States. Writing Group for the SEARCH for Diabetes in Youth Study Group. JAMA 2007; 297:2716–2724.

22. Scott CR, Smith JM, Cradock MM, et al. Characteristics of youth-onset noninsulin-dependent diabetes mellitus and insulin-dependent diabetes mellitus at diagnosis. Pediatrics 1997; 100:84–91.

23. Urakami T, Kubota S, Nitadori Y, et al. Annual incidence and clinical characteristics of type 2 diabetes in children as detected by urine glucose screening in the Tokyo metropolitan area. Diabetes Care 2005; 28:1876–1881.

24. Kitagawa T, Owada M, Urakami T, et al. Increased incidence of non-insulin dependent diabetes mellitus among Japanese schoolchildren correlates with an increased intake of animal protein and fat. Clin Pediatr (Phila) 1998; 37:111–115.

25. Lipton R, Keenan H, Onyemere KU, et al. Incidence and onset features of diabetes in African-American and Latino children in Chicago, 1985–1994. Diabetes Metab Res Rev 2002; 18:135–142.

26. Pinhas-Hamiel O, Dolan LM, Daniels SR, et al. Increased incidence of non-insulin-dependent diabetes mellitus among adolescents. J Pediatr 1996; 128, 608–615.

27. Macaluso CJ, Bauer UE, Deeb LC, et al. Type 2 diabetes mellitus among Florida children and adolescents, 1994 through 1998. Public Health Rep 2002; 117:373–379.

28. Acton K, Rios Burrows N, Moore K, et al. Trends in diabetes prevalence among American Indian and Alaska Native children, adolescents and young adults. Am J Public Health 2002; 92:1485–1490.

29. Likitmaskul S, Kiattisathavee P, Chaichanwatanakul K, et al. Increasing prevalence of type 2 diabetes mellitus in Thai children and adolescents associated with increasing prevalence of obesity. J Pediatr Endocrinol Metab 2003; 16:71–77.

30. Korner AM, Madacsy L. Rising tide of type 2 diabetes mellitus and impaired glucose tolerance among Hungarian children and adolescents. Diabetol Hung 2002; 10(suppl 2): 22–27.

31. Haines L, Wan KC, Lynn R, et al. Rising incidence of type 2 diabetes in children in the U.K. Diabetes Care 2007; 30:1097–1101.

32. EURODIAB ACE Study Group. Variation and trends in incidence of childhood diabetes in Europe. Lancet 2000; 355:873–876.
33. McMahon SK, Haynes A, Ratnam N, et al. Increase in type 2 diabetes in children and adolescents in Western Australia. Med J Aust 2004; 180:459–461.
34. Hotu S, Carter B, Watson PD, et al. Increasing prevalence of type 2 diabetes in adolescents. J Paediatr Child Health 2004; 40:201–204.
35. Schober E, Holl RW, Grabert M, et al. Diabetes mellitus type 2 in childhood and adolescence in Germany and parts of Austria. Eur J Pediatr 2005; 164:705–707.
36. Ortega-Rodriguez E, Levy-Marchal C, Tubiana N, et al. Emergence of type 2 diabetes in a hospital based cohort of children with diabetes mellitus. Diabetes Metab 2001; 27:574–578.
37. Feltbower RG, McKinney PA, Campbell FM, et al. Type 2 and other forms of diabetes in 0-30 year olds: a hospital based study in Leeds, UK. Arch Dis Child 2003; 88:676–679.
38. Ehtisham S, Hattersley AT, Dunger DB, et al. First UK survey of paediatric type 2 diabetes and MODY. Arch Dis Child 2004; 89:526–529.
39. Rami B, Schober E, Nachbauer E, et al. Type 2 diabetes mellitus is rare but not absent in children under 15 years of age in Austria. Eur J Pediatr 2003; 162:850–852.
40. Fagot-Campagna A, Pettitt DJ, Engelgau MM, et al. Type 2 diabetes among North American children and adolescents: an epidemiologic review and a public health perspective. J Pediatr 2000; 136:664–672.
41. Ford ES, Williamson DF, Liu SM. Weight change and diabetes incidence - findings from a national cohort of US adults. Am J Epidemiol 1997; 146:214–222.
42. Godsland IF, Walton C, Crook D, et al. Insulin resistance—modelling studies. Eur J Epidemiol 1992; 8(suppl 1):136–138.
43. Chan JM, Rimm EB, Colditz GA, et al. Obesity, fat distribution, and weight gain as risk factors for clinical diabetes in men. Diabetes Care 1994; 17:961–969.
44. Colditz GA, Willett WC, Rotnitzky A, et al. Weight gain as a risk factor for clinical diabetes mellitus in women. Ann Intern Med 1995; 122:481–486.
45. Colditz GA, Willett WC, Stampfer MJ, et al. Patterns of weight change and their relation to diet in a cohort of healthy women. Am J Clin Nutr 1990; 51:1100–1105.
46. Ford ES, Williamson DF, Liu SM. Weight change and diabetes incidence - findings from a national cohort of US adults. Am J Epidemiol 1997; 146:214–222.
47. Knowler WC, Pettitt DJ, Saad MF, et al. Diabetes mellitus in the Pima Indians: incidence, risk factors and pathogenesis. Diabetes Metab Rev 1990; 6:1–27.
48. Burchfiel CM, Curb JD, Rodriguez BL, et al. Incidence and predictors of diabetes in Japanese-American men. The Honolulu heart program. Ann Epidemiol 1995; 5:33–43.
49. Ohlson LO, Larsson B, Svardsudd K, et al. The influence of body fat distribution on the incidence of diabetes mellitus: 13.5 years of follow-up of the participants in the study of men born in 1913. Diabetes 1985; 34:1055–1058.
50. Cassano PA, Rosner B, Vokonas PS, et al. Obesity and body fat distribution in relation to the incidence of non-insulin-dependent diabetes mellitus: a prospective cohort study of men in the Normative Aging Study. Am J Epidemiol 1992; 136:1474–1486.
51. Haffner SM, Mitchell BD, Hazuda HP, et al. Greater influence of central distribution of adipose tissue on incidence of non-insulin-dependent diabetes in women than men. Am J Clin Nutr 1991; 53:1312–1317.
52. Feskens EJ, Kromhout D. Effects of body fat and its development over a ten-year period on glucose tolerance in euglycaemic men: the Zutphen Study. Int J Epidemiol 1989; 18:368–373.
53. Kuczmarski RJ, Flegal KM, Campbell SM, et al. Increasing prevalence of overweight among U.S. adults. JAMA 1994; 272:205–211.
54. NIH/NHLBI. Clinical Guidelines on the Identification, Evaluation and Treatment of Overweight and Obesity in Adults. Bethesda, MD: Author, 1998.
55. Harris MI, Flegal KM, Cowie CC, et al. Prevalence of diabetes, impaired fasting glucose, and impaired glucose tolerance in U.S. adults. The Third National Health and Nutrition Examination Survey, 1988-1994. Diabetes Care 1998; 21:518–524.
56. Mokdad AH, Ford ES, Bowman BA, et al. The continuing increase of diabetes in the US. Diabetes Care 2001; 24:412.
57. Dolan LM, Bean J, D'Alessio D, et al. Frequency of abnormal carbohydrate metabolism and diabetes in a population-based screening of adolescents. J Pediatr 2005; 146:751–758.

58. Atabek ME, Pirgon O, Kurtoglu S. Assessment of abnormal glucose homeostasis and insulin resistance in Turkish obese children and adolescents. Diabetes Obes Metab 2007; 9:304–310.
59. Anonymous. Type 2 diabetes in children and adolescents. American Diabetes Association Diabetes Care 2000; 23:381–389.
60. Pinhas-Hamiel O, Standiford D, Hamiel D, et al. The type 2 family: a setting for development and treatment of adolescent type 2 diabetes mellitus. Arch Pediatr Adolesc Med 1999; 153:1063–1067.
61. Kitagawa T, Owada M, Urakami T, et al. Epidemiology of type 1 (insulin-dependent) and type 2 (non-insulin-dependent) diabetes mellitus in Japanese children. Diabetes Res Clin Pract 1994; 24(suppl):S7–S13.
62. Troiano RP, Flegal KM. Overweight children and adolescents: description, epidemiology, and demographics. Pediatrics 1998; 101:497–504.
63. Malina RM, Zavaleta AN, Little BB. Body size, fatness, and leanness of Mexican American children in Brownsville, Texas: changes between 1972 and 1983. Am J Public Health 1987; 77:573–577.
64. Young TK, Dean HJ, Flett B, et al. Childhood obesity in a population at high risk for type 2 diabetes. J Pediatr 2000; 136:365–369.
65. Schonfeld-Warden N, Warden CH. Pediatric obesity. An overview of etiology and treatment. Pediatr Clin North Am 1997; 44:339–361.
66. Strauss RS, Pollack HA. Epidemic increase in childhood overweight, 1986–1998. JAMA 2001; 286:2845–2848.
67. Ogden CL, Flegal KM, Carroll MD, et al. Prevalence and trends in overweight among US children and adolescents, 1999–2000. JAMA 2002; 288:1728–1732.
68. Ogden CL, Carroll MD, Curtin LR, et al. Prevalence of overweight and obesity in the United States, 1999–2004. JAMA 2006; 295:1549–1555.
69. Update prevalence of overweight among children, adolescents, and adults—United States, 1988-1994 MMWR Morb Mortal Wkly Rep 1997; 46:198–202.
70. Booth ML, Chey T, Wake M, et al. Change in the prevalence of overweight and obesity among young Australians, 1969–1997. Am J Clin Nutr 2003; 77:29–36.
71. Ramachandran A, Snehalatha C, Vinitha R, et al. Prevalence of overweight in urban Indian adolescent school children. Diabetes Res Clin Pract 2002; 57:185–190.
72. Dean H. Diagnostic criteria for non-insulin dependent diabetes in youth (NIDDM-Y). Clin Pediatr (Phila) 1998; 37:67–71.
73. Pinhas-Hamiel O, Zeitler P. "Who is the wise man? The one who foresees consequences:" Childhood obesity, new associated comorbidity and prevention. Prev Med 2000; 31:702–705.
74. Ebbeling CB, Pawlak DB, Ludwig DS. Childhood obesity: public-health crisis, common sense cure. Lancet 2002; 360:473–482.
75. Tajima N. Type 2 diabetes in children and adolescents in Japan. International Diabetes Monitor 2002; 14:1–5.
76. Craypo L, Purcell A, Samuels SE, et al. Fast food sales on high school campuses: results from the 2000 California high school fast food survey. J Sch Health 2002; 72:78–82.
77. Jahns L, Siega-Riz AM, Popkin BM. The increasing prevalence of snacking among US children from 1977 to 1996. J Pediatr 2001; 138:493–498.
78. Nicklas TA, Elkasabany A, Srinivasan SR, et al. Trends in nutrient intake of 10-year-old children over two decades (1973–1994): The Bogalusa Heart Study. Am J Epidemiol 2001; 153:969–977.
79. Troiano RP, Briefel RR, Carroll MD, et al. Energy and fat intakes of children and adolescents in the United States: data from the national health and nutrition examination surveys. Am J Clin Nutr 2000; 72:1343S–1353S.
80. O'Loughlin J, Gray-Donald K, Paradis G, et al. One- and two-year predictors of excess weight gain among elementary schoolchildren in multiethnic, low-income, inner-city neighborhoods. Am J Epidemiol 2000; 152:739–746.
81. Wolf AM, Gortmaker SL, Cheung L, et al. Activity, inactivity, and obesity: racial, ethnic, and age differences among schoolgirls. Am J Public Health 1993; 83:1625–1627.

82. Gortmaker SL, Peterson K, Wiecha J, et al. Reducing obesity via a school-based interdisciplinary intervention among youth: Planet Health. Arch Pediatr Adolesc Med 1999; 153:409–418.
83. Gordon-Larsen P, McMurray RG, Popkin BM. Adolescent physical activity and inactivity vary by ethnicity: The National Longitudinal Study of Adolescent Health. J Pediatr 1999; 135:301–306.
84. Troiano RP. Physical inactivity among young people. N Engl J Med 2002; 347:706–707.
85. Kann L, Kinchen SA, Williams BI, et al. Youth risk behavior surveillance—United States 1999. MMWR 1999; 49:1–94.
86. Kimm SY, Glynn NW, Kriska AM, et al. Decline in physical activity in black girls and white girls during adolescence. N Engl J Med 2002; 347:709–715.
87. Nesmith JD. Type 2 diabetes mellitus in children and adolescents. Pediatr Rev 2001; 22:147–152.
88. Andersen LB, Harro M, Sardinha LB, et al. Physical activity and clustered cardiovascular risk in children: a cross-sectional study (The European Youth Heart Study). Lancet 2006; 368:299–304.
89. Hannon TS, Janosky J, Arslanian SA. Longitudinal study of physiologic insulin resistance and metabolic changes of puberty. Pediatr Res 2006; 60:759–663.
90. Goran MI, Gower BA. 50 Longitudinal study on pubertal insulin resistance. Diabetes 2001; 50:2444–2450.
91. Goran MI, Bergman RN, Cruz ML, et al. Insulin resistance and associated compensatory responses in African-American and Hispanic children. Diabetes Care 2002; 25:2184–2190.
92. Freedman DS, Dietz WH, Srinivasan SR, et al. The relation of overweight to cardiovascular risk factors among children and adolescents: the Bogalusa Heart Study. Pediatrics 1999; 103:1175–1182.
93. Freedman DS, Serdula MK, Srinivasan SR, et al. Relation of circumferences and skinfold thicknesses to lipid and insulin concentrations in children and adolescents: the Bogalusa Heart Study. Am J Clin Nutr 1999; 69:308–317.
94. Gutin B, Islam S, Manos T, et al. Relation of percentage of body fat and maximal aerobic capacity to risk factors for atherosclerosis and diabetes in black and white seven- to eleven-year-old children. J Pediatr 1994; 125:847–852.
95. Owens S, Gutin B, Barbeau P, et al. Visceral adipose tissue and markers of the insulin resistance syndrome in obese black and white teenagers. Obes Res 2000; 8:287–293.
96. Gower BA, Nagy TR, Goran MI. Visceral fat, insulin sensitivity, and lipids in prepubertal children. Diabetes 1999; 48:1515–1521.
97. Roemmich JN, Clark PA, Lusk M, et al. Pubertal alterations in growth and body composition. VI. Pubertal insulin resistance: relation to adiposity, body fat distribution and hormone release. Int J Obes Relat Metab Disord 2002; 26:701–709.
98. Travers SH, Jeffers BW, Bloch CA, et al. Gender and Tanner stage differences in body composition and insulin sensitivity in early pubertal children. J Clin Endocrinol Metab 1995; 80:172–178.
99. Svec F, Nastasi K, Hilton C, et al. Black-white contrasts in insulin levels during pubertal development. The Bogalusa Heart Study. Diabetes 1992; 41:313–317.
100. Arslanian SA, Saad R, Lewy V, et al. Hyperinsulinemia in African-American children: decreased insulin clearance and increased insulin secretion and its relationship to insulin sensitivity. Diabetes 2002; 51:3014–3019.
101. Goran MI, Bergman RN, Cruz ML, et al. Insulin resistance and associated compensatory responses in African-American and Hispanic children. Diabetes Care 2002; 25:2184–2190.
102. Narayan KM. Type 2 diabetes in children: a problem lurking for India? Indian Pediatr 2001; 38:701–704.
103. Mayer-Davis EJ, D'Agostino R Jr., Karter AJ, et al. Intensity and amount of physical activity in relation to insulin sensitivity: the Insulin Resistance Atherosclerosis Study. JAMA 1998; 279:669–674.
104. Manson JE, Nathan DM, Krolewski AS, et al. A prospective study of exercise and incidence of diabetes among US male physicians. JAMA 1992; 268:63–67.
105. Manson JE, Rimm EB, Stampfer MJ, et al. Physical activity and incidence of non-insulin-dependent diabetes mellitus in women. Lancet 1991; 338:774–778.

106. Hu FB, Sigal RJ, Rich-Edwards J, et al. Walking compared with vigorous physical activity and risk of type 2 diabetes in women. JAMA 1999; 282:1433–1439.

107. Crespo CJ, Smit E, Troiano RP, et al. Television watching, energy intake, and obesity in US children: results from the third National Health and Nutrition Examination Survey, 1988–1994. Arch Pediatr Adolesc Med 2001; 155:360–365.

108. Bonora E, Kiechl S, Willeit J, et al. Plasma glucose within the normal range is not associated with carotid atherosclerosis: prospective results in subjects with normal glucose tolerance from the Bruneck Study. Diabetes Care 1999; 22:1339–1346.

109. Hoffman RP, Stumbo PJ, Janz KF, et al. Altered insulin resistance is associated with increased dietary weight loss in obese children. Horm Res 1995; 44:17–22.

110. Delamarche P, Gratas-Delamarche A, Monnier M, et al. Glucoregulation and hormonal changes during prolonged exercise in boys and girls. Eur J Appl Physiol Occup Physiol 1994; 68:3–8.

111. Hardin DS, Hebert JD, Bayden T, et al. Treatment of childhood syndrome X. Pediatrics 1997; 100:E5.

112. Schmitz KH, Jacobs DR Jr., Hong CP, et al. Association of physical activity with insulin sensitivity in children. Int J Obes Relat Metab Disord 2002; 26:1310–1316.

113. Sinha AK, O'Rourke S, O Leonard D, et al. Early onset Type 2 diabetes (T2DM) in the indigenous communities of far north Queensland (FNQ). Australian Diabetes Society Annual Scientific Meeting, 2000, Cairns, Australia, 2000:90.

114. Glowinska B, Urban M, Koput A. Cardiovascular risk factors in children with obesity, hypertension and diabetes: lipoprotein(a) levels and body mass index correlate with family history of cardiovascular disease. Eur J Pediatr 2002; 161:511–518.

115. Berenson GS, Radhakrishnamurthy B, Bao W, et al. Does adult-onset diabetes mellitus begin in childhood? the Bogalusa Heart Study. Am J Med Sci 1995; 310(suppl 1): S77–S82.

116. McCance DR, Pettitt DJ, Hanson RL, et al. Glucose, insulin concentrations and obesity in childhood and adolescence as predictors of NIDDM. Diabetologia 1994; 37:617–623.

117. Britz B, Siegfried W, Ziegler A, et al. Rates of psychiatric disorders in a clinical study group of adolescents with extreme obesity and in obese adolescents ascertained via a population based study. Int J Obes Relat Metab Disord 2000; 24:1707–1714.

118. Pesa JA, Syre TR, Jones E. Psychosocial differences associated with body weight among female adolescents the importance of body image. J Adolesc Health 2000; 26:330–337.

119. Vila G, Robert JJ, Nollet-Clemencon C, et al. Eating and emotional disorders in adolescent obese girls with insulin-dependent diabetes mellitus. Eur Child Adolesc Psychiatry 1995; 4:270–279.

120. Stice E, Hayward C, Cameron RP, et al. Body-image and eating disturbances predict onset of depression among female adolescents: a longitudinal study. J Abnorm Psychol 2000; 109:438–444.

121. Erickson SJ, Robinson TN, Haydel KF, et al. Are overweight children unhappy? Body mass index, depressive symptoms, and overweight concerns in elementary school children. Arch Pediatr Adolesc Med 2000; 154:931–935.

122. Anderson RJ, Freedland KE, Clouse RE, et al. The prevalence of comorbid depression in adults with diabetes: a meta-analysis. Diabetes Care 2001; 24:1069–1078.

123. Carney C. Diabetes mellitus and major depressive disorder: an overview of prevalence, complications, and treatment. Depress Anxiety 1998; 7:149–157.

124. Jacobson AM. Depression and diabetes. Diabetes Care 1993; 16:1621–1623.

125. Okamura F, Tashiro A, Utumi A, et al. Insulin resistance in patients with depression and its changes during the clinical course of depression minimal model analysis. Metabolism 2000; 49:1255–1260.

126. Geringer ES. Affective disorders and diabetes mellitus. In: Holmes CS, ed. Neuropsychological and Behavioral Aspects of Diabetes. New York: Springer-Verlag, 1990:239–272.

127. Lawrence JM, Standiford DA, Loots B, et al. SEARCH for Diabetes in Youth Study. Prevalence and correlates of depressed mood among youth with diabetes: the SEARCH for Diabetes in Youth study. Pediatrics 2006; 117:1348–1358.

128. Littlefield CH, Craven JL, Rodin GM, et al. Relationship of self-efficacy and binging to adherence to diabetes regimen among adolescents. Diabetes Care 1992; 15:90–94.

129. Hauser ST, Jacobson AM, Lavori P, et al. Adherence among children and adolescents with insulin-dependent diabetes mellitus over a four-year longitudinal follow-up: II. Immediate and long-term linkages with the family milieu. J Pediatr Psychol 1990; 15:527–542.

130. Jacobson AM, Hauser ST, Lavori P, et al. Family environment and glycemic control: a four-year prospective study of children and adolescents with insulin-dependent diabetes mellitus. Psychosom Med 1994; 56:401–409.

131. Grey M, Davidson M, Boland EA, et al. Clinical and psychosocial factors associated with achievement of treatment goals in adolescents with diabetes mellitus. J Adolesc Health 2001; 28:377–385.

132. Liss DS, Waller DA, Kennard BD, et al. Psychiatric illness and family support in children and adolescents with diabetic ketoacidosis: a controlled study. J Am Acad Child Adolesc Psychiatry 1998; 37:536–544.

133. Crawford PB, Story M, Wang MC, et al. Ethnic issues in the epidemiology of childhood obesity. Pediatr Clin North Am 2001; 48:855–878.

134. Cubbin C, Hadden WC, Winkleby MA. Neighborhood context and cardiovascular disease risk factors: the contribution of material deprivation. Ethn Dis 2001; 11:687–700.

135. Guo SS, Roche AF, Chumlea WC, et al. The predictive value of childhood body mass index values for overweight at age 35 y. Am J Clin Nutr 1994; 59:810–819.

136. Ozanne SE, Hales CN. Early programming of glucose-insulin metabolism. Trends Endocrinol Metab 2002; 13:368–373.

137. Phillips DI. Birth weight and the future development of diabetes. A review of the evidence. Diabetes Care 1998; 21(suppl 2):B150–B155.

138. Dabelea D, Pettitt DJ, Hanson RL, et al. Birth weight, type 2 diabetes, and insulin resistance in Pima Indian children and young adults. Diabetes Care 1999; 22: 944–950.

139. Hales CN, Barker DJP, Clark PM, et al. Fetal and infant growth and impaired glucose tolerance at age 64. BMJ 1991; 303:1019–1022.

140. Phipps K, Barker DJ, Hales CN, et al. Fetal growth and impaired glucose tolerance in men and women. Diabetologia 1993; 36:225–228.

141. Valdez R, Athens MA, Thompson GH, et al. Birthweight and adult health outcomes in a biethnic population in the USA. Diabetologia 1994; 37:624–631.

142. McCance DR, Pettitt DJ, Hanson RL, et al. Birth weight and non-insulin dependent diabetes: thrifty genotype, thrifty phenotype, or surviving small baby genotype? BMJ 1994; 308:942–945.

143. Hales CN, Barker DJP. Type 2 (non-insulin-dependent) diabetes mellitus: the thrifty phenotype hypothesis. Diabetologia 1992; 35:595–601.

144. Hattersley AT, Beards F, Ballantyne E, et al. Mutations in the glucokinase gene of the fetus result in reduced birth weight. Nat Genet 1998; 19:268–270.

145. Dunger DB, Ong KK, Huxtable SJ, et al. Association of the INS VNTR with size at birth. ALSPAC Study Team. Avon Longitudinal Study of Pregnancy and Childhood. Nat Genet 1998; 19:98–100.

146. Poulsen P, Vaag AA, Kyvik KO, et al. Low birth weight is associated with NIDDM in discordant monozygotic and dizygotic twin pairs. Diabetologia 1997; 40:439–446.

147. Bo S, Cavallo-Perin P, Scaglione L, et al. Low birthweight and metabolic abnormalities in twins with increased susceptibility to Type 2 diabetes mellitus. Diabet Med 2000; 17:365–370.

148. Yajnik CS. The insulin resistance epidemic in India: fetal origins, later lifestyle, or both? Nutr Rev 2001; 59:1–9.

149. Yajnik CS, Fall CH, Coyaji KJ, et al. Neonatal anthropometry: the thin-fat Indian baby. The Pune Maternal Nutrition Study. Int J Obes Relat Metab Disord 2003; 27:173–180.

150. Yajnik CS, Lubree HG, Rege SS, et al. Adiposity and hyperinsulinemia in Indians are present at birth. J Clin Endocrinol Metab 2002; 87:5575–5580.

151. Peters J, Ulijaszek SJ. Population and sex differences in arm circumference and skinfold thicknesses among Indo-Pakistani children living in the East Midlands of Britain. Ann Hum Biol 1992; 19:17–22.

152. Crowther NJ, Cameron N, Trusler J, et al. Association between poor glucose tolerance and rapid post natal weight gain in seven-year-old children. Diabetologia 1998. 41:1163–1167.

153. Hypponen E, Smith GD, Power C. Parental diabetes and birth weight of offspring: intergenerational cohort study. BMJ 2003; 326:19–20.
154. Clausen JO, Borch-Johnsen K, Pedersen O. Relation between birth weight and the insulin sensitivity index in a population sample of 331 young, healthy Caucasians. Am J Epidemiol 1997; 146:23–31.
155. Leger J, Levy-Marchal C, Bloch J, et al. Reduced final height and indications for insulin resistance in 20 year olds born small for gestational age: regional cohort study. Brit Med J 1997; 315:341–347.
156. Jaquet D, Gaboriau A, Czernichow P, et al. Insulin resistance early in adulthood in subjects born with intrauterine growth retardation. J Clin Endocrinol Metab 2000; 85:1401–1406.
157. Wei JN, Sung FC, Li CY, et al. Low birth weight and high birth weight infants are both at an increased risk to have type 2 diabetes among schoolchildren in Taiwan. Diabetes Care 2003; 26:343–348.
158. Pfab T, Slowinski T, Godes M, et al. Low birth weight, a risk factor for cardiovascular diseases in later life, Is already associated with elevated fetal glycosylated hemoglobin at birth. Circulation 2006; 114:1687–1692.
159. Yajnik CS. Nutrition, growth, and body size in relation to insulin resistance and type 2 diabetes. Curr Diab Rep 2003; 3(2):108–114.
160. Hales CN, Barker DJ. The thrifty phenotype hypothesis. Br Med Bull 2001; 60:5–20.
161. Yajnik C. Interactions of perturbations in intrauterine growth and growth during childhood on the risk of adult-onset disease. Proc Nutr Soc 2000; 59:257–265.
162. Bhargava SK, Sachdev HS, Fall CH, et al. Relation of serial changes in childhood body-mass index to impaired glucose tolerance in young adulthood. N Engl J Med 2004; 350:865–875.
163. McCarthy M. Weighing in on diabetes risk. Nat Genet 1998; 19:209–210.
164. Lindsay RS, Dabelea D, Roumain J, et al. Type 2 diabetes and low birth weight: the role of paternal inheritance in the association of low birth weight and diabetes. Diabetes 2000; 49:445–449.
165. Huxtable SJ, Saker PJ, Haddad L, et al. Analysis of parent-offspring trios provides evidence for linkage and association between the insulin gene and type 2 diabetes mediated exclusively through paternally transmitted class III variable number tandem repeat alleles. Diabetes 2000; 49:126–130.
166. Fetita LS, Sobngwi E, Serradas P, et al. Review: consequences of fetal exposure to maternal diabetes in offspring. J Clin Endocrinol Metab 2006; 91:3718–3724.
167. Pettitt DJ, Baird HR, Aleck KA, et al. Excessive obesity in offspring of Pima Indian women with diabetes during pregnancy. New Engl J Med 1983; 308:242–245.
168. Pettitt DJ, Bennett PH, Knowler WC, et al. Gestational diabetes mellitus and impaired glucose tolerance during pregnancy. Long-term effects on obesity and glucose tolerance in the offspring. Diabetes 1985; 34(suppl 2); 119–122.
169. Pettitt DJ, Bennett PH, Saad MF, et al. Abnormal glucose tolerance during pregnancy in Pima Indian women. Long-term effects on offspring. Diabetes 1991; 40(suppl 2):126–130.
170. Dabelea D, Knowler WC, Pettitt DJ. Effect of diabetes in pregnancy on offspring: follow-up research in the Pima Indians. J Matern Fetal Med 2000; 9:83–88.
171. Pettitt DJ, Aleck KA, Baird HR, et al. Congenital susceptibility to NIDDM: role of intrauterine environment. Diabetes 1998; 37:622–628.
172. Pettitt DJ, Bennett PH, Everhart J, et al. High plasma glucose concentrations in normal weight offspring of diabetic women. Diabetes Res Clin Pract 1985, S445.
173. Silverman BL, Metzger BE, Cho NH, et al. Impaired glucose tolerance in adolescent offspring of diabetic mothers. Relationship to fetal hyperinsulinism. Diabetes Care 1995; 18(5):611–617.
174. Metzger BE, Silverman BL, Freinkel N, et al. Amniotic fluid insulin concentration as a predictor of obesity. Arch Dis Child 1990; 65:1050–1052.
175. Dabelea D, Hanson RL, Lindsay RS, et al. Intrauterine exposure to diabetes conveys risks for type 2 diabetes and obesity: a study of discordant sibships. Diabetes 2000; 49:2208–2211.
176. Heding LG, Persson B, Stangenberg M. B-cell function in newborn infants of diabetic mothers. Diabetologia 1980; 19:427–432.

177. Hultquist GT, Olding LB. Pancreatic-islet fibrosis in young infants of diabetic mothers. Lancet 1975; 2:1015–1016.
178. Gautier JF, Wilson C, Weyer C, et al. Low acute insulin secretory responses in adult offspring of people with early onset type 2 diabetes. Diabetes 2001; 50:1828–1833.
179. Sobngwi E, Boudou P, Mauvais-Jarvis F, et al. Effect of a diabetic environment in utero on predisposition to type 2 diabetes. Lancet 2003; 361:1861–1865.
180. Bihoreau MT, Ktorza A, Kinebanyan MF, et al. Impaired glucose homeostasis in adult rats from hyperglycemic mothers. Diabetes 1986; 35:979–984.
181. Aerts L, Sodoyez-Goffaux F, Sodoyez JC, et al. The diabetic intrauterine milieu has a long-lasting effect on insulin secretion by B cells and on insulin uptake by target tissues. Am J Obstet Gynecol 1998; 159:1287–1292.
182. Grill V, Johansson B, Jalkanen P, et al. Influence of severe diabetes mellitus early in pregnancy in the rat: effects on insulin sensitivity and insulin secretion in the offspring. Diabetologia 1991; 34:373–378.
183. Dorner G. Influence of early postnatal nutrition on body height in adolescence. Acta Biol Med Ger 1978; 37:1149–1151.
184. Kramer MS, Barr RG, Leduc DG, et al. Infant determinants of childhood weight and adiposity. J Pediatr 1985; 107:104–107.
185. Dewey KG, Heinig MJ, Nommsen LA, et al. Breast-fed infants are leaner than formula-fed infants at 1 y of age the DARLING study. Am J Clin Nutr 1993; 57:140–145.
186. Burke V, Beilin LJ, Simmer K, et al. Breastfeeding and overweight: longitudinal analysis in an Australian birth cohort. J Pediatr 2005; 147:56–61.
187. Lucas A, Sarson DL, Blackburn AM, et al. Breast vs bottle: endocrine responses are different with formula feeding. Lancet 1980; 1:1267–1269.
188. von Kries R, Koletzko B, Sauerwald T, et al. Breast feeding and obesity: cross sectional study. Br Med J 1999; 319:147–150.
189. Liese AD, Hirsch T, von Mutius E, et al. Inverse association of overweight and breast feeding in 9 to 10-y-old children in Germany. Int J Obes Relat Metab Disord 2001; 25:1644–1650.
190. Gillman MW, Rifas-Shiman SL, Camargo CA, et al. Risk of overweight among adolescents who were breastfed as infants. JAMA 2001; 285:2461–2467.
191. Hall B. Changing composition of human milk and early development of an appetite control. Lancet 1975; 1:779–781.
192. Pettitt DJ, Forman MR, Hanson RL, et al. Breastfeeding and incidence of non-insulin-dependent diabetes mellitus in Pima Indians. Lancet 1997; 350:166–168.
193. Pettitt DJ, Knowler WC. Long-term effects of the intrauterine environment, birth weight, and breast-feeding in Pima Indians. Diabetes Care 1998; 21(suppl 2):B138–B141.
194. Mayer-Davis EJ, Dabelea D, Pande A, et al. Breast Feeding is associated with lower odds of type 2 diabetes mellitus in youth: SEARCH Case-Control (SEARCH-CC) study. Diabetes 2007; 56(suppl 1):A487.
195. WHO. Life in the 21st century—a vision for all. The World Health Report 1998. Geneva, Switzerland WHO, 1998: 87.
196. Pavkov ME, Hanson RL, Knowler WC, et al. Changing patterns of type 2 diabetes incidence among Pima Indians. Diabetes Care 2007; 30:1758–1763.

8 Obesity and T2DM in Youth

Ram Weiss
Department of Human Nutrition and Metabolism, Hebrew University School of Medicine, Jerusalem, Israel

Sonia Caprio
Department of Pediatrics and the Children's General Clinical Research Center, Yale University School of Medicine, New Haven, Connecticut, U.S.A.

INTRODUCTION

Type 2 diabetes mellitus (T2DM) is strongly associated with increased risk of cardiovascular morbidity and mortality. Recently numerous reports have been published describing the alarming rise in the prevalence of T2DM in children and adolescents in both developed and developing countries (1,2). The increase in prevalence of T2DM parallels the increase in the prevalence of obesity (3) in this age group, and they are appropriately called the "twin epidemics."

The pathophysiology underlying the development of T2DM is multifactorial and the relative roles and sequence of development of defects in insulin secretion, insulin action, and hepatic glucose output are not clear (4,5). Until recently, little was known regarding the significance and temporal development of defects in the above mentioned factors early in the course of altered glucose metabolism in obese children. Moreover, the roles of discrete lipid depots in the development of altered glucose metabolism in childhood have not been defined.

Impaired glucose tolerance (IGT) is a reversible prediabetic condition. In adults, the progression rate of IGT to diabetes is estimated at 5–8% per year (6), yet little is known about the natural history of IGT in children. With lifestyle modifications and/or pharmacotherapy, the progression of IGT to diabetes in adults can be halted or completely prevented (7–9), making this condition highly attractive for early diagnosis and intervention. The early development of T2DM in childhood makes the investigation of IGT even more important, as the "window of opportunity" for intervention may be narrower in this age group. This review focuses on the intricate interrelations of specific obesity phenotypes and glucose metabolism in obese youth.

RELATION OF OBESITY, LIPID PARTITIONING, AND METABOLIC RISK

The close association of T2DM with cardiovascular disease (CVD) led to the hypothesis that the two may arise from a common antecedent (10,11). It was Reaven (12) who noticed that common risk factors of CVD and altered glucose metabolism tend to cluster in specific individuals and thus named this constellation of risk factors "the insulin resistance syndrome" [later named "the metabolic syndrome" (MS)], highlighting the critical role of peripheral insulin resistance as a driving force of the underlying pathological process. Individuals meeting at least three of the following five criteria qualify as having the MS: elevated blood pressure, a high triglyceride level, low HDL–cholesterol level, high fasting glucose, and central obesity (13). Because of its wide prevalence, the MS has enormous clinical and public health importance, even at its earliest stages, as it promotes athero-sclerosis and sets the stage for the development of diabetes (14), the component that appears early in obese youth. According to the paradigm presented herein, the impact of obesity is determined by the pattern of lipid partitioning, i.e., the specific depots in which excess fat is stored. The pattern of lipid storage has an impact on the adipocytokine secretion profile, on circulating concentrations of inflammatory cytokines, and on the free fatty acid flux. The combined effect of these factors determines the sensitivity of insulin target organs (such as muscle and liver) to insulin and impacts the vascular system by affecting endothelial function. Peripheral insulin resistance and endothelial dysfunction are the early promoters of future pathology, mainly of CVD and altered glucose metabolism, eventually manifesting as T2DM.

Degree of Obesity and Metabolic Risk

Classification of the degree of obesity in adults defines a BMI > 30 kg/m^2 as class 1 obesity, BMI of 35–39.9 kg/m^2 as class 2 obesity, and BMI ≥ 40 kg/m^2 as class 3 obesity (15). No similar classifications for the degree of obesity exist for children and adolescents, except for the definition of those whose BMI is between the 85th and 95th percentile as "at risk for overweight" and those at greater than the 95th per-centile as "overweight." Several studies have shown that the degree of obesity has an adverse impact on the metabolic profile of obese youth, although no sub-categorization of the degrees of obesity within the upper 5 percentiles, as described in adults, exists for children. When obese children were divided to moderately (BMI z score of 2–2.5, corresponding to the 97th to the 99.5 percentile) and severely (BMI z score > 2.5, corresponding to the 99.5 percentile) obese and compared with over-weight and nonobese children in regards to components of the MS (16), the impact of the degree of obesity was demonstrated. Increasing obesity categories in children and adolescents was associated with worsening of all components of the MS, specifically with an increase in fasting glucose, fasting insulin, triglycerides, and systolic blood pressure. An increasing prevalence of IGT and a decrease of HDL cholesterol were also observed with increasing adiposity. The prevalence of MS, using a modified conservative definition adjusted for the pediatric age group, was ~30% in the moderately obese and nearly 50% in severely obese participants. When the Bogalusa cohort participants (17) were stratified according to discrete percentiles above the 90th for BMI, those in the 99th percentile for age and gender had a significantly greater prevalence of biochemical components of the MS and being above the 99th percentile for age and gender during childhood had a very high predictive value for adult BMI of greater than 35 kg/m^2. The implication of these studies is that among obese children and adolescents, those at the 99th per-centile and above, in other words—the "severely obese," are an extremely high-risk group for the presence of components of the MS and for future class 2–3 obesity in adulthood. Importantly, the prevalence of the MS, regardless of the definition used, is significant even among overweight and mildly obese children and adolescents (18,19), and not limited to those with severe obesity.

Impact of Lipid Partitioning

Obesity does not necessarily implicate morbidity in childhood or adulthood. Although obesity is the most common cause of insulin resistance in children and adolescents, some obese youth may be very insulin sensitive and thus be at reduced risk for the development of the adverse cardiovascular and metabolic outcomes driven by insulin resistance. It has been clearly demonstrated that those obese youth with IGT are significantly more insulin resistant than those with normal glucose tolerance (NGT), despite having an overall equal degree of adiposity (20). The difference in insulin sensitivity was attributed to different patterns of lipid partitioning—where those with severe insulin resistance were characterized by increased deposition of lipid in the visceral and intramyocellular compartments.

Intramyocellular Lipid Deposition

Increased intramyocellular lipid (IMCL) deposition has been shown to occur early in childhood obesity and be directly associated with peripheral insulin sensitivity (21). Importantly, not all obese children have increased IMCL levels and those who do not are much more insulin sensitive (22). Why some individuals who are seemingly equally obese and share common lifestyle and dietary habits tend to accumulate more IMCL than others is a matter of intensive research. An excellent model to study this issue is lean offspring of patients with T2DM, as they lack the confounding factors of obesity and hyperglycemia seen in obese patients with diabetes. These individuals have been shown to have impaired insulin stimulated nonoxidative muscle glucose disposal, i.e., to possess significant skeletal muscle insulin resistance earlier than the development of any clinical manifestations of altered glucose metabolism (23). The best correlate of insulin resistance in these lean individuals is indeed IMCL content (24). A putative explanation for the tendency to accumulate lipids in skeletal muscle may be differences of quantity and functionality of the mitochondria within the myocyte. Indeed, when elderly lean insulin-resistant individuals were compared with younger body habitus and activity matched men using ^{13}C and ^{31}P magnetic resonance spectroscopy, they were found to have a ~40% reduction in oxidative phosphorylation (25). When offspring of diabetics were compared with age and activity matched insulin-sensitive controls, it was demonstrated that they had an ~30% reduction rate of ATP production in mitochondria of skeletal muscle (26). Lean offspring of diabetic parents have also been shown to have lower mitochondrial content in skeletal muscle and that is postulated to predispose them to increased lipid accumulation within the myocyte (27). A second factor leading to IMCL accumulation may be fat constituents of the diet. High-fat diets of varying durations have been shown to increase IMCL content by 36–90% depending on their duration and baseline IMCL levels (28,29). In physically inactive obese individuals, a continuous increased supply of fatty acids by way of excess energy intake, alongside a reduced capacity to oxidize fat may lead to overall fat storage, specifically in skeletal muscle. An obvious third source of increased IMCL is an increase in circulating free fatty acid (FFA) concentration, characteristic to obese insulin-resistant individuals. These observations indicate that the tendency to accumulate IMCL may be genetically determined as well is be influenced by diet and activity and result from reduced quantity and altered functionality of myocellular mitochondria. A tendency for increased IMCL deposition, which is partially genetically determined, predisposes individuals to greater insulin resistance while obesity with low IMCL deposition seems to be more "metabolically benign."

The effects of IMCL accumulation on the response of the myocyte to insulin stimulation are not caused by the stored triglyceride per se. Rather, fatty acid derivates of the accumulated IMCL cause a disturbance of the insulin signal transduction pathway, eventually leading to reduced glucose uptake (30). The insulin signal transduction pathway culminates in the trafficking of glucose transporter 4 (GLUT-4) to the cellular membrane, allowing transport of glucose into the myocyte. In brief, insulin stimulation causes phosphorylation of insulin receptor substrate 1 (IRS-1) leading to its binding and activation of phosphatidy-linositol-3 (PI3) kinase. Activation of PI3 kinase leads to GLUT-4 trafficking to the cell membrane, allowing glucose transport into the myocyte. Fatty acid derivates within the cell have been shown to inhibit this signal transduction pathway through activation of protein kinase C-θ, which in turn blunts IRS-1 tyrosine phosphorylation via a serine–threonine kinase cascade. Reduction of IRS-1 tyrosine phosphorylation leads to reduced PI3-kinase activation and reduced GLUT-4 trafficking to the cellular membrane (31).

Abdominal Lipid Deposition

Upper-body obesity, manifested clinically by increased waist circumference, is known to be associated with CVD and T2DM. The adverse impact of upper-body obesity is implicated on accumulation of intra-abdominal (visceral) fat, yet the adverse effects of abdominal subcutaneous tissue should not be overlooked. The major source of circulating FFAs is fat tissue and one can assume that with greater adiposity there is an increase in FFA flux. When FFA flux is expressed per units of fat mass (from where FFAs are released), thus enabling a comparison of lean and obese individuals, FFA turnover is ~50% lower in obese compared to lean individuals (32). This difference may be attributed to greater circulating insulin concentrations that may thus prevent an overflow of FFAs released from the increased lipid stores of obese persons. When FFA turnover is expressed per lean body (fat free) mass (where FFAs are mainly consumed)—FFA lipolysis is greater in obese compared to lean individuals by ~50% (33) and those with upper-body obesity have greater FFA lipolysis rates in comparison to those with lower body obesity (34). These observations suggest that there are differences in the regulation of lipolysis in adipose tissue in individuals with different obesity phenotypes.

Visceral fat has been suggested to cause insulin resistance (35). Whether this relation is due to the relative resistance of visceral fat to insulin resulting in increased FFA release is unclear. Elegant studies by Jensen et al. (36) revealed that increased visceral fat is indeed associated with increased delivery of FFAs to the liver, yet that this visceral FFA flux is responsible for only ~20–30% and that splanchnic bed contributes up to 15% of FFAs reaching the liver. This result implies that visceral fat is probably not the source of the majority of systemic circulating FFAs and its postulated effects on insulin resistance of tissues other than the liver cannot be attributed to increased discharge of FFAs. Thus, the abdominal subcutaneous fat is probably the source of increased circulating FFAs of lean and obese individuals. Indeed, upper-body fat (mainly from the subcutaneous abdominal tissue) is lipolytically more active than lower-body fat and contributes the majority of circulating FFAs in the postabsorptive state (37,38). This observation may explain the adverse metabolic implications of "male pattern obesity," characterized by greater upper body fat, in comparison to "female pattern obesity" which typically involves greater lower body fat. Thus, the contribution of visceral fat to altered glucose metabolism and decreased insulin sensitivity specifically may be related to elements other than FFA discharge and its presence may be only a surrogate of relatively increased upper body fat depots. A proposed mechanism by which visceral fat may cause its adverse effects is related to secretion of inflammatory cytokines. When examined in vitro, visceral fat has been shown to secrete increased amounts of inflammatory mediators, including CRP, IL-6, TNF-α, and PAI-1, in comparison with subcutaneous fat (39,40). Similarly, obese individuals with increased visceral adiposity have increased markers of systemic inflammation in comparison with equally obese subjects with increased subcutaneous fat (41). The contribution of visceral fat to the typical subclinical chronic inflammation seen in some obese individuals may thus be the causal link between visceral adiposity and the MS and its related morbidity.

Indeed, adults with visceral adiposity tend to manifest insulin resistance, hypertension, a hypercoagulable state, and dyslipidemia in comparison with equally obese subjects with lower levels of visceral fat (42,43). Increased visceral adiposity has also been shown to be related to a greater atherogenic metabolic profile in childhood (44). Visceral fat has been shown to be related to greater insulin resistance and lower insulin secretory response in obese children and adolescents (45), thus potentially promoting deteriorating glucose metabolism. Adiponectin levels are lower in obese children with increased visceral fat deposition (46), even when the comparison is made between those with similar overall adiposity (10).

Hepatic Lipid Deposition

Nonalcoholic fatty liver disease (NAFLD) represents fatty infiltration of the liver without excessive alcohol consumption (47). The spectrum of NAFLD ranges from isolated fatty infiltration (steatosis) to inflammation (steatohepatitis, also known as NASH) to fibrosis and even cirrhosis (48). While the majority of obese people with NAFLD do not progress to NASH or cirrhosis, some develop a local inflammatory process leading over a variable period to advanced liver disease. Lipid accumulation in the liver is characterized as macrovesicular hepatic steatosis and is the result of an imbalance between production and utilization of triglycerides. There are three sources that may increase the hepatic fatty acid pool: circulating FFAs from various adipose compartments discussed earlier, de novo lipogenesis within the liver, and dietary factors that promote lipogenesis. De novo lipogenesis, shown to be increased in NAFLD (49), is dependent on acetyl coenzyme A (coA), an intermediate that enables proteins and carbohydrates to be driven toward lipogenic pathways. The two main effectors that drive hepatic de novo lipogenesis are acetyl coA carboxylase and fatty acid synthase. Dietary factors that may promote hepatic lipogenesis include exogenous fatty acids as well as carbohydrates that can drive triglyceride formation by way of triose phosphate as a basis for glycerol formation and by way of fatty acid formation by acetyl coA. A specific dietary factor that promotes hepatic lipogenesis is fructose, which is an unregulated substrate for liver triglyceride synthesis. Factors that decrease the hepatic fatty acid pool are either synthesis of triglycerides and phospholipids or fatty acid oxidation. Very low density lipoprotein (VLDL) and chylomicron remnants have also been shown to contribute to hepatic triglyceride synthesis and storage (50). The rate-limiting step of mitochondrial β-oxidation is the transfer of fatty acids into the mitochondria, regulated by carnitine palmytoyl acyltransferase 1 (CPT-1), which is inhibited by insulin. The balance between lipogenesis and lipolysis in the liver is mainly affected by the ratio of insulin and glucagon. In the case of insulin resistance, fatty acid flux to the liver is increased from increased lipolysis in adipose tissue leading to increased fatty acid uptake. This process in turn increases hepatic glucose output and triggers increased insulin secretion in order to maintain euglycemia. Increased concentrations of insulin in the liver induce de novo lipogenesis, thus creating a vicious cycle. The dietary factors such as increased consumption of carbohydrates (specifically fructose) and saturated fats, typically seen in obese subjects, further contribute to hepatic lipogenesis.

NAFLD is not confined to adults and is now the most common liver disease among obese children and adolescents in North America (51,52) with similar reports coming from other countries (53,54). NAFLD was found in the NHANES III survey to be prevalent in obese African American and Hispanic males with T2DM, hypertension, and hyperlipidemia (55). These associations have led to the hypothesis that NAFLD may precede the onset of T2DM in some individuals. The natural history of NAFLD in children is unknown, yet it may progress to cirrhosis and related complications (56). The gold standard for the assessment of fatty liver is a liver biopsy, yet recently several noninvasive quantitative methods, such as specific magnetic resonance imaging protocols and NMR spectroscopy, have been developed to evaluate patients suspected to have NAFLD. A surrogate typically used in the clinical setting is screening alanine amino transferase (ALT) levels. In a study of 392 obese children and adolescents (57), elevated ALT levels (>35 U/L) were found in 14% of participants, with a predominance of male gender and of the white or Hispanic race or ethnicity. After adjusting for potential confounders, rising ALT was associated with reduced insulin sensitivity and glucose tolerance as well as increasing concentrations of FFAs and triglycerides. Worsening of glucose and lipid metabolism was already evident as ALT levels rose into the upper half of the normal range (18–35 U/L). When hepatic fat fraction was assessed using fast magnetic resonance imaging, 32% of subjects had an increased hepatic fat fraction, which was associated with decreased insulin sensitivity and adiponectin, and with increased triglycerides and visceral fat. The prevalence of the MS was significantly greater in those with fatty liver. These results implicate that fatty infiltration of the liver is a common finding among obese children and adolescents and is associated with the adverse components of the MS, namely insulin resistance, dyslipidemia, and altered glucose metabolism.

The Relation Between Insulin Resistance and Tissue Lipid Partitioning

In obese children and adolescents, insulin resistance is the best predictor of IGT. Moreover, increasing levels of insulin resistance are strongly associated with higher prevalence of the MS in obese youngsters. The observation that not all obese youth demonstrate altered glucose metabolism or other components of the MS highlights the fact that obesity per se is not the single determinant of the underlying pathophysiology. We performed a study to unravel the underlying mechanisms responsible for the changes in insulin sensitivity and secretion in the early stage of IGT in obese youth (58). We combined the hyperinsulinemic-euglycemic clamp with stable isotopes infusion, indirect calorimetry, and the hyperglycemic clamp in adolescents with NGT and IGT who were well matched for age and total body fat. ^{1}H-NMR and MRI techniques were used to noninvasively quantify skeletal muscle and abdominal fat partitioning.

The lipid composition of the skeletal muscle tissue, where most (70%) of the whole glucose disposal occurs, has attracted much attention recently as a major player in the development of muscle insulin resistance (59). Strong inverse correlations between insulin resistance and IMCL have been reported in offspring of T2DM adults, suggesting that a high-IMCL content might be involved in the development of insulin resistance (60). We found an excessive accumulation of IMCL in the soleus muscle of obese adolescents with IGT compared with age and adiposity matched obese adolescents with NGT. Abdominal MRI showed that subcutaneous fat in IGT subjects was significantly lower compared with NGT subjects, while visceral fat tended to be higher in the IGT group than in the NGT group. The ratio of visceral to subcutaneous fat was 50% higher in the IGT subjects compared with NGT. IMCL and visceral fat content were inversely correlated with the glucose disposal ($r = -0.51$ and $r = -0.63$, $p < 0.01$, respectively) and with nonoxidative glucose metabolism in the two groups together ($r = -0.45$ and $r = -0.47$, $p > 0.03$, respectively). These data are consistent with results obtained in both human and animal models of lipodystrophy, in which there is an absence of subcutaneous adipose tissue, leading to increased accumulation of lipids in both myocytes and the visceral depot. It appears that the ability of peripheral subcutaneous fat tissue to vary its storage capacity is critical for regulating insulin sensitivity and ultimately protecting against diabetes.

Lipid Deposition and Subclinical Inflammation

Recent accumulating evidence indicates that obesity and insulin resistance are associated with a "subclinical inflammatory status" (61). The immune and metabolic responses are tightly linked as both evolutionary evolved from common structures, still present in primitive organisms such as the Drosophila fat body, which shares the functions of the liver and the hematopoietic/immune system (62). It is thus reasonable to assume that regulatory signal transduction pathways are shared by the metabolic and immunological systems and respond to similar hormonal and environmental stimuli (63). The adipose tissue serves as an active secretory organ, releasing peptides and cytokines into the circulation (64). In the presence of obesity, the balance between these numerous molecules is altered, such that enlarged adipocytes, or potentially macrophages embedded within adipocytes (65), produces more proinflammatory cytokines (i.e., TNF-α, IL-6) and less anti-inflammatory peptides such as adiponectin (66). Such macrophages may be the major source of proinflammatory cytokines initiating a proinflammatory status that predates the development of insulin resistance and endothelial dysfunction (67). The relation of elevated circulating proinflammatory molecules and peripheral insulin resistance is mediated by the common interface of these signals and the insulin signal transduction pathway at the level of insulin receptor substrates through activation of several serine kinases (68). The dysregulated production of adipocytokines has been found to participate in the development of metabolic and vascular diseases related to obesity (69). Indeed, inflammation may be the missing link between obesity and insulin resistance. In obese children and adolescents, C reactive protein, a marker of systemic inflammation (70), and IL-6 levels are related to the degree and severity of obesity (71). In contrast, levels of adiponectin, an anti-inflammatory biomarker, decreased with increasing levels of obesity and insulin resistance. Importantly, despite observing increased visceral and hepatic lipid deposition in obese youth, the levels of the proinflammatory cytokines are far lower than those observed in adults with similar obesity phenotypes. This observation may indicate a smaller role of systemic inflammation in the development of obesity-related morbidity in childhood but does not rule out local prominent roles of inflammatory cytokines in the development of organ-specific insulin resistance by way of paracrine effects.

INSULIN SECRETION AND CLEARANCE IN THE OBESE CHILD

Overt diabetes or prediabetes does not develop until the β cells fail to compensate appropriately for the peripheral insulin-resistant milieu. The ability of the β cells to secrete sufficient insulin to overcome insulin resistance is dependent on multiple factors, including β-cell mass and secretory capacity. These factors are influenced by genetic, intrauterine, and postnatal factors. Thus, youth with predetermined risk factors, such as exposure to gestational diabetes, or those exposed to specific constituents of the diet may be more vulnerable and may fail to compensate appropriately for the deleterious effects of insulin resistance.

Using mathematical modeling of β-cell sensitivity to first- and second-phase insulin secretion, we demonstrated that obese youth with prediabetes have a significant defect in the sensitivity of first-phase secretion compared with their normal glucose-tolerant counterparts (72). A further significant deterioration of first-phase sensitivity was found in obese youth with T2DM. Sensitivity of the β cell to second-phase secretion was similar in subjects with NGT and IGT but was significantly reduced in subjects with overt T2DM. Thus, T2DM in obese children and adolescents is characterized by a major defect in both phases of insulin secretion, while in prediabetes, first-phase insulin secretion alone is compromised.

Using different methodologies, a lower disposition index has been shown in obese Hispanic subjects with IGT (73) and impaired fasting glucose, and in young nonobese offspring of patients with T2DM (74). The disposition index serves as an indicator of the β cell's ability to secrete insulin in the context of the measured insulin sensitivity; thus, a lower disposition index in the face of severe insulin resistance signifies a greater propensity to develop altered glucose metabolism. Studies in adults have shown that the disposition index is strongly genetically determined, thus making certain individuals more prone to developing altered glucose metabolism in the presence of marked insulin resistance. Using oral glucose tolerance tests, we have recently demonstrated that, as the two-hour glucose increases even within the NGT range, a significantly reduced early insulin response can be demonstrated in subjects with similar levels of insulin sensitivity (75). This response translates into a leftward shift of the insulin feedback loop, namely a reduced disposition index in obese youth with NGT and higher glucose levels.

A secondary mechanism of compensating for peripheral insulin resistance, in conjunction with increased insulin secretion, is reduced insulin clearance. Lower hepatic first-pass metabolism of insulin facilitates a greater systemic insulin concentration and is proportional to increasing insulin resistance in obese youth. When insulin resistance is marked, insulin clearance reaches a trough beyond which it does not decrease further. At this phase, increased insulin secretion remains the sole compensatory response, and hyperglycemia occurs when the amount of insulin required exceeds β-cell capacity. We performed a large number of oral glucose tolerance tests in obese children and adolescents with NGT and IGT (76). We then divided those with NGT into tertiles of insulin sensitivity and compared them with their counterparts with IGT. We demonstrated that those with IGT are as severely insulin resistant and have similar insulin clearance as the most resistant subjects with NGT. Early insulin secretion increases and insulin clearance decreases with worsening insulin resistance in subjects with NGT, yet in subjects with IGT, insulin secretion is reduced, indicating β-cell failure, and explains the observed hyperglycemia.

THE DYNAMICS OF ALTERED GLUCOSE METABOLISM IN CHILDHOOD

Data on longitudinal assessment of children and adolescents with insulin resistance with normal or IGT is scarce in the literature. We published our preliminary observations of repeated oral glucose tolerance tests in obese youth without pharmacologic intervention and demonstrated that IGT is a highly dynamic condition in this age group (77). During a follow-up period of less than two years, 25% of youth with IGT developed overt or silent T2D, while 45% converted to NGT. Importantly, those who developed T2D were more obese at baseline and continued to gain weight during follow-up, while those who converted to NGT maintained their body weight without further weight gain. Youth with the greatest degree of obesity at baseline tended to deteriorate their glucose metabolism (raised their two-hour glucose level over time) regardless of their weight change over time (78). When β-cell demand was compared between subjects with a similar disposition index and different levels of insulin sensitivity (implicating different degrees of insulin secretion)—it was clearly shown that those with greater β-cell demand at baseline tended to deteriorate their glucose metabolism over time, even when adjusted for weight changes during the follow-up period.

SUMMARY

Obese youth are at significant risk for the development of altered glucose metabolism and other elements of the MS. The degree of obesity and the pattern of lipid partitioning are strongly related to the metabolic phenotype of the obese child. Lipid deposition in insulin-responsive tissues (such as liver and muscle) and secretion of cytokines from other lipid depots (visceral and subcutaneous fat) have a strong impact on glucose metabolism and metabolic risk.

REFERENCES

1. Kaufman FR. T2DM in children and youth. Rev Endocr Metab Disord 2003; 4(1):33–42.
2. Fagot-Campagna A, Pettitt DJ, Engelgau MM, et al. T2DM among North American children and adolescents: an epidemiologic review and a public health perspective. J Pediatr 2000; 136(5):664–672.
3. Ogden CL, Flegal KM, Carroll MD, et al. Prevalence and trends in overweight among US children and adolescents, 1999–2000. JAMA 2002; 288(14):1728–1732.
4. Kahn SE. The relative contributions of insulin resistance and beta-cell dysfunction to the pathophysiology of T2DM. Diabetologia 2003; 46(1):3–19.
5. Bergman RN, Finegood DT, Kahn SE. The evolution of beta-cell dysfunction and insulin resistance in T2DM. Eur J Clin Invest 2002; 32(suppl 3):35–45.
6. Edelstein SL, Knowler WC, Bain RP. Predictors of progression from impaired glucose tolerance to NIDDM: an analysis of six prospective studies. Diabetes 1997; 46:701–710.
7. Diabetes Prevention Program Research Group. The diabetes prevention program: reduction in the incidence of T2DM with lifestyle intervention or metformin. N Engl J Med 2002; 346:393–403.

8. Tuomilehto J, Lindstrom J, Eriksson JG et al. Finnish Diabetes Prevention Study Group. Prevention of T2DM mellitus by changes in lifestyle among subjects with impaired glucose tolerance. N Engl J Med. 2001; 344(18):1343–1350.

9. Pan XR, Li GW, Hu YH, et al. Effects of diet and exercise in preventing NIDDM in people with impaired glucose tolerance. The Da Qing IGT and Diabetes Study. Diabetes Care 1997; 20(4):537–544.

10. Hu FB, Stampfer JM, Hafner SM, et al. Elevated risk of cardiovascular disease prior to clinical diagnosis of T2DM. Diabetes Care 2002; 25:1129–1134.

11. Haffner SM. Epidemiology of insulin resistance and its relation to coronary artery disease. Am J Cardiol 1999; 84(1A):11J–14J.

12. Reaven GM. Banting lecture 1988. Role of insulin resistance in human disease. Diabetes 1988; 37(12):1595–1607.

13. Third Report of the National Cholesterol Education Program Expert Panel on Detection, Evaluation and Treatment of High Blood Cholesterol in Adults (Adult Treatment Panel III): Executive Summary. Bethesda, MD: National Institutes of Health, 2001. NIH Publication N0 01–3670.

14. Cersosimo E, DeFronzo RA. Insulin resistance and endothelial dysfunction: the road map to cardiovascular diseases. Diabetes Metab Res Rev 2006; 22(6):423–436.

15. Kuczmarski RJ, Flegal KM. Criteria for definition of overweight in transition: background and recommendations for the United States. Am J Clin Nutr 2000; 72(5): 1074–1081.

16. Weiss R, Dziura J, Burgert TS, et al. Obesity and the metabolic syndrome in children and adolescents. N Engl J Med 2004; 350(23):2362–2374.

17. Freedman DS, Mei Z, Srinivasan SR, et al. Cardiovascular risk factors and excess adiposity among overweight children and adolescents: the Bogalusa Heart Study. J Pediatr 2007; 150(1):12–17.

18. Druet C, Dabbas M, Baltakse V, et al. Insulin resistance and the metabolic syndrome in obese French children. Clin Endocrinol 2006; 64(6):672–678.

19. de Ferranti SD, Gauvreau K, Ludwig DS, et al. Prevalence of the metabolic syndrome in American adolescents: findings from the Third National Health and Nutrition Examination Survey. Circulation 2004; 110(16):2494–2497.

20. Weiss R, Dufour S, Taksali SE, et al. Prediabetes in obese youth: a syndrome of impaired glucose tolerance, severe insulin resistance, and altered myocellular and abdominal fat partitioning. Lancet 2003; 362(9388):951–957.

21. Sinha R, Dufour S, Petersen KF, et al. Assessment of skeletal muscle triglyceride content by (1)H nuclear magnetic resonance spectroscopy in lean and obese adolescents: relationships to insulin sensitivity, total body fat, and central adiposity. Diabetes 2002; 51(4): 1022–1027.

22. Weiss R, Taksali SE, Dufour S, et al. The "obese insulin-sensitive" adolescent: importance of adiponectin and lipid partitioning. J Clin Endocrinol Metab 2005; 90(6): 3731–3737.

23. Rothman DL, Magnusson I, Cline G, et al. Decreased muscle glucose transport/phosphorylation is an early defect in the pathogenesis of non-insulin-dependent diabetes mellitus. Proc Natl Acad Sci U S A 1995; 92(4):983–987.

24. Krssak M, Falk Petersen K, Dresner A, et al. IMCL concentrations are correlated with insulin sensitivity in humans: a 1H NMR spectroscopy study. Diabetologia 1999; 42(1): 113–116.

25. Petersen KF, Befroy D, Dufour S, et al. Mitochondrial dysfunction in the elderly: possible role in insulin resistance. Science 2003; 300:1140–1142.

26. Petersen KF, Dufour S, Befroy D, et al. Impaired mitochondrial activity in the insulin-resistant offspring of patients with T2DM. N Engl J Med 2004; 350:664–671.

27. Morino K, Petersen KF, Dufour S, et al. Reduced mitochondrial density and increased IRS-1 serine phosphorylation in muscle of insulin-resistant offspring of type 2 diabetic parents. J Clin Invest 2005; 115(12):3587–3593.

28. Zderic TW, Davidson CJ, Schenk S, et al. High-fat diet elevates resting intramuscular triglyceride concentration and whole-body lipolysis during exercise. Am J Physiol Endocrinol Meta 2003; 286: E217–E225.

29. Helge JW, Watt PW, Richter EA, et al. Fat utilization during exercise: adaptation to a fat-rich diet increases utilization of plasma fatty acids and very low density lipoprotein-triacylglycerol in humans. J Physiol 2001; 537:1009–1020.
30. Shulman GI. Cellular mechanisms of insulin resistance. J Clin Invest 2000; 106(2): 171–176.
31. Griffin ME, Marcucci MJ, Cline GW, et al. Free fatty acid–induced insulin resistance is associated with activation of protein kinase C theta and alterations in the insulin signaling cascade. Diabetes 1999; 48:1270–1274.
32. Horowitz JF, Coppack SW, Paramore D, et al. Effect of short-term fasting on lipid kinetics in lean and obese women. Am J Physiol 1999; 276(2 pt 1):E278–E284.
33. Jensen MD, Haymond MW, Rizza RA, et al. Influence of body fat distribution on free fatty acid metabolism in obesity. Clin Invest 1989; 83(4):1168–1173.
34. Koutsari C, Jensen MD. Thematic review series: patient-oriented research. Free fatty acid metabolism in human obesity. J Lipid Res 2006; 47(8):1643–1650.
35. Lebovitz HE, Banerji MA. Point: visceral adiposity is causally related to insulin resistance. Diabetes Care 2005; 28(9):2322–2325.
36. Nielsen S, Guo Z, Johnson CM, et al. Splanchnic lipolysis in human obesity. J Clin Invest 2004; 113(11):1582–1588.
37. Tan GD, Goossens GH, Humphreys SM, et al. Upper and lower body adipose tissue function: a direct comparison of fat mobilization in humans. Obes Res 2004; 12(1): 114–118.
38. Guo Z, Hensrud DD, Johnson CM, et al. Regional postprandial fatty acid metabolism in different obesity phenotypes. Diabetes 1999; 48(8):1586–1592.
39. Fain JN, Madan AK, Hiler ML, et al. Comparison of the release of adipokines by adipose tissue, adipose tissue matrix, and adipocytes from visceral and subcutaneous abdominal adipose tissues of obese humans. Endocrinology 2004; 145:2273–2282.
40. Shimomura I, Funahashi T, Takahashi M, et al. Enhanced expression of PAI-1 in visceral fat: possible contributor to vascular disease in obesity. Nat Med 1996; 2:800–803.
41. Tsigos C, Kyrou I, Chala E, et al. Circulating tumor necrosis factor alpha concentrations are higher in abdominal versus peripheral obesity. Metabolism 1999; 48:1332–1335.
42. Yudkin JS, Juhan-Vague I, Hawe E, et al. Low-grade inflammation may play a role in the etiology of the metabolic syndrome in patients with coronary heart disease: the HIFMECH study. Metabolism 2004; 53:852–857.
43. Ridker PM, Cook N. Clinical usefulness of very high and very low levels of C-reactive protein across the full range of Framingham Risk Scores. Circulation 2004; 109: 1955–1959.
44. Bacha F, Saad R, Gungor N, et al. Obesity, regional fat distribution, and syndrome X in obese black versus white adolescents: race differential in diabetogenic and atherogenic risk factors. J Clin Endocrinol Metab 2003; 88(6):2534–2540.
45. Cruz ML, Bergman RN, Goran MI. Unique effect of visceral fat on insulin sensitivity in obese Hispanic children with a family history of T2DM. Diabetes Care 2002; 25(9): 1631–1636.
46. Lee S, Bacha F, Gungor N, et al. Racial differences in adiponectin in youth: relationship to visceral fat and insulin sensitivity. Diabetes Care 2006; 29(1):51–56.
47. Angulo P. Nonalcoholic fatty liver disease. N Eng J Med 2002; 346(16):1221–1231.
48. Ludwig J, Viggiano TR, McGill DB, et al. Nonalcoholic steatohepatitis: Mayo clinic experience with a hitherto unnamed disease. Mayo Clin Proc 1980; 55:434–438.
49. Diraison F, Moulin P, Beylot M. Contribution of hepatic de novo lipogenesis and reesterification of plasma non-esterified fatty acids to plasma triglyceride synthesis during non-alcoholic fatty liver disease. Diabetes Metab 2003; 29(5):478–485.
50. Parks EJ, Hellerstein MK. Thematic review series: patient-oriented research. Recent advances in liver triacylglycerol and fatty acid metabolism using stable isotope labeling techniques. J Lipid Res 2006; 47(8):1651–1660.
51. Roberts E. Nonalcoholic steatohepatitis in children. Curr Gastroenterol Rep 2003; 5: 253–259.
52. Lavine JE, Schwimmer JB. Nonalcoholic fatty liver disease in the pediatric population. Clin Liver Dis 2004; 8(3):549–558.

53. Tominaga K, Kurata JH, Chen YK, et al. Prevalence of fatty liver in Japanese children and relationship to obesity. An epidemiological ultrasonographic survey. Dig Dis Sci 1995; 40(9):2002–2009.
54. Franzese A, Vajro P, Argenziano A, et al. Liver involvement in obese children. Ultrasonography and liver enzyme levels at diagnosis and during follow-up in an Italian population. Dig Dis Sci 1997; 42(7):1428–1432.
55. Meltzer AA, Everhart JE. Association between diabetes and elevated serum alanine aminotransferase activity among Mexican Americans. Am J Epidemiol 1997; 146: 565–571.
56. Feldstein AE, Canbay A, Angulo P, et al. Hepatocyte apoptosis and fas expression are prominent features of human nonalcoholic steatohepatitis. Gastroenterology 2003; 125 (2):437–443.
57. Burgert TS, Taksali SE, Dziura J, et al. Alanine aminotransferase levels and fatty liver in childhood obesity: associations with insulin resistance, adiponectin, and visceral fat. J Clin Endocrinol Metab 2006; 91(11):4287–4294.
58. Weiss R, Dufour S, Taksali SE, et al. Prediabetes in obese youth: a syndrome of impaired glucose tolerance, severe insulin resistance, and altered myocellular and abdominal fat partitioning. Lancet 2003; 362(9388):951–957.
59. Kelley DE. Skeletal muscle triglycerides: an aspect of regional adiposity and insulin resistance. Ann N Y Acad Sci 2002; 967:135–145.
60. Petersen KF, Dufour S, Befroy D, et al. Impaired mitochondrial activity in the insulin-resistant offspring of patients with T2DM. N Engl J Med 2004; 350(7):664–671.
61. Wellen KE, Hotamisligil GS. Inflammation, stress, and diabetes. J Clin Invest 2005; 115 (5):1111–1119.
62. Leclerc V, Reichhart JM. The immune response of Drosophila melanogaster. Immunol Rev 2004; 198:59–71.
63. Beutler B. Innate immunity: an overview. Mol Immunol 2004; 40(12):845–859.
64. Rajala MW, Scherer PE. The adipocyte at the crossroads of energy homeostasis, inflammation and atherosclerosis. Endocrinology 2003; 144(9):3765–3773.
65. Weisberg SP, McCann D, Desai M, et al. Obesity is associated with macrophage accumulation in adipose tissue. J Clin Invest 2003; 112(12):1796–1808.
66. Matsuzawa Y, Funahashi T, Nakamura T. Molecular mechanism of metabolic syndromeX: contribution of adipocytokines adipocyte-derived bioactive substances. Ann N Y Acad Sci 1999; 892:146–154.
67. Pickup JC, Crook MA. Is type 2 diabetes mellitus a disease of the innate immune system? Diabetologia 1998; 41:1241–1248.
68. Taniguchi CM, Emanuelli B, Kahn CR. Critical nodes in signalling pathways: insights into insulin action. Nat Rev Mol Cell Biol 2006; 7(2):85–96.
69. Yudkin JS, Kumari M, Humphries SE, et al. Inflammation, obesity, stress and coronary heart disease: is interleukin-6 the link? Atherosclerosis 2000; 148:209–214.
70. Blake GJ, Ridker PM. Inflammatory biomarkers and cardiovascular risk prediction. J Intern Med 2002; 252:283–294.
71. Ford ES. National Health and Nutrition Examination Survey. C-reactive protein concentration and cardiovascular disease risk factors in children: findings from the National Health and Nutrition Examination Survey 1999–2000. Circulation 2003; 108(9):1053–1058.
72. Weiss R, Caprio S, Trombetta M, et al. Beta-cell function across the spectrum of glucose tolerance in obese youth. Diabetes 2005; 54(6):1735–1743.
73. Goran MI, Bergman RN, Avila Q, et al. Impaired glucose tolerance and reduced beta-cell function in overweight Latino children with a positive family history for type 2 diabetes. J Clin Endocrinol Metab 2004; 89(1):207–212.
74. Arslanian SA, Bacha F, Saad R, et al. Family history of type 2 diabetes is associated with decreased insulin sensitivity and an impaired balance between insulin sensitivity and insulin secretion in white youth. Diabetes Care 2005; 28(1):115–119.
75. Yeckel CW, Taksali SE, Dziura J, et al. The normal glucose tolerance continuum in obese youth: evidence for impairment in beta-cell function independent of insulin resistance. J Clin Endocrinol Metab 2005; 90(2):747–754.

76. Weiss R, Dziura JD, Burgert TS, et al. Ethnic differences in beta cell adaptation to insulin resistance in obese youth. Diabetologia 2006; 49(3):571–579.
77. Weiss R, Taksali SE, Tamborlane WV, et al. Predictors of changes in glucose tolerance status in obese youth. Diabetes Care 2005; 28(4):902–909.
78. Weiss R, Cali A, Dziura J, et al. Degree of obesity and glucose allostasis are major effectors of glucose tolerance dynamics in obese youth. Diabetes Care 2007; 30(7): 1845–1850.

9 Insulin Resistance and Insulin Secretion in the Pathophysiology of Youth Type 2 Diabetes

Fida Bacha
Division of Pediatric Endocrinology, Metabolism and Diabetes Mellitus, and Division of Weight Management and Wellness, Children's Hospital of Pittsburgh, Pittsburgh, Pennsylvania, U.S.A.

Silva Arslanian
Division of Weight Management and Wellness, Children's Hospital of Pittsburgh, Pittsburgh, Pennsylvania, U.S.A.

INTRODUCTION

Type 2 diabetes mellitus (T2DM), a diagnosis once restricted to the adult population, is now recognized as a disease of the pediatric age group with escalating numbers of new cases referred to as an "epidemic" by the American Diabetes Association (ADA) (1,2). A similar trend of increasing numbers has also been reported in children from around the world (3–12). T2DM is a heterogeneous condition in which social, behavioral, and environmental factors contribute to unravel the genetic susceptibility leading to the clinical expression of the disease. Insulin resistance and β-cell failure with inadequate insulin secretion are the pathophysiological abnormalities of T2DM. This chapter will review the physiology of insulin sensitivity and secretion during childhood growth and development, and the abnormalities in these that lead to T2DM.

PATHOPHYSIOLOGY OF TYPE 2 DIABETES

Type 2 diabetes is characterized by insulin resistance and relative insulin deficiency. Glucose homeostasis is maintained by a delicate balance between insulin secretion and insulin sensitivity of the peripheral tissues (muscle, liver, and adipose tissue) (13) so that the product of insulin sensitivity and β-cell function is constant for a given glucose tolerance in any one individual. This constant is referred to as the glucose disposition index (GDI) (Fig. 1) (14). Thus, when insulin sensitivity decreases, insulin secretion increases to maintain normoglycemia (15). Failure of this compensatory increase in insulin secretion may lead to the progression to glucose intolerance and diabetes.

Experience in adults indicate that both insulin resistance and impaired β-cell function are key components in the pathogenesis of T2DM (15,16). The sequence of development of these abnormalities in the pathogenesis of T2DM has been extensively debated. However, the overall consensus is that insulin resistance with compensatory hyperinsulinemia is the earliest abnormality with the subsequent step being impairment in insulin secretion, which leads to hyperglycemia and the clinical manifestation of diabetes (17,18). Consistent with the latter, our proposed hypothesis for the sequence of events leading to youth T2DM is depicted in Figure 2 (19). Even though pediatric data regarding the pathogenesis of youth T2DM remain

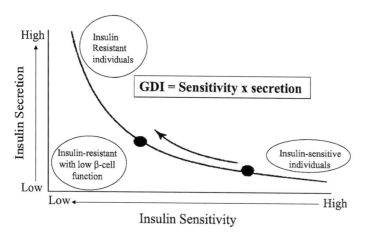

FIGURE 1 Hyperbolic relationship between insulin sensitivity and secretion. *Source*: Adapted from Ref. 14.

Proposed pathophysiology of youth-onset T2DM

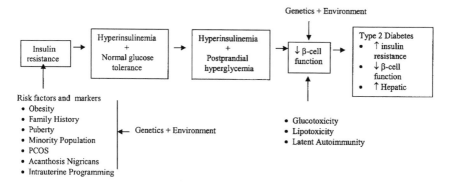

FIGURE 2 Proposed pathophysiology of youth-onset T2DM. *Source*: Adapted from Ref. 19.

fairly limited, this chapter summarizes the existing literature on the pathophysiology of youth T2DM and its risk factors.

INSULIN RESISTANCE VS. INSULIN SECRETION AS RISK FACTORS FOR YOUTH T2DM

Several risk factors, including obesity, particularly abdominal adiposity, minority ethnic background, family history of T2DM, puberty, polycystic ovary syndrome (PCOS), and intrauterine programming, predispose to youth T2DM. The common element among all these is insulin resistance. However, type 2 diabetes does not manifest unless these conditions are complicated by a defect in insulin secretion, leading to a disruption of the delicate balance that maintains glucose homeostasis. Below, we will discuss the current knowledge that supports this framework of thinking about the pathogenesis of T2DM in relationship to each of these risk factors.

Obesity

The increased prevalence of T2DM in childhood has been linked to the epidemic of childhood obesity in the United States and around the world (20,21). In the United States, the National Health and Nutrition Examination Survey (NHANES) update revealed that 31% of children aged 6 to 19 years are either overweight or at risk for overweight and 16% are overweight (BMI > 95%), with greater prevalence of overweight among non-Hispanic Black and Mexican-American adolescents (22). Not only overall obesity is on the rise but recent U.S. data indicate that waist circumference has increased by 1.4 inches between NHANES 1988–1994 and 1999–2004 among children aged 2 to 19 years (23). Similar data were reported in British youths (24). It is well established that obesity is associated with insulin resistance in all ethnic groups (25). This association is evident early in childhood with total body adiposity accounting for 55% of the variance in insulin sensitivity in Caucasian children (26). NHANES 1999–2002 data demonstrate that obesity is the most important risk factor for insulin resistance independent of age, sex, or ethnicity, with weight status accounting for 29.1% of the variance in homeostasis model assessment of insulin resistance (HOMA-IR) (27). The insulin resistance associated with obesity is manifested in lower insulin-stimulated glucose disposal, oxidation, and storage, as well as inability to suppress fat oxidation (28). However, not all obese adolescents have the same risk for insulin resistance. It appears that body fat topography plays a major role. In our studies, higher visceral adiposity was associated with ~40% lower in vivo insulin sensitivity in obese children independent of race (29) and was also related to significantly lower levels of the anti-diabetogenic hormone adiponectin (30). Thus, abdominally obese adolescents who have higher visceral adipose tissue and higher waist/hip ratio than their BMI and percent body fat matched obese peers are significantly more insulin resistant with a lower GDI indicative of an impaired β-cell compensation for the degree of insulin resistance (31). Moreover, waist circumference is a significant predictor of in vivo insulin sensitivity and the components of the metabolic syndrome after controlling for BMI percentiles (32,33). However, despite the presence of significant insulin resistance, the majority of these obese youths do not develop T2DM because of β-cell compensation as evidenced by elevated fasting and stimulated insulin levels in obese children (28,29,31,34). Therefore, although obesity, particularly abdominal adiposity, is a major risk factor for youth T2DM, the progression to T2DM does not occur unless there is β-cell failure.

Family History of T2DM

There is a strong evidence for a genetic component in T2DM, despite that relatively few susceptibility genes have thus far been identified (35,36). The genetic predisposition to T2DM is evidenced by the strong heritability of the disease (37). Studies in adult twins demonstrate a 50–76% concordance rate of T2DM in monozygotic twins and a heritability estimate of 61% for abnormal glucose tolerance and 26% for T2DM (38,39). A 40% lifetime risk of developing T2DM has been reported in first-degree relatives of T2DM patients (40).

A strong family history of T2DM is a consistent finding in the majority of youths with T2DM regardless of ethnic background (20,41–44). Adult studies have shown that markers of insulin resistance and β-cell dysfunction are present in high-risk adult populations one to two decades before the diagnosis of the disease (37,45,46) and predict the progression to T2DM (47). In adults, insulin secretion adjusted for the degree of insulin resistance is a more heritable trait than either insulin sensitivity or insulin secretion alone (48). Our studies demonstrate that family history of T2DM is associated with ~25% lower insulin sensitivity in pre-pubertal healthy African-American children compared with their peers without a family history of T2DM, despite similar body composition, abdominal adiposity, and fitness level (49). Also, healthy white children with a positive family history of T2DM have lower insulin sensitivity with an inadequate compensatory increase in insulin secretion resulting in a lower GDI compared with youth without a family history of the disease (50). Similarly, decreased β-cell function is reported in overweight pubertal Hispanic children with family history of T2DM (51). The superimposition of adverse environmental factors, such as excessive energy consumption and sedentary lifestyle, on this familial high risk profile of an impaired balance between insulin sensitivity and secretion may lead to T2DM.

Ethnic Background

The majority of the pediatric patients with T2DM in the United States belong to minority ethnic populations, including Native Americans, Pima Indians, Mexican-Americans, and African-Americans (1,20,52). In Pima Indian children, more than 5% of 15- to 19-year-old children are affected (20). The pathogenesis of T2DM in this population is attributed to a genetic predisposition to insulin resistance modified by lifestyle habits (43). Epidemiological and clinical studies indicate that black children are insulin resistant and hyperinsulinemic compared with their white peers (53–58). The hyperinsulinemia appears to be a compensatory response to the decreased insulin sensitivity, and is a result of both increased insulin secretion (55,56) and decreased insulin clearance (54,57,59). A study using genetic admixture analysis suggested that the higher insulin resistance in blacks may have a genetic basis, while the higher insulin secretion may be due to both genetic and environmental factors (60).

In the presence of obesity, there is a race differential in diabetogenic and atherogenic risk factors between black and white youths (29). Our studies demonstrate that black obese adolescents with high visceral fat have suboptimal compensatory increase in insulin secretion in the face of decreased insulin sensitivity, resulting in a lower GDI compared with their white peers (29). On the other hand, white obese adolescents with visceral adiposity appear to be more at risk for atherogenesis. Additionally, adiponectin levels have been reported to be lower in black compared with white healthy children of similar body composition (61,62). The lower adiponectin levels in black children may in part explain their lower insulin sensitivity (62). These findings suggest racial differences in diabetogenic profile with higher risk of progression to T2DM in blacks. Similar to the data in black children, insulin sensitivity was found to be significantly lower in Hispanic compared with non-Hispanic white children (63).

Puberty

The mean age of diagnosis of youth T2DM is 13.5 years, around the time of mid-puberty (19,20). Puberty is associated with transient physiologic insulin resistance manifesting as hyperinsulinemia in response to oral glucose tolerance test (OGTT) (64) and to intravenous glucose tolerance test (IVGTT) (65). In vivo measurement of insulin sensitivity using the hyperinsulinemic-euglycemic clamp technique demonstrated that insulin sensitivity is on average 30% lower in adolescents compared with both pre-pubertal children and young adults (66–69). This insulin resistance is compensated by increased insulin secretion (70), which leads to peripheral hyperinsulinemia. In addition, our longitudinal assessment of insulin sensitivity and secretion in healthy children who progressed from prepuberty to adolescence was consistent with the cross-sectional observations showing 50% decline in insulin sensitivity, compensated by a doubling of insulin secretion, maintaining glucose homeostasis (71).

The hormonal mechanisms responsible for pubertal insulin resistance have been investigated to demonstrate that sex steroids in males do not play a role, while growth hormone (GH) may. Administration of testosterone or dihydrotestosterone to adolescents with delayed puberty did not result in insulin resistance (56,72). On the other hand, studies have shown that insulin-stimulated glucose disposal cor-relates inversely with GH or insulin-like growth factor-I (IGF-I) levels (68,73,74). Administration of GH to non-GH-deficient adolescents with short stature resulted in hepatic insulin resistance and 17% deterioration in peripheral insulin sensitivity (75). Moreover, similar to cross-sectional observations, IGF-I levels explained 34% of the variance in insulin sensitivity with no correlation between sex steroids and measures of carbohydrate metabolism during puberty (71). Therefore, the well-known transient increase in GH secretion during normal puberty appears to be the cause of the pubertal insulin resistance, and not sex steroids (56,71,72,75). Both GH secretion and insulin resistance reverse to prepubertal levels with completion of puberty, while sex steroids remain elevated further supporting a role for GH and not sex hormones. It is therefore conceivable that the evolution of insulin resistance during adolescence may precipitate the imbalance between insulin action and secretion in a child with a predisposition to T2DM.

Polycystic Ovary Syndrome

PCOS affects 5–10% of the females in the reproductive age group and is charac-terized by hyperandrogenism and amenorrhea or oligomenorrhea secondary to chronic anovulation (76). Insulin resistance and/or hyperinsulinemia are major components of PCOS not only in obese but also in lean adult women affected by this condition (77). A similar profile is present in adolescent girls with PCOS (76). Moreover, 30–40% of women with PCOS have impaired glucose tolerance (IGT) and 7.5–10% have T2DM by the fourth decade (78,79). Among PCOS adolescents, a screening oral glucose tolerance test revealed that ~30% had IGT and ~4% were diabetic (80). Our studies in obese adolescents with PCOS revealed that insulin sensitivity is ~50% lower in PCOS versus obese matched controls (81). Moreover, adolescents with PCOS and IGT have 40% lower first-phase insulin secretion and thus lower GDI compared with those with normal glucose tolerance (NGT) (82). The presence of this metabolic profile in adolescents in the early stages of PCOS suggests a significant increase in the risk for T2DM.

Intrauterine Programming

Epidemiologic and clinical studies conducted largely in the adult population suggest a link between in utero events and subsequent risk of T2DM and cardio-vascular disease (CVD) (83–86). This led to the "Intrauterine Programming" or fetal origins hypothesis, which has been supported by some clinical studies (87–90) but not by others (91). Studies in young adults and in the pediatric age group are limited, with some suggesting decreased insulin resistance in children born small for gestational age (92–94), others demonstrating a defect in insulin secretion (95). Others suggest that obesity is a more powerful determinant of insulin resistance than size at birth (96,97). The picture is compounded by the influence of "catch-up" growth with the highest levels of insulin resistance reported in children of low birth weight but high BMI and fat mass in childhood (93,98). A major deficiency in many of these studies is the absence of body composition and abdominal fat determination, which significantly impact insulin resistance.

The other extreme of over nutrition of the fetus appears to have long-term effects on obesity and glucose tolerance (83,99) with offspring of mothers having diabetes during pregnancy reported to have a higher frequency of childhood obesity and earlier onset of IGT (100,101) and diabetes (99,102). Rates of IGT are around 20% in adolescent offsprings of mothers who had diabetes during pregnancy (101). Thus, a history of maternal diabetes during gestation imparts a high risk for T2DM in youth.

INSULIN RESISTANCE VS. INSULIN SECRETION IN PREDIABETES

Prediabetes defined as the presence of impaired fasting glucose (IFG) or IGT has been associated with greater risk for T2DM and CVD in adults (103,104). The debate continues in the literature about the significance of the prediabetic state (IFG vs. IGT) and whether it implies a defect in insulin secretion or insulin resistance.

The prevalence and significance of these conditions in terms of risk for progression to diabetes and risk for CVD in the pediatric population is largely unknown. The prevalence of IGT and T2DM in children varies depending on the population studied. An obesity clinic-based study found 25% IGT in 4- to 10-year-olds, and 21% in 11- to 18-year-olds, and around 4% T2DM (105). Another study in high-risk Latino children with positive family history of T2DM revealed that 28% of the children had IGT (106). However, much lower rates of IGT ranging from 4.1% to 4.5% were reported in children recruited from the community (107,108).

In longitudinal studies in populations at high risk for developing T2DM, such as the Pima Indians of Arizona (109), the progression from NGT to IGT was associated with an increase in body weight, worsening in insulin sensitivity, and a decrease in the acute insulin secretory response to intravenous glucose. Progression from IGT to diabetes was associated with further increase in body weight, impairment in insulin sensitivity, and β-cell function, as well as an increase in hepatic glucose output (109). Similar findings were reported by Festa et al. in a group of African American, Caucasian, and Hispanic adults (110). Longitudinal studies are not available in the pediatric age group. Studies using different methodologies have shown conflicting results. Obese children and adolescents with IGT compared with NGT were reported to have higher BMI, worse fasting indices of insulin resistance, and a tendency ($p = 0.09$) for lower insulinogenic index (105), but insulin secretion was estimated to be similar between the two groups. The same investigators subsequently reported, using mathematical modeling of the hyperglycemic clamp data, that obese adolescents with IGT had a defect in first-phase insulin secretion but not in second phase insulin secretion (111). In overweight Latino children with family history of type 2 diabetes, insulin sensitivity and acute insulin response were not different but GDI was lower in IGT (106).

In our studies, obese adolescent girls with PCOS, IGT versus NGT of similar body composition, and abdominal fat distribution had similar insulin sensitivity, but lower first-phase insulin secretion and lower GDI (82). The different findings in various studies can be explained by the different methodologies used and the different BMI and body composition between the NGT and IGT groups evaluated in some of the former studies. Our findings in PCOS girls were confirmed when we compared overweight adolescents with NGT to subjects with IGT and T2DM of similar body composition and abdominal adiposity, using the clamp methodology. Adolescents with diabetes or IGT compared with obese controls of similar body composition and abdominal adiposity had no significant difference in insulin sensitivity, lower first phase insulin secretion, and lower GDI (112). Type 2 diabetes was further characterized by a defect in second-phase insulin secretion (112).

Similar to the risk conferred by IGT status, IFG is recognized as an independent risk factor for progression T2DM in adults (113,114). The change in the definition of IFG (Fasting blood glucose 100–125 mg/dL) (104) has led to an almost fourfold increase in the prevalence of IFG in adults (115). A study of obese children with IGT showed that the prevalence of IFG (based on the former threshold of >110 mg/dL) was extremely low (<0.08%) (105). Our studies using the new ADA criterion for IFG (100–125 mg/dL) suggest a higher number of overweight children at risk for IFG, and that even at a young age, youth with IFG have worse CVD risk profiles than those with normal fasting glucose (116). These findings are consistent with those reported recently from the NHANES 1999–2000 data, which revealed a prevalence of IFG of 7% in U.S. adolescents who also had a worse CVD risk profile with higher total and low-density lipoprotein cholesterol, lower high-density lipoprotein cholesterol, and higher systolic blood pressure (117).

Epidemiologic studies suggest that insulin resistance measured by HOMA-IR is higher in subjects with IFG than in those with IGT (118,119). On the contrary, others reported that IFG is associated with β-cell dysfunction measured by HOMA (120), whereas IGT was associated with insulin resistance (120,121). However, the IGT groups also had a higher BMI in the latter two studies (120,121). In Pima-Indians, a study using euglycemic clamps and IVGTT revealed similar defect in insulin sensitivity in IFG and IGT but lower insulin secretion in IFG (122). In the Insulin Resistance Atherosclerosis Study (123) where insulin resistance was measured using the frequently sampled intravenous glucose tolerance test (FSIVGTT), it was found that adults with IGT had lower insulin sensitivity and increased acute insulin response (123). In overweight Latino children aged 8 to 13 years, those with IFG had lower GDI compared to those with NFG of similar BMI and body composition, evaluated by FSIVGTT (124). Our recent studies in adolescents with IFG compared to those with IGT and NGT of similar body composition and abdominal adiposity reveal that adolescents with IGT seem to have a greater impairment in insulin sensitivity whereas insulin secretion is more significantly impaired in those with IFG (125). This resulted in a similar reduction in GDI in IFG and IGT adolescents compared to those of NGT, suggesting increased risk for future type 2 diabetes in both.

INSULIN RESISTANCE VS. INSULIN SECRETION IN YOUTH WITH T2DM

Studies on the metabolic abnormalities in youth with type 2 diabetes are very limited. One study evaluated insulin and glucagon response to a mixed liquid meal (Sustacal) tolerance test in 24 patients with T2DM, and 24 control subjects (aged 9–20 years, matched for BMI and pubertal stage) (126). Children with T2DM had relative hypoinsulinemia and hyperglucagonemia indicating pancreatic β- and α-cell dysfunctions. However, insulin resistance was not measured. In a study from Japan (34), using FSIVGTT, obese nondiabetic and obese diabetic groups were equally insulin resistant. The diabetic group had lower, first-phase insulin release and thus lower GDI. However, there was no evaluation of body composition and body fat topography.

Our group recently demonstrated that both insulin sensitivity and insulin secretion are impaired in adolescents with T2DM, utilizing the hyperinsulinemic-euglycemic clamp technique to measure in vivo insulin sensitivity and the hyperglycemic clamp to measure in vivo insulin secretion, in addition to stable isotope methodology to measure hepatic glucose production (127). Obese adolescents with T2DM of short duration were compared with obese control subjects of similar age, BMI, body composition, and pubertal stage (127). Youth with T2DM compared with obese controls had ~1.3 times higher hepatic glucose production, ~50% lower in vivo insulin sensitivity, ~74% lower first-phase insulin secretion, and ~53% lower second-phase insulin secretion. Additionally, proinsulin to insulin ratio was significantly higher in T2DM in further support of a failing β cell. Thus, GDI was ~86% lower in adolescents with T2DM indicative of severe impairment in glucose homeostasis. Moreover, HbA1C levels correlated with first-phase insulin secretion (Fig. 3) (127). Our findings were in agreement with the

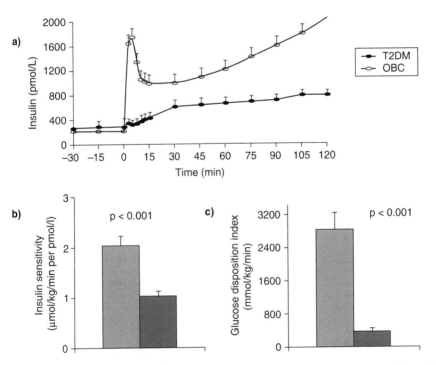

FIGURE 3 Insulin levels during the hyperglycemic clamp (*Panel a*); Insulin sensitivity during a three-hour hyperinsulinemic (80 μ/m²/min)-euglycemic clamp in adolescents with T2DM versus obese controls (*Panel b*); GDI in T2DM adolescents and obese controls (*Panel c*). *Source*: Adapted from Ref. 127.

literature in adults with T2DM (15). In a follow-up study to ours, another group of investigators using different methodologies reported on adolescents with T2DM of widely varying duration of diabetes. Their results were consistent with our findings with regards to insulin resistance (128). However, contrary to our observation, these authors did not show significant differences between diabetics and controls in proinsulin/insulin ratio, nor in glucagon levels which is in contrast to the finding by others (126). These contrasting findings could be attributed to the wide difference in duration of diabetes in the former study as well as the wide range of HbA1C levels of the patients, both of which are important factors that modulate islet cell function. In another very small study, it was demonstrated that there is remarkable variation in insulin secretion in adolescents with T2DM (129). This observation could have resulted from the fact that there were too many differences among the diabetic subjects, including the degree of obesity, ethnicity, duration of diabetes, and different therapeutic modalities, all of which could impact insulin secretion (130). In summary, the limited pediatric data in T2DM suggest severe impairment in insulin secretion early in the course of the disease. This could imply the potential need for starting insulin replacement therapy early in youth T2DM in order to maintain glycemic control and prevent diabetes-related complications (131).

Several adult studies, particularly the U.K. Prospective Diabetes Study (UKPDS), demonstrated that at the time of clinical diagnosis of adult T2DM there is already a 50% loss of β-cell function, with further deterioration on average by 7% per year (132). Limited observations by our group suggest that the deterioration in β-cell function in youth T2DM may be accelerated to ∼15% per year (133). This represents a threefold faster decline in β-cell function in youth compared with adults. Additional studies are needed, however, to explore whether or not there is an accelerated loss of β-cell function in youth with T2DM, and what are the determinants of it. Such an observation may indicate the need for earlier and more aggressive use of insulin therapy in youth with T2DM.

PANCREATIC AUTOANTIBODIES IN YOUTH WITH A CLINICAL PHENOTYPE OF T2DM

Type 2 diabetes and type 1 diabetes are classically viewed as having distinct clinical features at presentation and different pathogenesis. However, with the increasing epidemic of obesity in children in the general population, it is becoming hard to clinically distinguish T2DM from T1DM especially at the onset of the disease. Features that may be helpful in distinguishing T2DM from T1DM are obesity, signs of insulin resistance (acanthosis nigricans, hypertension, PCOS), family history of T2DM, minority ethnicity, and elevated C-peptide levels (2). However, the increase in the prevalence of obesity in children with T1DM (134) makes it even more difficult to distinguish T2DM from T1DM in obese children. Furthermore, T1DM-associated autoantibodies, including glutamic-acid decarboxylase (GADA), islet cell antibodies (ICA), islet antigen 2 (IA-2), and insulin antibodies (IAA) are relatively common in clinically diagnosed patients with T2DM, with different studies reporting frequencies from 30% to 75% (135–138). However, little is known whether the pathophysiological mechanisms are different in the presence of autoantibodies and/or other markers of autoimmunity in children who present with a clinical picture of T2DM, and whether or not their clinical course is different. Data from the UKPDS, which measured ICA and GADA at diagnosis of T2DM in 3672 patients between 25 and 65 years, revealed that 12% of patients had either ICA or GADA, and 4% had both. The presence of antibodies was the major predictor of subsequent need for insulin therapy. However, this was more noticeable in the younger age group. In the group aged 34 years or younger, 94% of patients with ICA and 84% of those with GADA required insulin therapy within 6 years, compared to only 44% with ICA and 34% among patients older than 55 years (139). Data from the Pittsburgh Cohort of the Cardiovascular Health Study, which measured GAD65 and IA-2 autoantibodies in 196 patients with T2DM and in 94 nondiabetic control subjects over the age of 65 years found that 12% of T2DM patients had autoantibodies against GAD65 and/or IA-2, significantly higher than the 1.1% prevalence in the nondiabetic individuals. No differences were seen in the percentage of insulin requirement in the two groups (140).

At the present, absence of islet autoimmune markers is a prerequisite for the accurate diagnosis of T2DM in children and adolescents (2). Clinically, the significance of the presence of autoantibodies in some youth with what appears to be T2DM is uncertain. However, observations of First Nation youth of Manitoba with T2DM revealed positive ICA titers in 4 of 14 children who did not require insulin during 10 years of follow-up (141). Recently, we evaluated the significance of the presence of autoantibodies (GADA and IA-2) in youth with a clinical diagnosis of T2DM with respect to insulin sensitivity and secretion. The antibody-positive and antibody-negative children with a clinical diagnosis of T2DM had similar age, body composition, abdominal adiposity, and HbA1C. The antibody-negative group had significantly lower insulin sensitivity but higher insulin secretion, while the antibody-positive group had severe impairment in insulin secretion but not in insulin sensitivity (142). Therefore, at the moment the limited metabolic findings in patients with a clinical phenotype of T2DM and positive pancreatic autoantibodies would suggest that these patients have T1DM against the backdrop of the obese phenotype. In these patients, insulin secretion is severely impaired or absent, but they lack the severe insulin resistance, which is the typical of the genetics of T2DM. Prospective studies are needed to identify the long-term consequences of these findings.

SUMMARY

Genetic as well as environmental factors modulate the risk for T2DM in youth. The interplay between insulin resistance and insulin secretion determines whether risk factors translate into a disorder of glucose regulation (IGT or IFG) and subsequent development of T2DM. Prevention efforts should aim at maintaining insulin secretion and improving insulin sensitivity in order to maintain normoglycemia. This is best achieved by early intervention in the pediatric age group to prevent the escalating epidemic of obesity and its consequent comorbidities, particularly T2DM. Future investigations are paramount to understanding the clinical course and the complications in youth with T2DM with careful attention to the presence or absence of pancreatic autoimmunity.

ACKNOWLEDGMENTS

This work was supported by the United States Public Health Service grant RO1 HD27503 (SA), K24 HD01357 (SA), the Thrasher Research Fund (NG & FB), MO1-RR00084 General Clinical Research Center, The Pediatric Clinical and Translational

Research Center at Children's Hospital of Pittsburgh UL1 RR024153, Eli Lilly and Company (SA), and the Renziehausen Trust Fund. We are indebted to the children and their parents participating in our research studies which facilitated our understanding of T2DM and related conditions.

REFERENCES

1. Fagot-Campagna A, Pettitt D, Engelgau MM, et al. Type 2 diabetes among North American children and adolescents: an epidemiologic review and a public health perspective. J Pediatr 2000; 136:664–672.
2. American Diabetes Association. Type 2 diabetes in children and adolescents. Diabetes Care 2000; 23:381–389.
3. Ehtisham S, Barrett TG, Shaw NJ. Type 2 diabetes mellitus in UK children—an emerging problem. Diabet Med 2000; 17:867–871.
4. Drake AJ, Smith A, Betts PR, et al. Type 2 diabetes in obese white children. Arch Dis Child 2002; 86:207–208.
5. Holl RW, Grabert M, Krause U, et al. Prevalence and Clinical characteristics of patients with non-type 1 diabetes in the pediatric age range: analysis of a multicenter database including 20,410 patietns from 148 centers in Germany and Austria. Diabetologia 2003; 46(suppl 2):A26.
6. Zachrisson I, Tibell C, Bang P, et al. Prevalence of type 2 diabetes among known cases of diabetes aged 0-18 years in Sweden. Diabetologia 2003; 46(suppl 2):A25.
7. Chan JC, Hawkins BR, Cockram CS. A Chinese family with non-insulin-dependent diabetes of early onset and severe diabetic complications. Diabet Med 1990; 7:211–214.
8. Kitagawa T, Owada M, Urakami T, et al. Epidemiology of type 1 (insulin-dependent) and type 2 (non-insulin-dependent) diabetes mellitus in Japanese children. Diabetes Res Clin Pract 1994; 24:S7–S13.
9. Tajima N. Type 2 diabetes in children and adolescents in Japan. Int Diab Monit 2002; 14:1–5.
10. Wei JN, Sung FC, Lin CC, et al. National surveillance for type 2 diabetes mellitus in Taiwanese children. JAMA 2003; 290:1345–1350.
11. Kadiki O, Reddy M, Marzouk A. Incidence of insulin-dependent diabetes (IDDM) and non insulin-dependent diabetes (NIDDM) (0–34 years at onset) in Benghazi, Libya. Diabetes Res Clin Prac 1996; 32:165–173.
12. Haines L, Wan KC, Lynn R, et al. Rising incidence of type 2 diabetes in children in the U.K. Diabetes Care 2007; 30:1097–1101.
13. Kahn SE. Regulation of β-cell function in vivo: from health to disease. Diabetes Rev 1996; 4:372–389.
14. Arslanian SA. Clamp techniques in pediatrics: what have we learned? Horm Res 2005; 64(suppl 3):16–24.
15. Kahn SE. The importance of β-cell failure in the development and progression of type 2 diabetes. J Clin Endocrinol Metab 2001; 86:4047–4058.
16. DeFronzo RA. Lilly Lecture 1987. The triumvirate: beta-cell, muscle, liver. A collusion responsible for NIDDM. Diabetes 1988; 37:667–687.
17. Kasuga M. Insulin resistance and pancreatic β cell failure. J Clin Invest 2006; 116: 1756–1760.
18. Kahn SE, Hull RL, Utzschneider KM. Mechanisms linking obesity to insulin resistance and type 2 diabetes. Nature 2006; 444:840–846.
19. Arslanian SA. Type 2 diabetes mellitus in children: clinical aspects and risk factors. Horm Res 2002; 57(suppl 1):19–28.
20. Dabelea D, Pettitt DJ, Jones KL, et al. Type 2 diabetes mellitus in minority children and adolescents. An emerging problem. Endocrinol Metab Cli North Am 1999; 28:709–729.
21. Rosenbloom AL, Joe JR, Young RS, et al. Emerging epidemic of type 2 diabetes in youth. Diabetes Care 1999; 22:345–354.
22. Hedley AA, Ogden CL, Johnson CL, et al. Prevalence of overweight and obesity among US children, adolescents, and adults, 1999–2002. JAMA 2004; 291:2847–2850.

23. Li C, Ford ES, Mokdad AH, et al. Recent trends in waist circumference and waist-height ratio among US children and adolescents. Pediatrics 2006; 118:1390–1398.
24. McCarthy HD, Ellis SM, Cole TJ. Central overweight and obesity in British youth aged 11-16 years: cross sectional surveys of waist circumference. BMJ 2003; 326:624–626.
25. Cossrow N, Falkner B. Race/ethnic issues in obesity and obesity-related comorbidities. J Clin Endocrinol Metab 2004; 89:2590–2594.
26. Arslanian SA, Suprasongsin C. Insulin sensitivity, lipids, and body composition in childhood: is "syndromeX" present? J Clin Endocrinol Metab 1996; 81:1058–1062.
27. Lee JM, Okumura MJ, Davis MM, et al. Prevalence and determinants of insulin resistance among U.S. adolescents. Diabetes Care 2006; 29:2427–2432.
28. Caprio S, Tamborlane WV. Metabolic impact of obesity in childhood. Endocrinol Metab Clin N Am 1999; 28:731–747.
29. Bacha F, Saad R, Gungor N, et al. Obesity, regional fat distribution and syndrome X in obese black vs white adolescents: race differential in diabetogenic and atherogenic risk factors. J Clin Endocrinol Metab 2003; 88:2534–2540.
30. Bacha F, Saad R, Gungor N, et al. Adiponectin in youth: relationship to visceral adiposity, insulin sensitivity, and beta-cell function. Diabetes Care 2004; 27:547–552.
31. Bacha F, Saad R, Gungor N, et al. Are obesity-related metabolic risk factors modulated by the degree of insulin resistance in adolescents? Diabetes Care 2006; 29:1613–1618.
32. Lee S, Bacha F, Gungor N, et al. Waist circumference is an independent predictor of insulin resistance in African-American and White youth. J Pediatr 2006; 148:188–194.
33. Lee S, Bacha F, Arslanian S. Waist circumference, blood pressure and lipid components of the metabolic syndrome. J Pediatr 2006; 149:809–816.
34. Kobayashi K, Amemiya S, Higashida K, et al. Pathogenic factors of glucose intolerance in obese Japanese adolescents with type 2 diabetes. Metabolism 2000; 49:186–191.
35. Hansen L, Pedersen O. Genetics of type 2 diabetes mellitus: status and perspectives. Diabetes Obes Metab 2005; 7:122–135.
36. Sladek R, Rocheleau G, Rung J, et al. A genome-wide association study identifies novel risk loci for type 2 diabetes. Nature 2007; 10:1–5.
37. Kahn CR. Banting lecture: insulin action, diabetogenes, and the cause of type II diabetes. Diabetes 1994; 43:1066–1084.
38. Poulsen P, Kyvik KO, Vaag A, et al. Heritability of type II (non-insulin-dependent) diabetes mellitus and abnormal glucose tolerance—a population-based twin study. Diabetologia 1999; 42:139–145.
39. Medici F, Hawa M, Ianari A, et al. Concordance rate for type II diabetes mellitus in monozygotic twins: actuarial analysis. Diabetologia 1999; 42:146–150.
40. Zimmet P, Turner R, McCarty D, et al. Crucial points at diagnosis. Type 2 diabetes or slow type 1 diabetes. Diabetes Care 1999; 22(suppl 2):B59–B64.
41. Pinhas-Hamiel O, Dolan LM, Daniels SR, et al. Increased incidence of non-insulin dependent diabetes mellitus among adolescents. J Pediatr 1996; 128:608–615.
42. Scott C, Smith J, Cradock M, et al. Characteristics of youth-onset non-insulin dependent diabetes mellitus and insulin-dependent diabetes mellitus at diagnosis. Pediatrics 1997; 100:84–91.
43. Knowler WC, Pettitt DJ, Saad MF. Diabetes mellitus in the Pima Indians: incidence, risk factors and pathogenesis. Diabetes Metab Rev 1990; 6:1–27.
44. Glaser NS. Non-insulin-dependent diabetes mellitus in childhood and adolescence. Pediatr Clin North Am 1997; 44:307–337.
45. Martin BC, Warram JH, Krolewski AS, et al. Role of glucose and insulin resistance in development of type 2 diabetes mellitus: results of a 25-year follow up study. Lancet 1992; 340:925–929.
46. Bonadonna RC, Stumvoll M, Fritsche A, et al. Altered homeostatic adaptation of first- and second-phase β-cell secretion in the offspring of patients with type 2 diabetes. Diabetes 2003; 52:470–480.
47. Lillioja S, Mott DM, Spraul M, et al. Insulin resistance and insulin secretory dysfunction as precursors of non-insulin-dependent diabetes mellitus: prospective studies of Pima Indians. N Engl J Med 1993; 329:1988–1992.

48. Elbein SC, Hasstedt SJ, Wegner K, et al. Heritability of pancreatic β-cell function among nondiabetic members of Caucasian familial type 2 diabetic kindreds. J Clin Endocrinol Metab 1999; 84:1398–1403.
49. Danadian K, Balasekaren G, Lewy V, et al. Insulin sensitivity in African-American children with and without family history of type 2 diabetes. Diabetes Care 1999; 22:1325–1329.
50. Arslanian SA, Bacha F, Saad R, et al. Family history of type 2 diabetes is associated with decreased insulin sensitivity and an impaired balance between insulin sensitivity and insulin secretion in white youth. Diabetes Care 2005; 28:127–131.
51. Ball GDC, Weigensberg MJ, Cruz ML, et al. Insulin sensitivity, insulin secretion and β-cell function during puberty in overweight Hispanic children with a family history of type 2 diabetes. Int J Obes 2005; 29:1471–1477.
52. Dean H. NIDDM-Y in First Nation children in Canada. Clin Pediatr 1998; 37:89–96.
53. Svec F, Nastasi K, Hilton C, et al. Black-White contrasts in insulin levels during pubertal development. The Bogalusa Heart Study. Diabetes 1992; 41:313–317.
54. Jiang X, Srinivasan SR, Radhakrishnamurthy B, et al. Racial (Black-White) differences in insulin secretion and clearance in adolescents: The Bogalusa Heart Study. Pediatrics 1996; 97:357–360.
55. Arslanian S, Suprasongsin C. Differences in the in vivo insulin secretion and sensitivity in healthy black vs white adolescents. J Pediatr 1996; 129:440–444.
56. Arslanian S, Suprasongsin C. Testosterone treatment in adolescents with delayed puberty: changes in body composition, protein, fat and glucose metabolism. J Clin Endocrinol Metab 1997; 82:3213–3220.
57. Arslanian SA, Saad R, Lewy V, et al. Hyperinsulinemia in African-American children: decreased insulin clearance and increased insulin secretion and its relationship to insulin sensitivity. Diabetes 2002; 51:3014–3019.
58. Gutin B, Islam S, Manos T, et al. Relation of percentage of body fat and maximal aerobic capacity to risk factors for atherosclerosis and diabetes in Black and White seven-to-eleven-year-old children. J Pediatr 1994; 125:847–852.
59. Gower B, Granger WM, Franklin F, et al. Contribution of insulin secretion and clearance to glucose-induced insulin concentration in african-american and Caucasian children. J Clin Endocrinol Metab 2002; 87:2218–2224.
60. Gower BA, Fernandez JR, Beasley TM, et al. Using genetic admixture to explain racial differences in insulin-related phenotypes. Diabetes 2003; 52:1047–1051.
61. Bacha F, Saad R, Gungor N, et al. Does adiponectin explain the lower insulin sensitivity and hyperinsulinemia of African-american children? Pediatr Diab 2005; 6:100–102.
62. Lee S, Bacha F, Gungor N, et al. Racial differences in adiponectin in youth: relationship to visceral fat and insulin sensitivity. Diabetes Care 2006; 29:51–56.
63. Goran MI, Bergman RN, Cruz ML, et al. Insulin resistance and associated compensatory responses in African American and Hispanic children. Diabetes Care 2002; 25:2184–2190.
64. Lestradet H, Deschamps I, Giron B. Insulin and free fatty acid levels during oral glucose tolerance tests and their relation to age in 70 healthy children. Diabetes 1976; 25:505–508.
65. Smith CP, Dunger DB, Williams AJ, et al. Relationship between insulin, insulin-like growth factor, I and dehydroepiandrosterone sulfate concentrations during childhood, puberty and adult life. J Clin Endocrinol Metab 1989; 68:932–937.
66. Amiel SA, Caprio S, Sherwin RS, et al. Insulin resistance of puberty: a defect restricted to peripheral glucose metabolism. J Clin Endocrinol Metab 1991; 72:277–282.
67. Bloch CA, Clemons P, Sperling MA. Puberty decreases insulin sensitivity. J Pediatr 1987; 110:481–487.
68. Arslanian SA, Kalhan SC. Correlations between fatty acid and glucose metabolism. Potential explanation of insulin resistance of puberty. Diabetes 1994; 43(7):908–914.
69. Moran A, Jacobs DR, Steinberger J, et al. Insulin resistance during puberty; results from clamp studies in 357 children. Diabetes 1999; 48:2039–2044.
70. Caprio S, Plewe G, Diamond MP, et al. Increased insulin secretion in puberty: a compensatory response to reductions in insulin sensitivity. J Pediatr 1989; 114:963–967.

71. Hannon T, Janosky J, Arslanian S. Longitudinal study of physiologic insulin resistance and metabolic changes of puberty. Pediatr Res 2006; 60:759–763.

72. Saad RJ, Keenan BS, Danadian K, et al. Dihydrotestosterone treatment in adolescents with delayed puberty: does it explain insulin resistance of puberty? J Clin Endocrinol Metab 2001; 86:4881–4886.

73. Amiel SA, Sherwin RS, Simenson DC, et al. Impaired insulin action in puberty. N Engl J Med 1986; 315:215–219.

74. Saad RJ, Danadian K, Lewy V, et al. Insulin resistance of puberty in African-American children: lack of a compensatory increase in insulin secretion. Pediatr Diab 2002; 3:4–9.

75. Hannon TS, Danadian K, Suprasongsin C, et al. Growth hormone treatment in adolescent males with idiopathic short stature: changes in body composition, protein, fat, and glucose metabolism. J Clin Endocrin Metab 2007; 92:3033–3039.

76. Arslanian SA, Witchel SF. Polycystic ovary syndrome in adolescents: is there an epidemic? Current Opinion in Endocrinology and Diabetes 2002; 9:32–42.

77. Dunaif A. Insulin action in the polycystic ovary syndrome. Endocrinol Metab Clin North Am 1999; 28:341–359.

78. Legro RS, Kunselman AR, Dodson WC, et al. Prevalence and predictors of risk for type 2 diabetes mellitus and impaired glucose tolerance in polycystic ovary syndrome: a prospective, controlled study in 254 affected women. J Clin Endocrinol Metab 1999; 84:165–169.

79. Ehrmann DA. Polycystic ovary syndrome. N Engl J Med 2005; 352:1223–1236.

80. Palmert MR, Gordon CM, Kartashov AI, et al. Screening for abnormal glucose tolerance in adolescents with polycystic ovary syndrome. J Clin Endocrinol Metab 2002; 87: 1017–1023.

81. Lewy VD, Danadian K, Witchel SF, et al. Early metabolic abnormalities in adolescent girls with polycystic ovarian syndrome. J Pediatr 2001; 138:38–44.

82. Arslanian SA, Lewy VD, Danadian K. Glucose intolerance in obese adolescents with polycystic ovary syndrome: roles of insulin resistance and beta-cell dysfunction and risk of cardiovascular disease. J Clin Endocrinol Metab 2001; 86:66–71.

83. Hales CN, Barker DJ. The thrifty phenotype hypothesis. Br Med Bull 2001; 60:5–20.

84. Hales CN, Barker DJ. Type 2 (non-insulin-dependent) diabetes mellitus: the thrifty phenotype hypothesis. Diabetologia 1992; 35:595–601.

85. Barker DJP, Hales CN, Fall CHD, et al. Type 2 (non-insulin-dependent) diabetes mellitus, hypertension and hyperlipidaemia (syndrome X): relation to reduced fetal growth. Diabetologia 1993; 36:62–67.

86. Rich-Edwards JW, Colditz GA, Stampfer MJ, et al. Birthweight and the risk for type 2 diabetes mellitus in adult women. Ann Intern Med 1999; 130:278–284.

87. Robinson S, Walton RJ, Clark PM, et al. The relation of fetal growth to plasma glucose in young men. Diabetologia 1992; 35:444–446.

88. Leger J, Levy-Marchal C, Bloch J, et al. Reduced final height and indications for insulin resistance in 20 year olds born small for gestational age: regional cohort study. Br Med J 1997; 315:341–349.

89. Jaquet D, Gaboriau A, Czernichow P, et al. Insulin resistance early in adulthood in subjects born with intrauterine growth retardation. J Clin Endocrinol Metab 2000; 85:1401–1406.

90. Valdez R, Athens MA, Thompsn GH, et al. Birthweight and adult health outcomes in a biethnic population in the USA. Diabetologia 1994; 37:624–631.

91. Hattersley A, Tooke J. The fetal insulin hypothesis: an alternative explanation of the association of low birth weight with diabetes and vascular disease. The Lancet 1999; 353:1789–1792.

92. Hofman PL, Cutfield WS, Robinson EM, et al. Insulin resistance in short children with intrauterine growth retardation. J Clin Endocrinol Metab 1997; 82:402–406.

93. Ong K, Petry C, Emmett P, et al. Insulin sensitivity and secretion in normal children related to size at birth, postnatal growth, and plasma insulin-like growth factor-I levels. Diabetologia 2004; 47:1064–1070.

94. Veening MA, van Weissenbruch MM, Delemarre-van de Waal HA. Glucose tolerance, insulin sensitivity, and insulin secretion in children born small for gestational age. J Clin Endocrinol Metab 2002; 87:4657–4661.

95. Jensen CB, Storgaard H, Dela F, et al. Early differential defects of insulin secretion and action in 19-year-old Caucasian men who had low birth weight. Diabetes 2002; 51: 1271–1280.
96. Whincup PH, Cook DG, Adshead F, et al. Childhood size is more strongly related than size at birth to glucose and insulin levels in 10-11 year old children. Diabetologia 1997; 40(3):319–326.
97. Wilkin TJ, Metcalf BS, Murphy MJ., et al. The relative contributions of birth weight, weight change, and current weight to insulin resistance in contemporary 5-year-olds. Diabetes 2002; 51:3468–3472.
98. Bavdekar A, Yajnik CS, Fall CHD, et al. Insulin resistance syndrome in 8-year-old Indian children. Diabetes 1999; 48:2422–2429.
99. Pettitt DJ, Baird HR, Aleck KA, et al. Diabetes mellitus in children following maternal diabetes during gestation. Diabetes 1982; 31:66A.
100. Silverman BL, Metzger BE, Cho NH, et al. Impaired glucose tolerance in adolescent offspring of diabetic mothers. Relationship to fetal hyperinsulinism. Diabetes Care 1995; 18:611–617.
101. Silverman BL, TA Rizzo, Cho NH, et al. Long-term effects of the intrauterine environment. The Northwestern University Diabetes in Pregnancy Center. Diabetes Care 1998; 21(suppl 2):B142–B149.
102. Pettitt DJ, Baird HR, Aleck KA, et al. Excessive obesity in offspring of Pima Indian women with diabetes during pregnancy. N Engl J Med 1983; 308:242–245.
103. The Expert Committee on the Diagnosis and Classification of Diabetes Mellitus. Report of the expert committee on the diagnosis and classification of diabetes mellitus. Diabetes Care 1997; 20:1183–1197.
104. The American Diabetes Association. Diagnosis and classification of diabetes mellitus. Diabetes Care 2004; 27(suppl 1):S5–S10.
105. Sinha R, Fisch G, Teague B, et al. Prevalence of impaired glucose tolerance among children and adolescents with marked obesity. N Engl J Med 2002; 346:802–810.
106. Goran MI, Bergman RN, Avila Q, et al. Impaired glucose tolerance and reduced β-cell function in overweight Latino children with a positive family history for type 2 diabetes. J Clin Endocrinol Metab 2004; 89:207–212.
107. Uwaifo GI, Elberg J, Yanovski JA. Impaired glucose tolerance in obese children and adolescents. N Eng J Med 2002; 347:290–292.
108. Invitti C, Gilardini L, Viberti G. Impaired glucose tolerance in obese children and adolescents. N Engl J Med 2002; 347:290–292.
109. Weyer C, Bogardus C, Mott DM, et al. The natural history of insulin secretory dysfunction and insulin resistance in the pathogenesis of type 2 diabetes mellitus. J Clin Invest 1999; 104:787–794.
110. Festa A, Williams K, D'Agostino R Jr., et al. The natural course of B-cell function in nondiabetic and diabetic individuals: The Insulin Resistance Atherosclerosis Study. Diabetes 2006; 55:1114–1120.
111. Weiss R, Caprio S, Trombetta M, et al. Beta-cell function across the spectrum of glucose tolerance in obese youth. Diabetes 2005; 54:1735–1743.
112. Bacha F, Gungor N, Arslanian S. Pre-diabetes in obese youth: a defect in insulin sensitivity (IS) or insulin secretion (ISC)? Diabetes 2006; 55(suppl 1):A68, 292–OR.
113. de Vegt F, Dekker JM, Jager A, et al. Relation of impaired fasting and postload glucose with incident type 2 diabetes in a Dutch population: the Hoorn Study. JAMA 2001; 285:2109–2113.
114. Qiao Q, Lindstrom J, Valle TT, et al. Progression to clinically diagnosed and treated diabetes from impaired glucose tolerance and impaired fasting glycaemia. Diabet Med 2003; 20:1027–1033.
115. Benjamin SM, Cadwell BL, Geiss LS, et al. A change in definition results in an increased number of adults with prediabetes in the United States. Arch Intern Med 2004; 164:2386.
116. Libman I, Marcus M, Kalarchian M, et al. Impaired fasting glucose according to the new ADA criteria: does it identify more youth at risk for cardiovascular disease? oral presentation at the American Diabetes Association Annual Meeting, Orlando, Florida, June 2004. Diabetes 2004; 53(suppl 2):294.

117. Williams DE, Cadwell BL, Cheng YJ, et al. Prevalence of impaired fasting glucose and its relationship with cardiovascular disease risk factors in US adolescents, 1999–2000. Pediatrics 2005; 116:1122–1126.
118. Tripathy D, Carlsson M, Almgren P, et al. Insulin secretion and insulin sensitivity in relation to glucose tolerance: lessons from the Botnia Study. Diabetes 2000; 49:975–980.
119. Hanefeld M, Koehler C, Fuecker K, et al. Insulin secretion and insulin sensitivity pattern is different in isolated impaired glucose tolerance and impaired fasting glucose. Diabetes Care 2003; 26:868–874.
120. Davies MJ, Raymond NT, Day JL, et al. Impaired glucose tolerance and fasting hyperglycaemia have different characteristics. Diabet Med 2000; 17:433–440.
121. Schianca GPC, Rossi A, Sainaghi PP, et al. The significance of impaired fasting glucose versus impaired glucose tolerance. Diabetes Care 2003; 26:1333–1337.
122. Weyer C, Bogardus C, Pratley RE. Metabolic characteristics of individuals with impaired fasting glucose and/or impaired glucose tolerance. Diabetes 1999; 48: 2197–2203.
123. Festa A, D'Agostino R Jr., Hanley AJG, et al. Differences in insulin resistance in non-diabetic subjects with isolated impaired glucose tolerance or isolated impaired fasting glucose. Diabetes 2004; 53:1549–1555.
124. Weigensberg MJ, Ball GDC, Shaibi GQ, et al. Decreased β-cell function in overweight Latino children with impaired fasting glucose. Diabetes Care 2005; 28:2519–2524.
125. Bacha F, Gungor N, Lee S, et al. Impaired fasting glucose vs impaired glucose tolerance in obese youth: what are the pathophysiological differences? 2007; 56(suppl 1): 292–OR.
126. Umpaichitra V, Bastian W, Taha D, et al. C-peptide and glucagon profiles in minority children with type 2 diabetes mellitus. J Clin Endocrinol Metab 2001; 86:1605–1609.
127. Gungor N, Bacha F, Saad R, et al. Youth type 2 diabetes: insulin resistance, beta-cell failure, or both? Diabetes Care 2005; 28:638–644.
128. Elder DA, Prigeon RL, Wadwa RP, et al. β-Cell function, insulin sensitivity, and glucose tolerance in obese diabetic and nondiabetic adolescents and young adults. J Clin Endocrinol Metab 2006; 91:185–191.
129. Druet C, Tubiana-Rufi N, Chevenne D, et al. Characterization of insulin secretion and resistance in Type 2 Diabetes of adolescents. J Clin Endocrinol Metab 2006; 91:401–404.
130. Arslanian SA. Youth with type 2 diabetes: insulin resistance and insulin secretion. Int Diab Monit 2007; 19:2–5.
131. Sellers EAC. Dean HJ: Short-term insulin therapy in adolescents with type 2 diabetes mellitus. J Pediatr Endocrinol Metab 2004; 17:1561–1564.
132. Matthews DR, Cull CA, Stratton IM, et al. UKPDS 26: sulfonylurea failure in non-insulin dependent diabetic patients over six years. UK Prospective Diabetes Study (UKPDS) Group. Diabet Med 1998; 15:297–303.
133. Gungor N, Arslanian S. Progressive beta cell failure in Type 2 diabetes mellitus of youth. J Pediatr 2004; 144:656–659.
134. Libman IM, Pietropaolo M, Arslanian SA, et al. Changing prevalence of overweight children and adolescents at onset of insulin-treated diabetes. Diabetes Care 2003; 26:2871–2875.
135. Littorin B, Sundkvist G, Hagopian W, et al. Islet cell and glutamic acid decarboxylase antibodies present at diagnosis of diabetes predict the need for insulin treatment. A cohort study in young adults whose disease was initially labeled as type 2 or unclassifiable diabetes. Diabetes Care 1999; 22(3):409–412.
136. Brooks-Worrell BM, Greenbaum CJ, Palmer JP, et al. Autoimmunity to islet proteins in children diagnosed with new-onset diabetes. J Clin Endocrinol Metab 2004; 89(5): 2222–2227.
137. Hathout EH, Thomas W, El-Shahawy M. Diabetic autoimmune markers in children and adolescents with type 2 diabetes. Pediatrics 2001; 107(6):E102.
138. Reinehr T, Schober E, Wiegand S, et al. β-cell autoantibodies in children with type 2 diabetes mellitus: subgroup or misclassification? DPV-Wiss Study Group. Arch Dis Child 2006; 91:473–477.

139. Turner R, Stratton I, Horton V, et al. UKPDS 25: autoantibodies to islet-cell cytoplasm and glutamic acid decarboxylase for prediction of insulin requirement in type 2 diabetes. Lancet 1997; 350:1288–1293.
140. Pietropaolo M, Barinas-Mitchell E, Pietropaolo SL, et al. Evidence of islet cell auto-immunity in elderly patients with type 2 diabetes. Diabetes 2000; 49:32–38.
141. Dean HE, Mandy RLL, Miffed M. Non-insulin dependent diabetes mellitus in Indian children in Manitoba. Can Med Assoc J 1992; 147:52–57.
142. Arslanian S, Bacha F, Gungor N. Phenotypic type 2 diabetes (T2DM) in youth: meta-bolic characteristics of islet-cell antibody negative vs. antibody positive patients 2007; 56(suppl 1):294–OR.

High and Low Birth Weights as Risk Factors for Diabetes

Rachel Pessah
Department of Medicine, Mount Sinai Medical Center, New York, New York, U.S.A.

Lois Jovanovic and David J. Pettitt
Department of Clinical Research, Sansum Diabetes Research Institute, Santa Barbara, California, U.S.A.

INTRODUCTION

There has been an increasing prevalence of childhood and adolescent type 2 diabetes over the past few decades (1,2), and recent studies have sparked interest in both low and high birth weight as risk factors for this disorder. In certain populations, low birth weight has been recognized as a risk factor for type 2 diabetes (3–8). Other diseases such as hypertension and dyslipidemia, which do not typically present until adulthood, have also been found in association with low birth weight (9). Studies have shown that shorter stature is associated with a higher rate of gestational diabetes (10), believed to be due to intrauterine malnutrition causing both low birth weight and short stature (11).

THRIFTY GENOTYPE AND THRIFTY PHENOTYPE HYPOTHESES

The thrifty genotype hypothesis, proposed by Neel in 1962 (12), states that anthropologically, individuals who were able to store calories as fat during periods of surplus could survive during periods of famine. Natural selection would select for this thrifty gene in populations exposed to famine, and result in mortality in people who lacked this gene.

Hales and Barker proposed the thrifty phenotype hypothesis as the etiology of type 2 diabetes mellitus (3). The underlying hypothesis relates to inadequate early nutrition in utero and during infancy adversely affects the development of the endocrine pancreas and β-cell function of the pancreatic islets of Langerhans. This undernutrition, known to result in infants of low birth weight and subsequent short stature, is expected to result in an increased susceptibility to developing type 2 diabetes. Genetic predisposition to diabetes is excluded from this hypothesis, as the direct cause of the adult problems are thought to be the intrauterine insult, but a genetic predisposition to diabetes may magnify the effect.

McCance et al. (4) used the thrifty genotype to explain the higher rates of diabetes in low birth weight babies. Given the high mortality of low birth weight infants, selective survival in infancy of those genetically predisposed to cope with adverse nutritional conditions in utero through insulin resistance and diabetes provides an explanation for the observation of low birth weight and diabetes. The same genetic makeup that permitted survival of adults during famine but is harmful during periods of extended abundance, may explain fetal survival under similarly adverse conditions. Hales and Barker (3) proposed that malnutrition of the fetus and infant would have permanent effects on organ system functioning and growth. As a result of varying deficiencies in growth, the fetus would develop adult diseases later in life such as diabetes and hypertension. Specifically, impaired development of β cells could result in type 2 diabetes once the nutritional status of the individual improved (3). Selective survival of small babies genetically predisposed to developing type 2 diabetes could account for the higher diabetes rates among surviving adults with known low birth weights.

Fetal mortality as opposed to survival of low birth weight babies was more common prior to the advent of newborn intensive care units (13–15). At that time, in order for a low birth weight infant to survive malnutrition in utero, there needed to be an exceptional factor to facilitate survival. The question remains as to what factor or factors contribute to this survival. The thrifty gene fits with this observation, and the efficient use of limited nutrients in utero could subsequently lead to insulin resistance and type 2 diabetes. This observation fits well with current studies noting the development of adult diseases in association with low birth weights. The question remains whether in the future, with more survival among infants lacking the thrifty gene who would have succumbed in the past, we will see a decrease in diabetes among surviving small babies or whether the small baby itself is at a nongenetic risk for diabetes in which case we will see an increase.

U-SHAPED ASSOCIATION BETWEEN BIRTH WEIGHT AND DIABETES

McCance et al. (4) examined birth weight as a risk factor for diabetes among the Pima Indian residents of the Gila River Indian community in Arizona. The Pima Indians have the highest reported prevalence and incidence of type 2 diabetes, often with a young age of onset (16–18). McCance et al. noted a U-shaped association in the diabetes rates among people with low birth weight (<2500 g) and high birth weight (≥4500 g) being nearly twice as high as among those with an intermediate birth weight between 2500 and 4500 g. While numerous hypotheses exist regarding the relationship between low birth weight and diabetes, it appears that high birth weight and diabetes are both related to intrauterine overnutrition. Therefore, fetal overgrowth during pregnancy is a major risk factor for the development of type 2 diabetes in the Pima Indians (19).

In the Pima study, diabetic pregnancy accounted for much of the diabetes in high birth weight individuals. When mothers who may have had diabetes during pregnancy were excluded, the diabetes rate in the highest birth weight category was no longer significantly higher than among those with a normal birth weight (4). The transmission of diabetes to the offspring of women with gestational diabetes increases the likelihood that their children will also have diabetes when they become pregnant (20).

McCance et al. discussed another hypothesis to explain the high prevalence of diabetes in the Pima population (4). While the thrifty genotype and thrifty phenotype explain the high prevalence of diabetes as a result of in utero nutritional deficiencies, they advance the surviving small baby genotype theory. This alternative suggests that the increase in rates of diabetes among low birth weight subjects is due to the selective ability for survival of low birth weight infants genetically susceptible to developing diabetes. Insulin resistance is a precursor of type 2 diabetes. In the Pima Indians, low birth weight might be associated with insulin resistance as well, which could explain the increased prevalence of diabetes among subjects with low birth weights. McCance et al. proposed that a genetic predisposition to developing insulin resistance may facilitate survival as well as increase the future risk of diabetes in that population.

Evidence for the role of transmission not solely due to genetics came from Dabelea et al. (21). They studied the prevalence of diabetes in siblings born before or after their mothers were diagnosed with diabetes. There was a significantly higher risk of developing diabetes in siblings born after the mother developed diabetes than among those born before the mother's diagnosis of diabetes (odds ratio 3.7, $p = 0.02$). A similar analysis of differences in risk of diabetes between offspring born before and after the father was diagnosed with diabetes, revealed no significant differences. In addition, those authors noted higher body mass indexes (BMIs) in the offspring of diabetic than nondiabetic pregnancies.

After the initial studies on the Pima Indian population, the incidence of diabetes was studied in Pima Indian children and in pregnant women (22–24). In this population, there were higher diabetes rates in pregnant women who had either high birth weight or low birth weight (23). This observation was subsequently reported during pregnancy in other populations as well (25). As populations become more affluent and with subsequent improvement in perinatal nutrition, we may expect to see women who were malnourished in utero years ago become obese during their childbearing years. As a result of obesity, the insulin resistance would predispose these women to a higher risk of developing diabetes (26).

In Taiwan, with the initiation of a mass urine screening program for diabetes in schoolchildren, Wei et al. examined the relationship between birth weight and the development of type 2 diabetes among adolescents (27). Interestingly, in this study, there appeared to be a U-shaped relationship between birth weight and risk of type 2 diabetes with subjects born with the lowest (<2500 g) and highest (>4000 g) birth weight at greatest risk for type 2 diabetes. The risk of diabetes in high birth weight babies was reduced to a nonsignificant level when adjusted for maternal diabetes; however, additional factors other than gestational diabetes, such as obesity and family history, are likely contributing to the high risk of diabetes among the high birth weight group.

Low birth weight schoolchildren with type 2 diabetes had different metabolic phenotypes than those born with high birth weights. Specifically, the authors noted that the type 2 diabetic subjects born with high birth weight also had higher blood pressure values, BMI, and positive family history of diabetes. This study also noted an association with childhood type 2 diabetes and obesity (27), consistent with prior studies (28–30).

While there are reports of an inverse association between stature and prevalence of type 2 diabetes mellitus, a positive association exists in California women from the Latino population who have gestational diabetes. Jovanovic et al. (31) postulated that early-life overnutrition could result in taller women at an increased risk of worse gestational diabetes. They examined this relationship in a Latino population of women in California, who failed the 50-g oral glucose load screening test for gestational diabetes. Upon returning for the definitive diagnostic glucose tolerance test with a 100-g oral glucose load, the authors noted a significant positive association between a woman's height and her glucose tolerance test results. These women with larger statures were associated with higher plasma glucose concentrations during an oral glucose tolerance test. Jovanovic et al. explain this finding by the geographic mixture of families into California from less affluent countries. Many families who arrived generations ago are now more affluent. As a result, this mixed population also has varying degrees of intrauterine nutrient consumption, and the likely variation in heights is directly associated with the quality of early-life nutrition (26). Moreover, the insulin resistance in this population will be associated with stature and intrauterine nutrient intake, resulting in the observed findings in this study of a positive association between stature and the oral glucose tolerance test.

LOW BIRTH WEIGHT AND ADULT DISEASES

There is evidence to suggest that low birth weight is related to glucose intolerance as well as other adult diseases. In 1986, Barker and Osmond suggested that the link between being born during a period of high infant mortality and later ischemic heart disease in the survivors was due to restraint of growth during fetal life (32). According to this theory, cardiovascular disease is a "programmed" effect of interference with early growth and development and is defined as long-term change in structure or function secondary to an insult during a critical period of early life.

Barker et al. studied 5654 men who were underweight at birth and two years after birth, and noted a high rate of death secondary to ischemic cardiac disease (33), and further noted in later studies that higher blood pressure and plasma fibrinogen levels were noted in adults with low body weight compared with placenta weight (34,35). These studies suggest that maternal malnutrition during critical periods of growth for the fetus may have systemic effects in the fetus and determine the metabolic impairment injury of the fetus such as diabetes, hypertension, and dyslipidemia (36).

In addition to glucose intolerance, low birth weight has been associated with hypertension (37). Phillips et al. investigated the relationship between birth weight and fasting plasma cortisol concentrations in subjects from Australia and the United Kingdom and reported a statistically significant correlation between fasting plasma cortisol concentrations and current blood pressure as well as low birth weight and raised fasting plasma cortisol concentrations.

Jeffery et al., in a recent study, found that there was no correlation between a woman's glucose during pregnancy and her child's weight or insulin resistance at age eight years (38). Limitations of that study were that it had only 26 mother-child pairs and utilized only fasting glucose rather than postprandial hyperglycemia that has been shown to be of importance during pregnancy and ignored other variables that might impact on early-accelerated weight gain of the children. Others have shown that even macrosomic infants normalize their weight during the first two years of life but thereafter initiate the accelerated grow rate (39).

In adults with a low birth weight, there is an increased risk of insulin resistance and likelihood of developing type 2 diabetes. In Hertfordshire, England, in men aged 64 years old, impaired glucose tolerance was noted to be 14% in the population with a birth weight greater or equal to 4310 g, but 40% in those who weighed less than 2500 g (36). This study supports the relationship between low birth weight and impaired glucose tolerance. Type 2 diabetes mellitus, a predominantly adult disease, appears to have fetal origins in many populations.

EARLY FETAL EVENTS PREDICT ADULT HEALTH

There is much evidence documenting the effect of prenatal events on long-term health. If the fetus is exposed to malnutrition during the active proliferation of pancreatic β-cells, the developing fetus must adapt to these changes (40). The disruption in development of the pancreas cannot recover subsequently, and the resulting impaired insulin secretion, requiring an increase in amount of insulin in adults, may result in the development of diabetes.

Some authors have questioned whether there is a potential role for fetal amino acid deficiency in the etiology of type 2 diabetes. Since amino acids are substrates for fetal energy production and maturation, amino acid deficiency could result in impairment of fetal growth. During fetal growth, insulin is regulated predominantly by amino acids, as is the growth of β-cells. In civilizations without access to protein, it is conceivable to envision nutritional deficiencies at this level.

LOW BIRTH WEIGHT AND INSULIN RESISTANCE

Low birth weight has been associated with lower socioeconomic circumstances (8). While it is widely accepted that folate deficiency during pregnancy can lead to neural tube defects, the data suggesting that inadequate fetal nutrition can result in insulin resistance are less clear despite many studies suggesting this relationship.

In a systematic review of the relationship between birth weight and insulin resistance, most studies show that low birth weight infants have increased insulin resistance as adults (41). Kim et al. examined the relationship between birth weight and insulin resistance in Korean adolescents (42). Subjects with a family history of diabetes were excluded from the study. The results indicated that low birth weight was related to insulin resistance in adolescence. In addition, in the lower birth weight tertile, there were higher levels of insulin, C-peptide, and homeostasis model assessment method for insulin resistance (HOMA-IR), suggesting a negative correlation between birth weight and these variables. There was also a negative correlation between birth weight and diastolic blood pressure, although no significant relationship to systolic blood pressure.

RELATIONSHIP BETWEEN BIRTH SIZE AND GENOTYPES

There have been associations described between birth weight, risk of diabetes, and genotypes. Type 1 diabetes is a result of immune-mediated destruction of the pancreatic β cells, developing from both genetic and nongenetic factors (43). Of the genes influencing the risk of type 1 diabetes, two of the most important are the HLA class II region and the insulin gene (44). There are some data associating high birth weight with a statistically significant increase in the risk of childhood-onset type 1 diabetes (45–47). Stene et al. performed a population-based case-control study in Norway to assess whether the relationship between size at birth and risk of type 1 diabetes is strengthened after adjusting for both the INS and HLA genotypes. While there was a tendency for those with the lowest birth weight to have a higher risk of type 1 diabetes, this relationship was not statistically significant even when adjusted for potential confounders (48). However this study had incomplete participation and a shift toward higher birth weights in the controls.

CONCLUSIONS

There are different rates of diabetes in populations that cannot be explained solely by genetics. The inverse association between birth weight and diabetes and stature in some populations, the U-shaped association with birth weight in Pima Indians, and a positive association between glucose and stature among women of Latino populations with an abnormal gestational diabetes screening test appears contradictory.

However, altered nutrition within different populations may have similar lasting effects on the developing fetus.

There are numerous studies associating low birth weight with an increased risk of diabetes; however, whether these defects are genetic or acquired in utero remain unanswered. It is difficult to estimate the degree to which type 2 diabetes could be reduced by preventing both low and high birth weight babies. However, this deductive thinking may lead to solutions to the vicious cycle.

The fact that malnutrition during fetal growth predicts development of adult diseases, specifically type 2 diabetes, has been well supported by the evidence. As a result of altered fetal growth, the infant is more likely to develop diabetes as an adult, regardless of the side of the U-shaped curve (i.e., intrauterine undernutrition or overnutrition from gestational diabetes). It is urgent to study this phenomenon further in order to find ways to reduce this perpetuating vicious cycle, potentially resulting in increasing numbers of individuals with diabetes across generations.

ACKNOWLEDGMENT

Dr. Pessah was the recipient of The Society for Experimental Biology and Medicine Mentoring Award that allowed her to study with Dr. Jovanovic at the Sansum Diabetes Research Institute.

REFERENCES

1. Dabelea D, Hanson RL, Bennett PH, et al. Increasing prevalence of type II diabetes in American Indian children. Diabetologia 1998; 41:904–910.
2. Fagot-Campagna A, Pettitt DJ, Engelgau MM, et al. Type 2 diabetes among North American children and adolescents: an epidemiologic review and a public health perspective. J Pediatr 2000; 136:664–672.
3. Hales CN, Barker D. Type 2 (non-insulin-dependent) diabetes mellitus: the thrifty phenotype hypothesis. Diabetologia 1992; 35:595–601.
4. McCance DR, Pettitt DJ, Hanson RL, et al. Birth weight and non-insulin dependent diabetes: thrifty genotype, thrifty phenotype, or surviving small baby genotype? Br Med J 1994; 308(6934):942–945.
5. Hales CN. Fetal nutrition and adult diabetes. Sci Am Sci Med 1994; 1:54–63.
6. Valdez R, Athens MA, Thompson GH, et al. Birthweight and adult health outcomes in a biethnic population in the USA. Diabetologia 1994; 37:624–631.
7. Lithell HO, McKeigue PM, Berglund L, et al. Relation of size at birth to non-insulin dependent diabetes and insulin concentrations in men aged 50–60 years. BMJ 1996; 312:406–410.
8. Clausen JO, Borch-Johnsen K, Pedersen O. Relation between birth weight and the insulin sensitivity index in a population sample of 331 young, healthy Caucasians. Am J Epidemiol 1997; 146:23–31.
9. Barker, DJP, Hales CN, Fall CH, et al. Type 2 (non-insulin dependent) diabetes mellitus, hypertension and hyperlipidemia (syndrome X): relation to reduced fetal growth. Diabetologia 1993; 36:62–67.
10. Anastasiou E, Alevizaki M, Grigorakis SJ, et al. Decreased stature in gestational diabetes mellitus. Diabetologia 1998; 41:997–1001.
11. Persson I, Ahlsson F, Ewald U, et al. Influence of perinatal factors on the onset of puberty in boys and girls: implications for interpretation of link with risk of long term diseases. Am J Epidemiol 1999; 150:747–755.
12. Neel J. Diabetes mellitus: a "thrifty" genotype rendered detrimental by "progress"? Am J Hum Genet 1962; 14(4):353–362.
13. Vanlandingham MJ, Buehler JW, Hogue CJR, et al. Birthweight-specific infant mortality for native Americans compared with whites, six states, 1980. Am J Public Health 1988; 78:499–503.

14. Alo CJ, Howe HL, Nelson MR. Birth-weight-specific infant mortality risk and leading causes of death: Illinois, 1980–1989. Am J Dis Child 1993; 147:1085–1089.
15. Rees JM, Lederman SA, Kiely JL. Birth weight associated with lowest neonatal mortality: infants of adolescent and adult mothers. Pediatrics 1996; 98:1161–1166.
16. Knowler WC, Bennett PH, Hamman RF, et al. Diabetes incidence and prevalence in Pima Indians: a 19-fold greater incidence than in Rochester, Minnesota. Am J Epidemiol 1978; 108:497–505.
17. Knowler WC, Pettitt DJ, Saad MF, et al. Diabetes mellitus in the Pima Indians: incidence, risk factors and pathogenesis. Diabetes Metab Rev 1990; 6:1–27.
18. Savage PJ, Bennett PH, Senter RG, et al. High prevalence of diabetes in young Pima Indians: evidence of phenotypic variation in a genetically isolated population. Diabetes 1979; 28:939–942.
19. Dabelea D, Pettitt DJ, Hanson RL, et al. Birth weight, type 2 diabetes and insulin resistance in Pima Indian children and young adults. Diabetes Care 1999, 22:944–950.
20. Pettitt DJ, Bennett PH, Saad MF, et al. Abnormal glucose tolerance during pregnancy in Pima Indian women: long-term effects on the offspring. Diabetes 1991; 40(suppl 2): 126–130.
21. Dabelea D, Hanson R, Lindsay R, et al. Intrauterine exposure to diabetes conveys risks for type 2 diabetes and obesity: a study of discordant sibships. Diabetes 2000; 49:2208–2211.
22. Pettitt DJ, Aleck KA, Baird HR, et al. Congenital susceptibility to NIDDM: role of intrauterine environment. Diabetes 1988; 37:622–628.
23. Pettitt DJ, Knowler WC. Long-term effects of the intrauterine environment, birth weight, and breast-feeding in Pima Indians. Diabetes Care 1988; 21:B138–B141.
24. Dabelea D, Knowler WC, Pettitt DJ. Effect of diabetes in pregnancy on offspring: follow-up research in the Pima Indians. J Matern Fetal Med 2000; 9:83–88.
25. Pettitt DJ, Jovanovic L. Low birth weight as a risk factor for gestational diabetes, diabetes and impaired glucose tolerance during pregnancy. Diabetes Care 2007; 30(Suppl 2):S147–S149.
26. Pettitt DJ, Jovanovic L. Birth weight as a predictor of type 2 diabetes mellitus: the U-shaped curve. Curr Diab Rep 2001; 1:78–81.
27. Wei JN, Sung FC, Li CY, et al. Low birth weight and high birth weight infants are both at an increased risk to have type 2 diabetes among schoolchildren in Taiwan. Diabetes Care 2003; 26(2):343–348.
28. Rich-Edwards JW, Colditz GA, Stampfer MJ, et al. Birthweight and the risk for type 2 diabetes mellitus in adult women. Ann Intern Med 1999; 130:278–284.
29. Bavdekar A, Yajnik CS, Fall CH, et al. Insulin resistance syndrome in 8-year-old Indian children: small at birth, big at 8 years, or both? Diabetes 1999; 48:2422–2429.
30. Curhan GC, Willett WC, Rimm EB, et al. Birth weight and adult hypertension, diabetes mellitus, and obesity in US men. Circulation 1996; 94:3246–3250.
31. Jovanovic L, Ilic S, Noyyen M, Pettitt DJ. Short stature in Latina women with gestational diabetes mellitus (GDM) is not associated with higher glucose. Diabetes 2000; 49(suppl 1): A443–A444.
32. Barker DJ, Osmond C. Diet and coronary heart disease in England and Wales during and after the second world war. Epidemiol Community Health 1986; 40:37–44.
33. Barker DJ, Winter PD, Osmond C, et al. Weight in infancy and death from ischemic heart disease. Lancet 1989; 2:577–580.
34. Barker DJ, Bull AR, Osmond C, et al. Fetal and placental size and risk of hypertension in adult life. Br Med J 1990; 301:259–262.
35. Barker DJ, Meade TW, Fall CH, et al. Relation of fetal and infant growth to plasma fibrinogen and factor VII concentrations in a adult life. Br Med J 1992; 304:148–152.
36. Hales CN, Barker DJP, Clark PMS, et al. Fetal and infant growth and impaired glucose tolerance at age 64. BMJ 1991; 303:1019–1022.
37. Phillips D, Walker B, Reynolds R, et al. Low birth weight predicts elevated plasma cortisol concentrations in adults from 3 populations. Hypertension 2000; 35:1301–1306.
38. Jeffery AN, Metcalf BS, Hosking J, et al. Little evidence for early programming of weight and insulin resistance for contemporary children: EarlyBird Diabetes Study report 19. Pediatrics 2006; 118:1118–1123.

39. Silverman BL, Rizzo TA, Cho NH, et al. Long-term effects of the intrauterine environment. The Northwestern University Diabetes in Pregnancy Center. Diabetes Care 1998; 21(suppl 2):B142–B149.
40. Hoet JJ. Influence of dietary changes on the development of the fetal pancreas—consequences later in life. Isr J Med Sci 1991; 27:423–424.
41. Newsome CA, Shiell AW, Fal C, et al. Is birth weight related to later glucose and insulin metabolism?—a systemic review. Diabet Med 2003; 20:339–348.
42. Kim CS, Park JS, Park J, et al. The relation between birth weight and insulin resistance in Korean adolescents. Yonsei Med J 2006; 47(1):85–92.
43. Atkinson MA, Eisenbarth GS. Type 1 diabetes: new perspectives on disease pathogenesis and treatment. Lancet 2001; 358:221–229.
44. Concannon P, Erlich HA, Julier C, et al. Type 1 diabetes: evidence for susceptibility loci from four genome-wide linkage scans in 1,435 multiplex families. Diabetes 2005; 54:995–1001.
45. Dahlquist G, Patterson C, Stoltesz G. Perinatal risk factors for childhood type 1 diabetes in Europe: the EURO DIAB Substudy 2 Study Group. Diabetes Care 1999; 22:1698–1702.
46. Stene LC, Magnus P, Lie RT, et al. The Norwegian Childhood Diabetes Study Group Birth weight and childhood onset type 1 diabetes: population based cohort study. BMJ 2001; 322:889–892.
47. Dahlquist GG, Pundziute-Lycka A, Nystrom L. Birth weight and risk of type 1 diabetes in children and young adults: a population-based register study. Diabetologia 2005; 48:1114–1117.
48. Stene, LC, Thorsby, PM, Berg, JP, et al. The relation between size at birth and risk of type 1 diabetes is not influenced by adjustment for the insulin gene (-23Hphl) polymorphism or *HLA-DQ* genotype. Diabetologia 2006; 49:2068–2073.

11 Monogenic Forms of Diabetes in the Young

Martine Vaxillaire
CNRS UMR 8090, Institute of Biology and Pasteur Institute, Lille, France

Philippe Froguel
Section of Genomic Medicine, Imperial College London, London, U.K.

INTRODUCTION

Type 2 diabetes mellitus (T2DM) is a heterogeneous metabolic disease occurring with concomitant or interdependent defects of both insulin secretion and action (1). T2DM results from a complex interplay of genetic and environmental factors influencing a number of intermediate traits of relevance to the diabetic phenotype (such as β-cell mass, insulin secretion, insulin action, fat distribution, and obesity) (2). It is now well recognized that T2DM is composed of many different subtypes where genetic susceptibility is strongly associated with environmental factors at one end of the spectrum, which are common polygenic T2DM forms, and highly genetic forms, defined as monogenic diabetes, at the other end (3). Although the current rise in T2DM prevalence is greatly driven by lifestyle changes, the inherent susceptibility to T2DM is well established and attributable to complex genetic determinants (4). In polygenic T2DM, the simultaneous action of several susceptibility alleles or multiple combinations of frequent variants at several loci may have deleterious effects when predisposing environmental factors are present. At the opposite side of human T2DM genetics, several monogenic forms of diabetes have been identified, such as maturity-onset diabetes of the young (MODY) (5), maternally inherited diabetes and deafness (MIDD) (6), and neonatal diabetes mellitus (NDM) (7). Moreover, retrospective studies showed that low birth weight is associated with insulin resistance and T2DM in adulthood, likely resulting from a metabolic adaptation to poor fetal nutrition (8). However, the identification of gene variants contributing both to variation in fetal growth and to the susceptibility to T2DM suggest that this metabolic "programing" could also be partly genetically determined (9).

The interactions between genes and environment complicate the task of identifying any single genetic susceptibility factor to T2DM. Indeed, common T2DM in the adults is a "complex" polygenic disease that arises as predisposing environmental factors interact with many genetic variants ("susceptibility" alleles) interspersed through the genome. Each susceptibility allele, considered in isolation, confers only a very small increased risk of disease (typically in the 1- to 1.5-fold range); this fact implies the need to use large population-based samples and cases enriched for familiality and early onset to reliably detect such modest effect. Most of the diabetes-associated genes with strong effects on the disease appearance were discovered so far by studying the highly familial and/or monogenic forms of diabetes with neonatal or early onset like NDM and MODY (5). In this chapter, we are reviewing the clinical features and the genetic and molecular bases of these varied monogenic conditions of diabetes in the young. We will also underline how the molecular understanding of these monogenic forms of diabetes led to pharmacogenomic approaches of the disease.

DEFINITION AND DIAGNOSTIC CRITERIA FOR MODY

The term MODY was based on the old classification of diabetes into juvenile-onset and maturity-onset diabetes. Both the American Diabetes Association (ADA) and the World Health Organization (WHO) have introduced a revised, etiology-based classification for diabetes. MODY is now defined as a "genetic defect in β-cell function" with subclassification according to the gene involved.

MODY is a familial form of non-insulin-dependent diabetes with autosomal-dominant inheritance, which usually develops at childhood, adolescence, or young adulthood, and presents primary insulin-secretion defects (5). The main diagnostic criteria for MODY are:

- Early onset of diabetes, frequently diagnosed before age 25 years in at least one and ideally two family members; it is to note that "anticipation" or progressive reduction in the age of diagnosis in succeeding generations was reported in almost all reported MODY pedigrees (probably because of enhanced awareness of diabetes leading to earlier testing).
- Non-insulin dependence shown by absence of insulin treatment five years after diagnosis or significant C-peptide even in a patient on insulin treatment.
- Autosomal-dominant inheritance, i.e., vertical transmission of diabetes through at least two, or ideally three, generations, with a similar phenotype in diabetic family members.
- Obesity is rarely associated with the MODY phenotype (and not required for the development of this form of diabetes).
- Diabetes results from β-cell dysfunction (insulin levels are often in the normal range, though inappropriately low for the degree of hyperglycemia).

The prevalence of MODY is estimated at less than 5% of patients with T2DM in most populations (10).

MOLECULAR GENETICS OF MODY

The well-defined mode of inheritance with high penetrance and the early age of onset of diabetes allow the collection of multigenerational pedigrees making MODY an attractive model for genetic studies. MODY is not a single entity but is a heterogeneous disease with regard to genetic, metabolic, and clinical features. All MODY genes have not been identified, but heterozygous mutations in six genes cause the majority of the MODY cases (Table 1). These genes encode the enzyme glucokinase (GCK/*MODY2*) (11) and the transcription factors hepatocyte nuclear factor 4α (HNF-4α/*MODY1*) (12), HNF-1α/*MODY3* (13,14), insulin promoter factor 1 (IPF-1/*MODY4*) (15), HNF-1β/*MODY5* (16), and neurogenic differentiation factor 1 (*NeuroD1*/Beta2, *MODY6*) (17). Moreover additional *MODY* genes may remain to be discovered, since there are families in which MODY co-segregates with markers outside the known *MODY* loci (18–19).

The relative prevalence of the different subtypes of MODY has been shown to vary greatly in studying British, French, German, and Spanish family cohorts (20–23). MODY2 represents from 10% to 60% of cases (the most prevalent form in French families) and MODY3 from 20% to 65% of cases (the most prevalent form in British families). The other MODY subtypes are rare disorders in all these populations, having been described only in a few families, while additional unknown MODY loci (MODY-X) may represent 20–50% of the cases (the most prevalent form

TABLE 1 Subtypes of MODY and Genes Involved

MODY subtype	Gene locus	Gene name	Year of discovery (references)	Distribution	Onset of diabetes	Primary defect	Severity of diabetes	Complications
MODY1	20q	*HNF4A*	1996 (12)	Rare	Adolescence Early adulthood	Pancreas/other	Severe	Frequent
MODY2	7p	*GCK*	1992 (11)	10–65%[a]	Early childhood Adolescence	Pancreas/liver	Mild	Rare
MODY3	12q	*TCF1*	1996 (13,14)	20–75%[a]	Early adulthood	Pancreas/kidney	Severe	Frequent
MODY4	13q	*IPF-1*	1997 (15)	Rare	Early adulthood	Pancreas/other	Severe	Unknown
MODY5	17q	*TCF2*	1997 (16)	Rare	Early adulthood	Kidney/pancreas	Severe	Kidney disease
MODY6	2q32	*NeuroD1*	1999 (17)	Rare	Early adulthood	Pancreas	Severe	Unknown

[a]Different distributions in different populations.

Abbreviations: GCK, glucokinase; HNF, hepatocyte nuclear factor; IPF-1, insulin promoter factor 1; MODY, maturity-onset diabetes of the young; NeuroD1, neurogenic differentiation factor 1; TCF, transcription factor 1.

in German and Spanish families). These contrasting results may be due to differences in the genetic background of these populations, or may reflect, at least partly, ascertainment bias in the recruitment of families.

GCK Mutations and MODY2

GCK phosphorylates glucose to glucose-6-phosphate in pancreatic β cells and hepatocytes, and plays a major role in the regulation and integration of glucose metabolism (24). More than 150 different *GCK* mutations have been observed. The kinetic properties of recombinant GCK proteins have shown that the relative enzymatic activity of the mutant proteins was impaired, resulting in decreased glycolytic flux in pancreatic β cells. This defect translates in vivo as a glucose-sensing defect leading to an increase in the blood glucose threshold that triggers insulin secretion (25), and a right shift in the dose-response curve of glucose-induced insulin secretion (26). Decreased net accumulation of hepatic glycogen and increased hepatic gluconeogenesis following standard meals were observed in GCK-deficient subjects and contribute to the postprandial hyperglycemia of MODY2 patients (27). Despite these multiple defects in the pancreas and the liver, the hyperglycemia associated with *GCK* mutations is often mild, usually responsive to diet, with fewer than 50% of subjects presenting with overt diabetes. There is a lower prevalence of diabetes microvascular complications (retinopathy and proteinuria) in MODY2 than in other subtypes of MODY and late-onset T2DM (28). It was observed that *GCK* mutations in the fetus result in reduced birth weight, probably by affecting insulin-mediated fetal growth, whereas maternal *GCK* mutations indirectly increase the birth weight by increasing fetal insulin secretion, as a consequence of maternal hyperglycemia during fetal life. None of these effects persists, however, into adult life (29,30). There is growing evidence that a common variant upstream of *GCK*, located –30 G/A in the β-cell-specific promoter, influence fasting glucose levels and birth weight, and is associated with gestational diabetes (31), with impaired glucose regulation and a higher prevalence of T2DM in patients with coronary artery disease (32).

Mutations in β-Cell-Expressed Transcription Factor Genes

Positional cloning of *MODY* loci and studies in candidate genes have led to the identification of mutations in five transcription factors: HNF-1α, HNF-4α, HNF-1β, IPF-1/PDX-1 and NeuroD1/Beta2. Gene-targeting experiments in animals have demonstrated that many of these islet-expressed genes have a key role in the fetal pancreas development and neogenesis, as well as, in the β-cell differentiation and function (33).

TCF1/HNF-1α

Mutations in *TCF1/HNF-1α* account for most of the MODY linked with a defect in nuclear factors. More than 150 different mutations located in the coding or promoter regions were found in various populations (24). An insulin-secretory defect in the absence of insulin resistance was observed in diabetic and nondiabetic carriers of *MODY3* mutations (34). In contrast to the usually mild hyperglycemia due to GCK deficiency, MODY3 is a more severe form of diabetes, often evolving toward insulin dependency. Microvascular complications of diabetes are observed as frequently in MODY3 as in late age of onset diabetic subjects (35). HNF-1α is also expressed in the kidney, and a defect in the renal reabsorption of glucose is often associated to the pancreatic β-cell defect in MODY3 subjects (36). Heterozygous knockout mice lacking one copy of HNF-1α have a normal phenotype, while MODY3 subjects are all heterozygous for their mutations and fully express the diabetes phenotype (37). Experimental data showed that only the mutations located in the transactivation domain of the protein exhibit a dominant negative effect on HNF-1α transactivation potential (38). The target genes associated with the β-cell defect of MODY3/HNF-1α were partly characterized from knockout mice studies (39–40).

HNF4A/HNF-4α

MODY1 is much less prevalent, and only a few kindred were described with HNF-4α mutations-associated diabetes (24). HNF-4α is a member of the steroid/thyroid hormone receptor superfamily and initially known as an upstream regulator of HNF-1α expression. Interestingly, it was demonstrated that long-chain fatty acids directly modulates the transcriptional activity of HNF-4α by binding as acyl-CoA thioesters to the ligand-binding domain of HNF-4α (41). This observation could contribute important data to the understanding of the role of dietary fats in the control of insulin secretion. Here again, a few target genes of HNF-4α associated with β-cell defect have been defined in insulin-secretion pathway, glucose transport, and metabolism (42,43). The recent discovery of a genetic interaction between the two transcriptional regulators, HNF-1α and -4α, which occurs specifically in differentiated pancreatic β cells can help modeling some molecular pathogenic events in the development of the MODY phenotype (44,45). HNF-4α controls the expression of HNF-1α in embryonic endoderm, liver, and pancreatic cells, whereas the HNF-1α control of HNF-4α is restricted to pancreatic cells and in part to intestinal cells. This cellular specificity is explained by the existence of an alternate promoter of HNF4A (known as P2). HNF-1β and IPF-1 may also regulate HNF-4α through the P2 promoter in the pancreas. Furthermore, in a large MODY family, a nucleotide substitution in the IPF-1/PDX-1 binding site, which co-segregated with diabetes, was shown to cause a threefold reduction in transcriptional activity (44). Current evidence indicates that there is interdependence between HNF-1α and HNF-4α in a positive cross-regulatory loop occurring specifically in pancreatic cells and essential for the differentiated β-cell function. Such a model would propose that loss of one functional allele results in insufficient activator concentration required to elicit normal target gene responses in islets.

Interestingly, the in utero and neonatal role of two key regulators of pancreatic insulin secretion, HNF-1α and HNF-4α, was assessed by studying birth weight and the incidence of neonatal hypoglycemia in patients with heterozygous mutations in these two MODY genes, and it was shown that HNF4A mutations are associated with a considerable increase in birth weight and macrosomia, and are a novel cause of neonatal hypoglycemia (46). This study establishes a key role for HNF-4α in determining fetal birth weight, and uncovers an unanticipated feature of the natural history of HNF-4α-deficient diabetes, with hyperinsulinemia at birth evolving to decreased insulin secretion and diabetes later in life.

TCF2/HNF-1β

Mutations in HNF-1β/TCF2 were also described in a few families with early-onset diabetes consistent with MODY. In these pedigrees, HNF-1β mutations are associated with both diabetes and severe kidney disease, which may appear before the impairment of glucose tolerance. Polycystic renal disease and/or particular histological abnormalities showing meganephrons are present in some subjects. This has led to the recognition of a discrete clinical syndrome associated with HNF-1β mutations, the renal cysts and early-onset diabetes (RCAD) syndrome (47). Indeed, this nuclear factor plays a major role in kidney development and nephron differentiation. In addition, internal genital abnormalities have been described in some female carriers (47). Altogether, point mutations, small deletions/insertions, and large genomic rearrangements of TCF2 account for 70% of the cases presenting with a clinical phenotype consistent with MODY5 (48).

IPF-1/PDX-1

All of these genetic defects in transcription factors lead to abnormalities of glucose homeostasis, and thereby promote the development of chronic hyperglycemia, through alterations in insulin secretion and possibly in the development of the pancreatic islets. In this regard, a deletion in the homeodomain transcription factor IPF-1 (also named IDX-1, PDX-1, STF-1), was found to co-segregate with MODY in a large kindred presenting a consanguineous link (49). The phenotype of the subjects who are heterozygous for the mutation ranges from normal to impaired glucose tolerance to overt non-insulin-dependent diabetes. One child who is homozygous for the mutation was born with pancreatic agenesis and suffers from diabetes as well as exocrine insufficiency. IPF-1 is critical for the embryonic development of the pancreatic islets as well as for transcriptional regulation of endocrine pancreatic tissue-specific genes in adults, such as the insulin, glucose transporter 2 (GLUT2), GCK genes in β cells, and the somatostatin gene in δ cells. IPF-1 is normally expressed in all cells of the pancreatic bud, and its absence in mice arrests development at the bud stage leading to pancreatic agenesis.

NeuroD1/Beta2

The transcription factor NeuroD1/Beta2 is involved in the regulation of endocrine pancreas development. In *NeuroD1* null mice, pancreatic islet morphogenesis is abnormal and hyperglycemia develops, due in part to inadequate expression of the insulin gene. Mutations in *NeuroD1* were shown to co-segregate with early-onset T2DM and autosomal dominant-like transmission (50). This observation suggests that NeuroD1 might also play an important role in endocrine pancreas development and/or insulin gene expression in humans.

Clinical Impact and Pharmacogenetics

Altogether, mutations in *GCK* and *TCF1*/HNF-1α account for around two-thirds of all MODY cases, the other MODY subtypes being infrequent disorders described only in a couple of families (24). These distinct molecular etiologies are associated with substantial differences in clinical course, explaining the clinical heterogeneity. Heterozygous *GCK* mutations cause fasting hyperglycemia, present from birth, which is only slowly progressive, usually responsive to diet and leads to few complications. In contrast, *HNF-1α* and *HNF-4α* mutations are associated with diabetes onset in early adulthood and a more severe deterioration in glucose homeostasis, which requires hypoglycemic treatment even at a middle age. Physiological studies have shown that initially insulin secretion is maintained at normal glucose values, but fails to rise adequately as the glucose concentration is increased. Therefore, these patients are at high risk of developing microvascular and macrovascular complications. Patients with *HNF-1α* mutations also show a particular sensitivity to the hypoglycemic effects of sulfonylureas (51). This pharmacogenetic effect is consistent with models of HNF-1α deficiency, which show that the β-cell defect is upstream of the sulfonylurea receptor (SUR), and also highlights that definition of the genetic basis of hyperglycemia has strong implications for patient management. The difference in pathophysiology between *HNF-1α* and *HNF-1β* is also clearly seen in the response to therapy. Patients with *HNF-1β* mutations are more frequently treated with insulin (67%) compared with *HNF-1α* mutation patients (31%) (20), and most patients rapidly require insulin treatment. This therapeutic response is consistent with a generalized reduction in β-cell mass. It is important to identify the different subtypes in patients presenting with early-onset diabetes, given that a precise molecular diagnosis may offer valuable prognostic and therapeutic benefits.

Furthermore, the identification of activating mutations within the heterotropic allosteric activator site of human β-cell GCK has validated the structural and functional models of GCK and the putative allosteric activator site (52), which is a potential drug target for the treatment of T2DM. These activating mutations are responsible of hyperinsulinism with hypoglycemia of infancy (HI). Other mutations that cause hyperglycemia are not necessarily kinetically inactivating but may exert their effects by other complex mechanisms. A drug-discovery process aimed at increasing the activity of GCK has received considerable attention, as several compounds that activate the enzyme, so-called GK activators (GKAs), have been discovered (53). The dual mechanism of action of GKAs in pancreatic β cells and liver suggest that these molecules will exert their biological effects in T2DM patients by improving overall β-cell function coupled with a suppression of hepatic glucose production. The net effect of their mechanism of action is a decrease of fasting plasma glucose and improved glucose tolerance. Since the discovery of the first orally active GKA (RO0281675), a number of research groups have reported the identification of novel potent GKAs. This excellent example of translational research has important outcomes for a new class of therapeutic agents useful in the treatment of T2DM, and also for understanding how these agents attack such a complicated system as the regulation of GCK. The therapeutic benefit to safety ratio must be high for these agents to be used long term in man.

MOLECULAR GENETICS OF NDM

NDM is a rare (1:300,000 to 1:400,000 newborns) but potentially devastating metabolic disorder characterized by mild to severe hyperglycemia combined with low levels of insulin within the first months of life (7). Two forms have been recognized on clinical grounds, transient NDM (TNDM) and permanent NDM (PNDM), which differ in the duration of insulin dependence early in the disease. TNDM infants develop diabetes in the first few weeks of life but go into remission in a few months, with possible relapse to a permanent diabetes state usually in adolescence or early adulthood. TNDM represents 50–60% of NDM cases. The pancreatic dysfunction in this condition may be maintained throughout life, with relapse initiated at times of metabolic stress such as puberty or pregnancy. In PNDM, insulin secretory failure occurs in the late fetal or early postnatal period and does not go into remission. Considerable overlap exists between the two groups, so that they cannot be distinguished on the basis of clinical features, although patients with TNDM are more likely to have intrauterine growth retardation and less likely to develop ketoacidosis than patients with PNDM. In most instances, very early-onset diabetes mellitus seems to be unrelated to autoimmunity.

Genetic Anomalies Linked to TNDM

TNDM is usually sporadic, but paternal transmission has been documented in about one-third of reported patients, some of whom had nondiabetic fathers (7). Paternal isodisomy of chromosome 6 has been demonstrated in several unrelated patients with TNDM. Other patients had partial duplications of the long arm of the paternal chromosome 6. These unbalanced duplications are inherited within families. TNDM arises only if the duplication is inherited from the father suggesting an imprinting disorder. A region in which methylation differs between the maternal and the paternal chromosome 6q24 has been identified (54), and two paternally expressed genes are located in the region: ZAC (also known as *LOT1* and *PLAGL-1*) encoding a transcription factor that regulates cell cycle arrest and apoptosis, and also the pituitary adenylate cyclase activating polypeptide 1 (PACAP1) receptor being a potent insulin secretagogue; and the hydatidiform mole associated and imprinted (*HYMAI*) gene whose function is unknown. No other loci have been implicated in TNDM to date. An animal model of TNDM has been generated by the insertion of the human TNDM locus into a mouse. Mice overexpressing the TNDM locus display many, but not all, of the features of human TNDM, and interestingly, have a reduced expression of the key transcription factor PDX-1 in the embryonic pancreas (55). Nevertheless, the precise link between those genetic anomalies and the insulin-secreting cell-impaired function remained to be established.

Mutations in K_{ATP} Channel Genes: A Common Molecular Origin for TNDM and PNDM

More recently, new advances have been made in the understanding of molecular mechanisms relevant to pancreas dysfunction in both PNDM and TNDM (56). This was achieved by the identification of mutations in the ATP-gated potassium (K_{ATP}) channel expressed at the surface of the pancreatic β cell, which is a hetero-octamer assembled from $K_{IR}6.2$ (encoded by potassium inwardly-rectifying channel, subfamily J, member 11 [*KCNJ11*]) and the high-affinity sulfonylurea receptor-1, SUR1 (encoded by *ABCC8*), and their characterization as a frequent cause of NDM, both by genetic and functional studies (57–60). The K_{ATP} channels link nutrient metabolism with membrane electrical activity by responding to changes in ATP/ADP levels, which reflect the energy status of the cell (61). Adenine nucleotides exert a dual action on K_{ATP} channels: ATP binding to the pore reduces channel activity, the mean open probability, P_O, while Mg-nucleotide binding and/or hydrolysis on SUR1 counterbalances this inhibition to increase P_O (62). Metabolism increases the ATP/ADP ratio which reduces the mean P_O of the channel via ATP binding to $K_{IR}6.2$ and by reducing the Mg-dependent stimulatory action of nucleotides that interact with the nucleotide-binding domains (NBD1 and 2) of SUR1 (63). This combined action closes K_{ATP} channels allowing membrane depolarization, Ca^{2+} channel activation and Ca^{2+} influx, which stimulates insulin secretion.

Indeed, 30–50% of the currently identified PNDM cases, and a few cases of TNDM, are attributable to mutations in the *KCNJ11* gene (57–59), which encodes the pore-forming $K_{IR}6.2$ subunit of the K_{ATP} channel expressed at the surface of the pancreatic β cell. The severity of the disease has been correlated with the degree of channel activity with several transient cases being attributed to attenuated ATP inhibition of mutant channels, whereas mutations that severely compromise inhibitory gating can result in marked developmental delay, muscle weakness, epilepsy, and neonatal diabetes, known as the developmental delay, epilepsy and neonatal diabetes (DEND) syndrome (56). This fact is also illustrated by the fact that transgenic mice expressing a mutant $K_{IR}6.2$, with reduced sensitivity to inhibitory ATP, succumb to hyperglycemia, hypoinsulinemia, and ketoacidosis within the first week of life (64).

Activating mutations in *ABCC8*, which encodes SUR1 have also been identified in NDM patients (60,65,66), accounting for $\sim 17\%$ of NDM in the French case series, and mostly in the transient form ($\sim 30\%$ of TNDM patients) (60,66). Interestingly, five mutations exhibited vertical transmission of neonatal and apparent adult-onset diabetes, implying that NDM has relevance for understanding T2DM physiopathology. A previous report identified a mild dominant form of hypoglycemia due to a mutation in the *ABCC8* gene, E1507K, which reduces channel activity and produces hyperinsulinism at an early age, followed by a decreasing insulin secretory capacity in early adulthood and diabetes in middle age (67). This mutation is responsible for a subtype of autosomal dominant diabetes, which underlines close relationships between a progressive deterioration of insulin secretion and decrease in insulin sensibility both involved in the pathogenesis of diabetes, thus leading to frank diabetes over time.

Functional analysis of some de novo *ABCC8* mutations, from both PNDM and TNDM subjects presenting with severe hyperglycemia and ketoacidosis, demonstrated a novel molecular mechanism by which mutant SUR1 receptors exhibit a marked increase in their Mg-nucleotide-dependent stimulatory action on the wild-type $K_{IR}6.2$ pore without altering sensitivity to inhibitory ATP (60,65). These new findings demonstrate that mutations in SUR1 can cause both PNDM and TNDM, accounting for a significant fraction of ND cases (60,66).

Therefore K_{ATP} channels play a key role in the regulation of insulin release and the expression of a small number of "overactive" mutant channels can hyperpolarize insulin-secreting pancreatic β cells, reduce Ca^{2+} influx through voltage-gated calcium channels, and reduce insulin secretion. In vitro experiments demonstrated that most of the mutant channels retain their sensitivity to inhibitory sulfonylureas (60). Importantly, glibenclamide and glipizide, instead of insulin therapy, provided good metabolic control in both PNDM and TNDM cases with separate *ABCC8* mutations (60), and in 44 out of 49 PNDM patients with *KCNJ11* mutations, who were successfully transferred from insulin to sulfonylureas (68). Young children and toddlers with mutations in either subunit of the K_{ATP} channel are therefore being treated now with sulfonylureas, a drug that modifies the activity of the K_{ATP} channel leading to changes in the membrane potential. In such young children, the long-term impact of those drugs on the insulin-secreting cell remains to be studied.

Several studies highlighted the heterogeneity of extrapancreatic symptoms associated with $K_{IR}6.2$ mutations potentially reflecting the sharing of $K_{IR}6.2$ pores by SUR1/$K_{IR}6.2$ neuroendocrine and SUR2A/$K_{IR}6.2$ sarcolemmal channels (56,57). Neurological abnormalities were also seen in NDM patients with SUR1 mutations and are most probably related to the expression of SUR1 in several populations of neurons. However, the neuromotor and neuropsychological phenotypes of patients with both SUR1 and $K_{IR}6.2$ mutations remained to be further defined and quantified.

Rare Syndromes Associated with PNDM

A number of rare clinical syndromes have been identified as associated with PNDM (Table 2).

TABLE 2 Molecular Etiologies for NDM

TNDM	PNDM
■ Chromosome 6 anomalies with imprinting mechanisms 　■ paternal duplications 　■ paternal isodisomy (paternal UPD 6) 　■ methylation defects ■ Others without chromosome 6 anomalies	■ Heterozygous activating mutations in *KCNJ11* and *ABCC8* genes ($K_{IR}6.2$ and SUR1 subunits of the pancreatic K_{ATP} channel) ■ Homozygous *GCK* mutations (insensitivity to glucose; dysregulation of glycemia in parents, like *MODY2*) ■ Severe pancreatic hypoplasia linked to homozygous *IPF-1/PDX-1* mutation ■ IPEX syndrome (with diffuse autoimmunity) ■ Mitochondrial disease ■ Association with epiphyseal dysplasia: Wolcott-Rallison syndrome ■ Association with hypothyroidism, glaucoma, and *GLIS3* mutation ■ Possibly associated with enterovirus infection ■ Association with cerebellar hypoplasia and *PTF1A* mutation

Abbreviations: GCK, glucokinase; GLIS, GLI-similar; IPF-1, insulin promoter factor 1; IPEX, immune dysregulation, polyendocrinopathy, enteropathy, X-linked; MODY, maturity-onset diabetes mellitus; NDM, neonatal diabetes mellitus; PNDM, permanent NDM; PTF1A, pancreas specific transcription factor, 1a; TNDM, transient NDM.

Pancreas Agenesis and the IPF-1 Gene
A child described with pancreatic agenesis was homozygous for a single nucleotide deletion within codon 63 of *IPF-1* (Pro63fsdelC) (49). Furthermore, eight individuals with early-onset diabetes have been identified in the extended family as heterozygotes for the same mutation, with the mutant-truncated isoform of *IPF-1* acting as a dominant-negative inhibitor of wild-type *IPF-1* activity.

Anomalies at the Homozygous State in the GCK gene
A few homozygous missense mutations within the *GCK* gene are responsible for complete deficiency in glycolytic activity of the GCK enzyme, yielding to PNDM in neonates, whereas their mild to moderately glucose-intolerant parents were heterozygous for the same mutations (69).

Wolcott-Rallison Syndrome (OMIM 226980)
Wolcott-Rallison syndrome (WRS or MED-IDDM) is an autosomal-recessive disorder characterized by infancy-onset (within the neonatal period) diabetes associated with a spondyloepiphyseal dysplasia. In addition, there is a constellation of other features such as hepatomegaly, mental retardation, renal failure, and early death (70). Further analysis of two consanguineous WRS families led to the identification of frameshift or amino acid–substitution mutations occurring in the *EIF2AK3* gene and segregating with the disorder in each family. The EIF2AK3/PERK kinase is highly expressed in islet cells and participates in protein synthesis regulation and endoplasmic reticulum folding machinery.

IPEX Syndrome (OMIM 304790) and Mutation in the FOXP3 Gene
An X-linked syndrome with a combination of exfoliative dermatitis, intractable diarrhea with villous atrophy, hemolytic anemia, autoimmune thyroid disease, and

NDM has been reported. Most children die in the first year of life with over-whelming sepsis. In some of these cases, agenesis of the islets of Langerhans has been described. The mutation in this condition lies in the forkhead box P3 (*FOXP3*) gene that encodes a forkhead domain–containing protein (71). It has now been demonstrated that the protein product "scurfin" is essential for normal immune homeostasis.

PNDM Associated with Cerebellar Hypoplasia (OMIM 609069) and Mutation in the PTF1A Gene

Another severe syndrome was described in three members of a consanguineous family, with an autosomal-recessive inheritance pattern, who developed NDM associated with pancreatic hypoplasia and microcephaly linked to cerebellar hypoplasia (72). All the infants died within a few months of birth from a combination of metabolic dysfunction, respiratory compromise, and sepsis. This syndrome was found to be linked to mutations in the *PTF1A* gene, encoding for a major transcription factor involved in pancreatic development and also expressed in the cerebellum.

Diabetes and Pancreatic Exocrine Dysfunction (OMIM 609812)

In two families with diabetes and exocrine pancreatic dysfunction (DPED), genetic, physiological, and in vitro functional studies identified that single-base deletions in the carboxyl ester lipase (CEL) gene, a major component of pancreatic juice responsible for the duodenal hydrolysis of cholesterol esters, are responsible for a similar phenotype with β-cell failure and pancreatic exocrine disease (73). The mutant enzyme was less stable and secreted at a lower rate compared with the wild-type CEL protein. These findings link diabetes to the disrupted function of a lipase in the pancreatic acinar cells. Pancreatic lipomatosis was shown to be a structural marker in nondiabetic children with CEL mutations reflecting early events involved in the pathogenesis of this syndrome (74).

OTHER FORMS OF FAMILIAL T2DM

In addition to the established MODY and NDM genes, mutations in additional genes and genetic defects have been implicated in other familial forms of T2DM.

Diabetes Associated with Mitochondrial Defects

Mitochondria contain their own genetic information in the form of a circular DNA molecule of 16,569 base pairs that encodes 13 subunits of the oxidative phosphorylation complex, 2 ribosomal RNAs, and 22 transfer RNAs (tRNA) needed for mitochondrial protein synthesis. Several mitochondrial cytopathies and syndromes caused by point mutations, deletions, or duplications of mitochondrial DNA (mtDNA) and characterized by decreased oxidative phosphorylation are associated with diabetes (75). One of these mutations, an A to G transition in the mitochondrial tRNALeu(UUR) gene at base-pair 3243, has been systematically tested and phenotypically characterized in several populations (75,76). The tRNALeu[3243] mutation co-segregates in families with diabetes and sensorineural deafness of maternal transmission, a syndrome known as MIDD (OMIM 520000). In some populations, MIDD might represent less than 1% of all cases of T2DM. The same mutation was also observed in patients with MELAS, a syndrome of mitochondrial myopathy, encephalopathy, lactic acidosis, and stroke-like episodes, which is often accompanied by diabetes and deafness (77). The mechanisms underlying the different phenotypic expression (MIDD or MELAS) might be related to the variable degree of heteroplasmy in different tissues. The carriers of the tRNALeu^{3243} mutation may present with variable clinical features, ranging from normal glucose tolerance to insulin-requiring diabetes. However, abnormalities in insulin secretion were found in all MIDD subjects that were tested, including those with normal glucose tolerance (78). A defect of glucose-regulated insulin secretion is an early, possible primary abnormality in carriers of the mutation, and it probably results from the progressive reduction of oxidative phosphorylation in β cells caused by the accumulation of mutant mtDNA in the cells (75).

Wolfram Syndrome (OMIM 22233)

Wolfram syndrome (WS) is a rare, autosomal recessive, and neurodegenerative disease. The syndrome is also known as DIDMOAD (diabetes insipidus, diabetes mellitus, optic atrophy, and deafness), which are the main clinical features in WS patients. The gene associated with the syndrome, called *WFS1*, encodes for the wolframin transmembrane protein located in the endoplasmic reticulum (79). The pattern of presentation of WS suggested the existence of mitochondrial impairment, and mtDNA rearrangements were detected in some patients. Although the function of the WFS1 protein remains unknown, it is thought to be related with intracellular calcium homeostasis. All WFS1 mutations resulted in highly unstable proteins, which were delivered to proteasomal degradation. No wolframin aggregates were found in patient cells, suggesting that WS is not a disease of protein aggregation. Rather, WFS1 mutations cause loss of function by cellular depletion of wolframin.

Other Candidate Genes in Familial Diabetes with Later Age of Onset

A mutation in Islet Brain-1 (IB1) was found to be associated with diabetes in one family (80). IB1 is a homologue of the c-jun amino-terminal kinase interacting protein 1 (JIP-1), which plays a role in the modulation of apoptosis. IB1 is also a transactivator of the islet-GLUT2. As the mutant IB1 was found to be unable to prevent apoptosis in vitro, abnormal function of IB1 may render the β cells more susceptible to apoptotic stimuli, thus decreasing β-cell mass. A nonsense mutation (Q310X) in the *MAPK8IP1* gene, coding for another β-cell transcription factor, Islet-1 (Isl-1), was described in a Japanese family with strong family history of diabetes (81).

Three nonsynonymous mutations in the TGF-β-inducible transcription factor kruppel-like factor 11 (KLF11), encoded by the transforming growth factor-beta-inducible early growth response (*TIEG2*) gene, associate with both monogenic early-onset (MODY-like diabetes) and polygenic middle-age-onset T2DM (82). These mutations are responsible for altered KLF11 transcriptional regulation activity (e.g., on insulin and PDX-1 expression). These results strongly suggest a role for the TGF-β signaling pathway in pancreatic diseases affecting endocrine islets (diabetes) or exocrine cells (cancer).

A missense mutation (N333S) in the active site of the enzyme transglutaminase 2 (TGase 2) was identified in a MODY patient and his father who is diabetic and moderately overweight. Assessment of in vivo fast insulin release and glucose-stimulated insulin secretion from isolated islets of TGase 2$^{-/-}$ mice revealed mild impairment of β-cell insulin secretory ability (83). Though the substitution is highly indicative of a role for TGase 2 in the disease and in keeping with the TGase 2 knockout mouse phenotype, the definitive involvement of the enzyme in the pathophysiology of MODY still requires further substantiation.

CONTRIBUTION OF MONOGENIC DIABETES TO MULTIFACTORIAL FORMS OF T2DM

There is now increasing evidence that variants in the genes implicated in monogenic and syndromic forms of diabetes are also involved in susceptibility to more common multifactorial forms of the disease. Indeed, if major mutations (i.e., causing a substantial functional defect and normally rare or absent in the general population) lead to a highly penetrant form of diabetes, it seems plausible that more subtle genetic changes affecting the structure or expression of proteins might play a role in determining (minor) susceptibility to T2DM. Our current understanding of genetic variants influencing T2DM strongly supports this hypothesis (3,24, and Table 3). However, common variants in the six known MODY genes contribute very modestly, if at all, to the common form of T2DM, as recently assessed in a staged case-control study from multiple clinical samples (84). In this study, the strongest effects were found for an intronic variant of *TCF2*/HNF-1β and for the −30 G/A variant of *GCK*.

Of note, private mutations in *HNF-1α* were identified in African-Americans and Japanese subjects with atypical nonautoimmune diabetes with acute onset (85,86); and in the Oji-Cree native Canadian population in which the G319S mutation in *HNF-1α* found in ∼40% of diabetic patients accelerates the onset of T2DM by seven years (87). Such findings also show that *HNF-1α* mutations can be associated with typical adult-onset insulin-resistant obesity-related diabetes in addition to MODY. Mutations in *HNF-4α* and *IPF-1* genes were also identified in a number of families with late-onset T2DM (88). IPF-1/PDX-1 has a dosage-dependent regulatory effect on the expression of β-cell-specific genes, and therefore assists

TABLE 3 Human Genes Identified as Responsible for Monogenic T2DM and for Which Large and/or Replicated Case-Control Studies have Shown Association Between Common Variants in or Close to the Gene and Increased Risk of Diabetes

Gene	Monogenic disease	OMIM	Polygenic T2DM	References
HNF4A	MODY1	125850	5′SNPs (P2 promoter) increased risk in Finnish (OR = 1.33) and Ashkenazim (OR = 1.4)	90,91
GCK	MODY2	125851	variant −30G/A (β-cell promoter) allele frequency: 20%	31,32
TCF1/HNF-1α	MODY3	600496	G319S, OR = 1.97 in Oji-Cree	87
IPF-1	MODY4	606392	5′SNPs and coding variants, increased risk in Caucasian populations	88
TIEG2/KLF11	Early-onset T2DM (T220M, A347S)	603301	G62R, OR = 1.29 in North European populations	82
KCNJ11	PNDM	606176	E23K, OR = 1.2	94,95
ABCC8	CHI, PNDM, dominant T2DM	256450	L270V, OR = 1.15	96,98

Abbreviations: CHI, congenital hyperinsulinism; GCK, glucokinase; HNF, hepatocyte nuclear factor; IPF-1, insulin promoter factor 1; MODY, maturity-onset diabetes of the young; OMIM, online mendelian inheritance in man; OR, odds ratio; PNDM, permanent neonatal diabetes mellitus; SNP, single nucleotide polymorphisms; T2DM, type 2 diabetes mellitus.

in the maintenance of euglycemia. As a consequence, frequent variants in the regulatory sequences controlling IPF-1/PDX-1 expression in the β cell, or in genes coding for transcription factors known to regulate IPF-1, could contribute to common T2DM susceptibility.

More recent studies showed that frequent variants at the *HNF-1α* and *HNF-4α* gene locus may be associated to T2DM in different ethnic groups (89–91). In two independent studies, from Ashkenazim (90) and Finnish (91) populations, convincing associations were reported between common variants adjacent to the *HNF-4α* P2 promoter and T2DM. Interestingly, some of the diabetes-associated variants account for most of the evidence for linkage to chromosome 20q13 reported in both these populations. Consistent with these results, genetic variation near the P2 region of *HNF-4α* is associated with T2DM in other Danish and U.K. populations, but not in French and other Caucasian populations (92), which argues for genetic heterogeneity in *HNF-4α* variant susceptibility. The causal variant(s) affecting the expression or function of HNF-4α are still unknown and could result in a combination of relative insulin deficiency and defective regulation of the hepatic gluconeogenesis.

One study in the Swedish/Finnish population provides in vitro and in vivo evidence that common variants in *HNF-1α* influence transcriptional activity and insulin secretion in vivo. Some of these variants are associated with a modestly increased risk of late-onset T2DM in subsets of elderly overweight individuals (93).

A common variant in *KCNJ11*/$K_{IR}6.2$, E23K, was also associated to an increased risk of diabetes and decreased insulin secretion in glucose-tolerant subjects (94,95). A modest gain of channel activity was attributed to the E23K-$K_{IR}6.2$ polymorphism. Given the functional interaction between the two subunits of the K_{ATP} channel, a mild dominant form of hypoglycemia due to a mutation in *ABCC8*, E1507K, which reduces channel activity, is reported to produce hyperinsulinism at an early age followed by a decreasing insulin secretory capacity in early adulthood and diabetes in middle-age (96).

A major lesson learned from monogenic diabetes is the interest to identify functional mutations co-segregating with early-onset diabetes as a proof of concept of a given gene pivotal role for the establishment and maintenance of adequate β-cell mass and functional capacity (some pathways are shown in Fig. 1), as it was revealed by the discovery of the IPF-1–HNFs regulatory network in β cells. Whether such gene also contributes to the genetic risk for multifactorial T2DM is another issue, dealing with epidemiology and with the search of biomarkers for diabetes. It is likely that other β-cell-expressed genes, when mutated, can increase T2DM risk, and their identification should provide a better understanding of diabetes physiopathology. This later issue can now be largely assessed in several phenotypes; thanks to the newly obtained huge data from the genome-wide association (GWA) studies for T2DM (97, and ongoing studies).

CONCLUSIONS AND PERSPECTIVES

The recent advent of GWA studies, involving the genotyping of hundreds of thousands of single nucleotide polymorphisms (SNPs) spanning the entire genome in patients with polygenic T2DM and controls, promises to greatly speed up the identification of novel T2DM susceptibility genes. The discovery of new T2DM genes will improve our understanding of the molecular mechanisms that maintain glucose homeostasis and of the precise molecular defects leading to

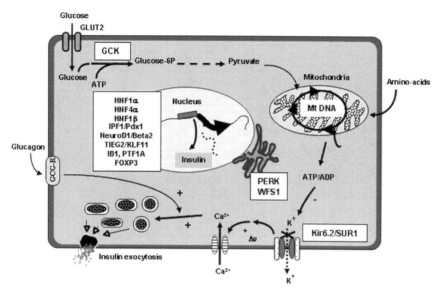

FIGURE 1 Pancreatic β-cell genes known as targets of monogenic diabetes. Human genes identified as responsible for monogenic T2DM are indicated within a white square. *Abbreviations*: GCG-R, glucagon receptor; GCK, glucokinase; Glucose-6P, glucose-6 phosphate; GLUT2, glucose transporter 2; FOXP3, Forkhead box protein P3; HNF, hepatocyte nuclear factor; IB1, Islet Brain-1; IPF-1, insulin promoter factor-1; KLF11, Kruppel-like factor 11; mtDNA, mitochondrial DNA; NeuroD1, neurogenic differentiation factor 1; PERK, pancreatic eIF2-alpha kinase; PTF1A, pancreas-specific transcription factor 1a; TIEG2, TGF-β-inducible early growth response protein 2; WFS1, wolframin transmembrane protein.

chronic hyperglycemia. A nosological classification of T2DM based on primary pathophysiological mechanisms will then be possible. This could lead to the development of more specifically targeted antidiabetic drugs or even gene-based therapies. Moreover, pharmacogenetic testing might then be used to predict for each patient the therapeutic response to different classes of drugs. These novel findings will also provide the tools for the timely identification of high-risk individuals, who might benefit from early behavioral or medical intervention for preventing the development of diabetes. An important reduction in diabetes-related morbidity and mortality could then be expected, along with a reduction in the costs of the treatment of diabetes and its complications.

REFERENCES

1. Ferrannini E. Insulin resistance versus insulin deficiency in non-insulin-dependent diabetes mellitus: problems and prospects. Endocr Rev 1998; 19(4):477–490.
2. Bonadonna RC. Alterations of glucose metabolism in type 2 diabetes mellitus. An overview. Rev Endocr Metab Disord 2004; 5:89–97.
3. Permutt MA, Wasson J, Cox N. Genetic epidemiology of diabetes. J Clin Invest 2005; 115 (6):1431–1439.
4. Zimmet P, Alberti KG, Shaw J. Global and societal implications of the diabetes epidemic. Nature 2001; 414(6865):782–787.

5. Vaxillaire M, Froguel P. Genetic basis of maturity-onset diabetes of the young. Endocrinol Metab Clin North Am 2006; 35(2):371–384.
6. van den Ouweland JM, Lemkes HH, Trembath RC, et al. Maternally inherited diabetes and deafness is a distinct subtype of diabetes and associates with a single point mutation in the mitochondrial tRNA(Leu(UUR)) gene. Diabetes 1994; 43(6):746–751.
7. Polak M, Shield J. Neonatal and very-early-onset diabetes mellitus. Semin Neonatol 2004; 9:59–65.
8. Barker DJ. The fetal and infant origins of disease. Eur J Clin Invest 1995; 25(7):457–463.
9. Hattersley AT, Tooke JE. The fetal insulin hypothesis: an alternative explanation of the association of low birthweight with diabetes and vascular disease. Lancet 1999; 353 (9166):1789–1792.
10. Ledermann HM. Is maturity onset diabetes at young age (MODY) more common in Europe than previously assumed? Lancet 1995; 345(8950):648.
11. Froguel P, Zouali H, Vionnet N, et al. Familial hyperglycemia due to mutations in glucokinase. Definition of a subtype of diabetes mellitus. N Engl J Med 1993; 328 (10):697–702.
12. Yamagata K, Furuta H, Oda N, et al. Mutations in the hepatocyte nuclear factor-4alpha gene in maturity-onset diabetes of the young (MODY1). Nature 1996; 384(6608):458–460.
13. Vaxillaire M, Boccio V, Philippi A, et al. A gene for maturity onset diabetes of the young (MODY) maps to chromosome 12q. Nat Genet 1995; 9(4):418–423.
14. Yamagata K, Oda N, Kaisaki PJ, et al. Mutations in the hepatocyte nuclear factor-1 alpha gene in maturity-onset diabetes of the young (MODY3). Nature 1996; 384(6608): 455–458.
15. Stoffers DA, Ferrer J, Clarke WL, et al. Early-onset type-II diabetes mellitus (MODY4) linked to IPF1. Nat Genet 1997; 17(2):138–139.
16. Horikawa Y, Iwasaki N, Hara M, et al. Mutation in hepatocyte nuclear factor-1 beta gene (TCF2) associated with MODY. Nat Genet 1997; 17(4):384–385.
17. Malecki MT, Jhala US, Antonellis A, et al. Mutations in NEUROD1 are associated with the development of type 2 diabetes mellitus. Nat Genet 1999; 23(3):323–328.
18. Frayling TM, Lindgren CM, Chevre JC, et al. A genome-wide scan in families with maturity-onset diabetes of the young: evidence for further genetic heterogeneity. Diabetes 2003; 52(3):872–881.
19. Kim SH, Ma X, Weremowicz S, et al. Identification of a locus for maturity-onset diabetes of the young on chromosome 8p23. Diabetes 2004; 53(5):1375–1384.
20. Pearson ER, Velho G, Clark P, et al. Beta-cell genes and diabetes: quantitative and qualitative differences in the pathophysiology of hepatic nuclear factor-1 alpha and glucokinase mutations. Diabetes 2001; 50(S1):S101–107.
21. Chevre JC, Hani EH, Boutin P, et al. Mutation screening in 18 Caucasian families suggest the existence of other MODY genes. Diabetologia 1998; 41(9):1017–1023.
22. Costa A, Bescos M, Velho G, et al. Genetic and clinical characterisation of maturity-onset diabetes of the young in Spanish families. Eur J Endocrinol 2000; 142(4):380–386.
23. Lindner TH, Cockburn BN, Bell GI. Molecular genetics of MODY in Germany. Diabetologia 1999; 42(1):121–123.
24. Fajans SS, Bell GI, Polonsky KS. Molecular mechanisms and clinical pathophysiology of maturity-onset diabetes of the young. N Engl J Med 2001; 345(13):971–980.
25. Velho G, Froguel P, Clement K, et al. Primary pancreatic beta-cell secretory defect caused by mutations in glucokinase gene in kindreds of maturity onset diabetes of the young. Lancet 1992; 340(8817):444–448.
26. Byrne MM, Sturis J, Clement K, et al. Insulin secretory abnormalities in subjects with hyperglycemia due to glucokinase mutations. J Clin Invest 1994; 93(3):1120–1130.
27. Velho G, Petersen KF, Perseghin G, et al. Impaired hepatic glycogen synthesis in glucokinase-deficient (MODY-2) subjects. J Clin Invest 1996; 98(8):1755–1761.
28. Velho G, Vaxillaire M, Boccio V, et al. Diabetes complications in NIDDM kindreds linked to the MODY3 locus on chromosome 12q. Diabetes Care 1996; 19(9):915–919.
29. Hattersley AT, Beards F, Ballantyne E, et al. Mutations in the glucokinase gene of the fetus result in reduced birth weight. Nat Genet 1998; 19(3):268–270.

30. Velho G, Hattersley AT, Froguel P. Maternal diabetes alters birth weight in glucokinase-deficient (MODY2) kindred but has no influence on adult weight, height, insulin secretion or insulin sensitivity. Diabetologia 2000; 43(8):1060–1063.
31. Weedon MN, Frayling TM, Shields B, et al. Genetic regulation of birth weight and fasting glucose by a common polymorphism in the islet cell promoter of the glucokinase gene. Diabetes 2005; 54(2):576–581.
32. Marz W, Nauck M, Hoffmann MM, et al. G(-30)A polymorphism in the pancreatic promoter of the glucokinase gene associated with angiographic coronary artery disease and type 2 diabetes mellitus. Circulation 2004; 109:2844–2849.
33. Shih DQ, Stoffel M. Dissecting the transcriptional network of pancreatic islets during development and differentiation. Proc Natl Acad Sci U S A 2001; 98(25):14189–14191.
34. Vaxillaire M, Pueyo ME, Clement K, et al. Insulin secretion and insulin sensitivity in diabetic and non-diabetic subjects with hepatic nuclear factor-1alpha (maturity-onset diabetes of the young-3) mutations. Eur J Endocrinol 1999; 141(6):609–618.
35. Isomaa B, Henricsson M, Lehto M, et al. Chronic diabetic complications in patients with MODY3 diabetes. Diabetologia 1998; 41(4):467–473.
36. Velho G, Benqué-Blanchet F, Vaxillaire M, et al. Renal proximal tubular defects associated to the MODY3 phenotype. Diabetologia 1998; 41(suppl 1):A108.
37. Pontoglio M, Sreenan S, Roe M, et al. Defective insulin secretion in hepatocyte nuclear factor 1alpha-deficient mice. J Clin Invest 1998; 101(10):2215–2222.
38. Vaxillaire M, Abderrahmani A, Boutin P, et al. Anatomy of a homeoprotein revealed by the analysis of human MODY3 mutations. J Biol Chem 1999; 274(50):35639–35646.
39. Wang H, Maechler P, Hagenfeldt KA, et al. Dominant-negative suppression of HNF-1 alpha function results in defective insulin gene transcription and impaired metabolism-secretion coupling in a pancreatic beta-cell line. EMBO J 1998; 17(22):6701–6713.
40. Akpinar P, Kuwajima S, Krutzfeldt J, et al. Tmem27: A cleaved and shed plasma membrane protein that stimulates pancreatic beta cell proliferation. Cell Metab 2005; 2(6):385–397.
41. Hertz R, Magenheim J, Berman I, et al. Fatty acyl-CoA thioesters are ligands of hepatic nuclear factor-4alpha. Nature 1998; 392(6675):512–516.
42. Stoffel M, Duncan SA. The maturity-onset diabetes of the young (MODY1) transcription factor HNF4alpha regulates expression of genes required for glucose transport and metabolism. Proc Natl Acad Sci U S A 1997; 94(24):13209–13214.
43. Gupta RK, Vatamaniuk MZ, Lee CS, et al. The MODY1 gene HNF-4alpha regulates selected genes involved in insulin secretion. J Clin Invest 2005; 115(4):1006–1015.
44. Thomas H, Jaschkowitz K, Bulman M, et al. A distant upstream promoter of the HNF4α gene connects the transcription factors involved in maturity-onset diabetes of the young. Hum Mol Genet 2001; 10(19):2089–2097.
45. Boj SF, Parrizas M, Maestro MA, et al. A transcription factor regulatory circuit in differentiated pancreatic cells. Proc Natl Acad Sci U S A 2001; 98(25):14481–14486.
46. Pearson ER, Boj SF, Steele AM, et al. Macrosomia and hyperinsulinaemic hypoglycaemia in patients with heterozygous mutations in the HNF4A gene. PLoS Med 2007; 4(4):e118.
47. Lindner TH, Njolstad PR, Horikawa Y, et al. A novel syndrome of diabetes mellitus, renal dysfunction and genital malformation associated with a partial deletion of the pseudo-POU domain of hepatocyte nuclear factor-1beta. Hum Mol Genet 1999; 8(11):2001–2008.
48. Bellanne-Chantelot C, Clauin S, Chauveau D, et al. Large genomic rearrangements in the hepatocyte nuclear factor-1{beta} (TCF2) gene are the most frequent cause of maturity-onset diabetes of the young type 5. Diabetes 2005; 54(11):3126–3132.
49. Stoffers DA, Ferrer J, Clarke WL, et al. Early-onset type-II diabetes mellitus (MODY4) linked to IPF1. Nat Genet 1997; 17(2):138–139.
50. Malecki MT, Jhala US, Antonellis A, et al. Mutations in NEUROD1 are associated with the development of type 2 diabetes mellitus. Nat Genet 1999; 23(3):323–328.
51. Pearson ER, Starkey BJ, Powell RJ, et al. Genetic cause of hyperglycaemia and response to treatment in diabetes. Lancet 2003; 362(9392):1275–1281.

52. Gloyn AL, Noordam K, Willemsen MA, et al. Insights into the biochemical and genetic basis of glucokinase activation from naturally occurring hypoglycemia mutations. Diabetes 2003; 52(9):2433–2440.
53. Guertin KR, Grimsby J. Small molecule glucokinase activators as glucose lowering agents: a new paradigm for diabetes therapy. Curr Med Chem 2006; 13(15):1839–1843.
54. Gardner RJ, Mackay DJ, Mungall AJ, et al. An imprinted locus associated with transient neonatal diabetes mellitus. Hum Mol Genet 2000; 9(4):589–596.
55. Ma D, Shield JP, Dean W, et al. Impaired glucose homeostasis in transgenic mice expressing the human transient neonatal diabetes mellitus locus, TNDM. J Clin Invest 2004; 114(3):339–348.
56. Hattersley AT, Ashcroft FM. Activating mutations in Kir6.2 and neonatal diabetes: new clinical syndromes, new scientific insights, and new therapy. Diabetes 2005; 54:2503–2513.
57. Gloyn AL, Pearson ER, Antcliff JF, et al. Activating mutations in the gene encoding the ATP-sensitive potassium-channel subunit Kir6.2 and permanent neonatal diabetes. N Engl J Med 2004; 350(18):1838–1849.
58. Vaxillaire M, Populaire C, Busiah K, et al. Kir6.2 mutations are a common cause of permanent neonatal diabetes in a large cohort of French patients. Diabetes 2004; 53 (10):2719–2722.
59. Flanagan SE, Edghill EL, Gloyn AL, et al. Mutations in KCNJ11, which encodes Kir6.2, are a common cause of diabetes diagnosed in the first 6 months of life, with the phenotype determined by genotype. Diabetologia 2006; 49(6):1190–1197.
60. Babenko AP, Polak M, Cavé H, et al. Activating mutations in ABCC8 cause neonatal diabetes mellitus. N Engl J Med 2006; 355(5):456–466.
61. Babenko AP, Gonzalez G, Aguilar-Bryan L, et al. Sulfonylurea receptors set the maximal open probability, ATP sensitivity and plasma membrane density of K_{ATP} channels. FEBS Lett 1999; 445:131–136.
62. Aguilar-Bryan L, Bryan J. Molecular biology of adenosine triphosphate-sensitive potassium channels. Endocr Rev 1999; 20(2):101–135.
63. Babenko AP. K_{ATP} channels "vingt ans apres": ATG to PDB to mechanism. J Mol Cell Cardiol 2005; 39:79–98.
64. Koster JC, Marshall BA, Ensor N, et al. Targeted overactivity of beta cell K_{ATP} channels induces profound neonatal diabetes. Cell 2000; 100:645–654.
65. Masia R, Deleon DD, Macmullen C, et al. A mutation in the TMD0-L0 region of SUR1 (L225P) causes permanent neonatal diabetes mellitus (PNDM). Diabetes 2007; 56:1357–1362.
66. Vaxillaire M, Dechaume A, Busiah K, et al. New ABCC8 mutations in relapsing neonatal diabetes and clinical features. Diabetes 2007; 56:1737–1741.
67. Huopio H, Otonkoski T, Vauhkonen I, et al. A new subtype of autosomal dominant diabetes attributable to a mutation in the gene for sulfonylurea receptor 1. Lancet 2003; 361(9354):301–307.
68. Pearson ER, Flechtner I, Njolstad PR, et al. Neonatal diabetes international collaborative group. switching from insulin to oral sulfonylureas in patients with diabetes due to Kir6.2. N Engl J Med 2006; 355:467–477.
69. Njolstad PR, Sovik O, Cuesta-Munoz A, et al. Neonatal diabetes mellitus due to complete glucokinase deficiency. N Engl J Med 2001; 344(21):1588–1592.
70. Senee V, Vattem KM, Delepine M, et al. Wolcott-Rallison Syndrome: clinical, genetic, and functional study of EIF2AK3 mutations and suggestion of genetic heterogeneity. Diabetes 2004; 53(7):1876–1883.
71. Bennett CL, Christie J, Ramsdell F, et al. The immune dysregulation, polyendocrinopathy, enteropathy, X-linked syndrome (IPEX) is caused by mutations of FOXP3. Nat Genet 2001; 27(1):20–21.
72. Sellick GS, Barker KT, Stolte-Dijkstra I, et al. Mutations in PTF1A cause pancreatic and cerebellar agenesis. Nat Genet 2004; 36(12):1301–1305.
73. Raeder H, Johansson S, Holm PI, et al. Mutations in the CEL VNTR cause a syndrome of diabetes and pancreatic exocrine dysfunction. Nat Genet 2006; 38(1):54–62.

74. Raeder H, Haldorsen IS, Ersland L, et al. Pancreatic lipomatosis is a structural marker in nondiabetic children with mutations in carboxyl-ester lipase. Diabetes 2007; 56 (2):444–449.
75. Maassen JA, Janssen GM, 't Hart LM. Molecular mechanisms of mitochondrial diabetes (MIDD). Ann Med 2005; 37(3):213–221.
76. Vionnet N, Passa P, Froguel P. Prevalence of mitochondrial gene mutations in families with diabetes mellitus. Lancet 1993; 342:1429–1430.
77. Ciafaloni E, Ricci E, Shanske S, et al. MELAS: clinical features, biochemistry, and molecular genetics. Ann Neurol 1992; 31:391–398.
78. Velho G, Byrne MM, Clement K, et al. Clinical phenotypes, insulin secretion, and insulin sensitivity in kindreds with maternally inherited diabetes and deafness due to mitochondrial tRNALeu(UUR) gene mutation. Diabetes 1996; 45:478–487.
79. Domenech E, Gomez-Zaera M, Nunes V. Wolfram/DIDMOAD syndrome, a heterogenic and molecularly complex neurodegenerative disease. Pediatr Endocrinol Rev 2006; 3(3):249–257.
80. Waeber G, Delplanque J, Bonny C, et al. The gene MAPK8IP1, encoding islet-brain-1, is a candidate for type 2 diabetes. Nat Genet 2000; 24(3):291–295.
81. Shimomura H, Sanke T, Hanabusa T, et al. Nonsense mutation of islet-1 gene (Q310X) found in a type 2 diabetic patient with a strong family history. Diabetes 2000; 49 (9):1597–1600.
82. Neve B, Fernandez-Zapico ME, Ashkenazi-Katalan V, et al. Role of transcription factor KLF11 and its diabetes-associated gene variants in pancreatic beta cell function. Proc Natl Acad Sci U S A 2005; 102(13):4807–4812.
83. Bernassola F, Federici M, Corazzari M, et al. Role of transglutaminase 2 in glucose tolerance: knockout mice studies and a putative mutation in a MODY patient. FASEB J 2002; 16(11):1371–1378.
84. Winckler W, Weedon MN, Graham RR, et al. Evaluation of common variants in the six known maturity-onset diabetes of the young (MODY) genes for association with type 2 diabetes. Diabetes 2007; 56(3):685–693.
85. Boutin P, Gresh L, Cisse A, et al. Missense mutation Gly574Ser in the transcription factor HNF-1alpha is a marker of atypical diabetes mellitus in African-American children. Diabetologia 1999; 42(3):380–381.
86. Iwasaki N, Oda N, Ogata M, et al. Mutations in the hepatocyte nuclear factor-1alpha/MODY3 gene in Japanese subjects with early- and late-onset NIDDM. Diabetes 1997; 46 (9):1504–1508.
87. Triggs-Raine BL, Kirkpatrick RD, Kelly SL, et al. HNF-1alpha G319S, a transactivation-deficient mutant, is associated with altered dynamics of diabetes onset in an Oji-Cree community. Proc Natl Acad Sci U S A 2002; 99(7):4614–4619.
88. Hani EH, Stoffers DA, Chevre JC, et al. Defective mutations in the insulin promoter factor-1 (IPF1) gene in late-onset type 2 diabetes mellitus. J Clin Invest 1999; 104(9):R41–R48.
89. Winckler W, Burtt NP, Holmkvist J, et al. Association of common variation in the HNF1alpha gene region with risk of type 2 diabetes. Diabetes 2005; 54(8):2336–2342.
90. Love-Gregory LD, Wasson J, Ma J, et al. A common polymorphism in the upstream promoter region of the hepatocyte nuclear factor-4α gene on chromosome 20q is associated with type 2 diabetes and appears to contribute to the evidence for linkage in an Ashkenazi Jewish population. Diabetes 2004; 53(4):1134–1140.
91. Silander K, Mohlke KL, Scott LJ, et al. Genetic variation near the hepatocyte nuclear factor-4alpha gene predicts susceptibility to type 2 diabetes. Diabetes 2004; 53(4): 1141–1149.
92. Vaxillaire M, Dina C, Lobbens S, et al. Effect of common polymorphisms in the HNF4α promoter on Type 2 diabetes susceptibility in the French Caucasian population. Diabetologia 2005; 48(3):440–444.
93. Holmkvist J, Cervin C, Lyssenko V, et al. Common variants in HNF-1 alpha and risk of type 2 diabetes. Diabetologia 2006; 49(12):2882–2891.
94. Love-Gregory L, Wasson K, Lin J, et al. An E23K single nucleotide polymorphism in the islet ATP-sensitive potassium channel gene (Kir6.2) contributes as much to the risk of type II diabetes in Caucasians as the PPARgamma. Diabetologia 2003; 46(1):136–137.

95. Gloyn AL, Weedon MN, Owen KR, et al. Large scale association studies of variants in genes encoding the pancreatic beta-cell K-ATP channel subunits Kir6.2 (KCNJ11) and SUR1 (ABCC8) confirm that the KCNJ11 E23K variant is associated with increased risk of type 2. Diabetes 2003; 52(2):568–572.

96. Huopio H, Otonkoski T, Vauhkonen I, et al. A new subtype of autosomal dominant diabetes attributable to a mutation in the gene for sulfonylurea receptor 1. Lancet 2003; 361:301–307.

97. Sladek R, Rocheleau G, Rung J, et al. A genome-wide association study identifies novel risk loci for type 2 diabetes. Nature 2007; 445(7130):881–885.

98. Florez JC, Burtt N, de Bakker PI, et al. Haplotype structure and genotype–phenotype correlations of the sulfonylurea receptor and the islet ATP-sensitive potassium channel gene region. Diabetes 2004; 53(5):1360–1368.

12 | Natural Evolution, Prediction, and Prevention of Type 1 Diabetes in Youth

Craig E. Taplin and Jennifer M. Barker
Barbara Davis Center for Childhood Diabetes, Aurora, Colorado, U.S.A.

INTRODUCTION

The autoimmune process underlying type 1 diabetes mellitus (T1DM) has been hypothesized to be chronic and progressive (1). In this model, people born with a genetic risk for diabetes experience an as yet undefined insult, initiating a cascade of events leading to the activation of autoreactive T cells, their migration to the pancreatic islet, and eventual destruction of β cells. This process is marked by the production of islet autoantibodies, which can be detected in the serum prior to the development of clinically significant hyperglycemia (2).

β-CELL AUTOIMMUNITY, ANTIBODIES, AND THE DEVELOPMENT OF T1DM

The first antibodies described in association with β-cell autoimmunity and the development of T1DM were islet-cell autoantibodies (ICA) (3), discovered upon the investigation of the association between Addison's disease (a disorder known to be associated with a lymphocytic infiltrative process) and diabetes. Subsequently, antibodies to insulin (IAA) (4,5), glutamic acid decarboxylase (GAA or GAD) (2), and protein tyrosine phosphatase (IA2 or ICA512) (6) have all been defined and are used in the clinical setting to confirm T1DM, as well as in research studies aimed at prediction and prevention of T1DM. They may be present years before the development of symptomatic hyperglycemia (7), and the presence of more than one persistently positive antibody has been shown to reliably predict the development of T1DM (8,9).

ANTIBODIES AND PROGRESSION TO TYPE 1 DIABETES

Intense investigation in recent years of the temporal relationship between islet autoantibodies and the development of T1DM has expanded the understanding of the evolution of β-cell destruction, and importantly, improved the ability to predict diabetes. The predictive value of measuring these antibodies in patients prior to the onset of hyperglycemia is now well established.

Prospective population-based studies, such as the diabetes autoimmunity study in the young (DAISY) (8), the German BabyDIAB study (10), and the Finnish diabetes prediction and prevention study (DIPP) study (11,12), have established that markers of β-cell destruction appear months or years before the onset of diabetes and can occur as early as the first year of life (8,13).

Islet Autoantibodies May Appear and Then Disappear

A subgroup of patients in the above-mentioned DAISY study of high-risk individuals developed markers of autoimmunity that subsequently waned on repeat testing months or years later (8). Falsely positive results were excluded as an explanation for this finding through rigorous study design and blinded repeat sampling. In the DAISY study, 50 of 162 confirmed positives were transient, with many positive at more than one visit before autoimmunity markers waned. In a mean follow-up period of four years, none of these patients went on to develop T1DM. These results suggest islet-cell autoimmunity is not always an inevitable and inexorable road toward absolute insulin deficiency, and there may be factors or characteristics in these patients that are associated with the "switching off" of islet-cell destruction. The identification of these factors might shed light on possible therapeutic interventions.

Markers of Islet Autoimmunity Develop Sequentially

Research suggests that humoral autoimmunity to islet antigens develops sequentially over months or years. This does not exclude the possibility that a precipitating event or insult occurs at one point in time, but evidence suggests that autoimmune β-cell destruction is chronic and progressive.

Samples from 155 young first-degree relatives of subjects with T1DM in the DAISY study, along with a separate group of older first-degree relatives, were studied yearly for appearance of IAA, IA2, and GAA and then at three to six months' intervals once one antibody became positive (14). In the childhood group, none showed evidence of simultaneous seroconversion for more than one antibody. The acquisition of a second or third islet autoantibody may occur months to years after the appearance of the first antibody, showing significant variability. Higher risk genotypes do not seem to be a factor in the tempo of sequential antibody acquisition. All those who eventually developed diabetes had multiple antibodies present before a diagnosis of T1DM was made. One child was persistently positive for three antibodies for eight years before presenting with symptoms of hyperglycemia, but most develop diabetes within two years of acquiring a third antibody.

Of the three commonly measured islet autoantibodies, GAA or IAA tends to appear first, followed by IA2. Of those patients above who eventually expressed multiple autoantibodies, two-thirds acquired GAA first and one-third acquired IAA first.

Number of Islet Autoantibodies Predicts T1DM

Research in the last 10 to 15 years has shown that the number of antibodies, rather than the type of individual antibody or combination of antibodies, is most predictive of progression to overt diabetes. Verge et al. analyzed samples from 45 new-onset T1DM patients along with a large number of first-degree relatives and controls (9). Of those with new-onset T1DM, 98% had at least one antibody and more than 75% had at least two antibodies at the time of diagnosis. No control subjects had more than one antibody. In the high-risk cohort, no difference in the diabetes-free period was found between those who acquired IAA first and those who acquired GAA first.

The same group quantified the five-year risk for developing T1DM in people with a first-degree relative with T1DM (7). 882 first-degree relatives were analyzed with GAA, IAA, and IA2 measured, and then followed for up to 11 years. For each extra autoantibody acquired, the risk for developing T1DM was significantly increased. For those with two or more antibodies, the three-year risk was 39%, and five-year risk 68%. Those subjects positive for all three islet antibodies had a five-year risk for developing T1DM of 100%. Later data from DAISY has shown that during a mean four-year follow-up period (range 0.17–9 years), 41% (24 of 58) patients persistently positive for at least one antibody developed overt T1DM (8).

Characteristics of Islet Autoimmunity Markers are Associated with an Increased Risk for T1DM

Autoantibody titers correlate with persistence of islet autoimmunity and development of overt diabetes. Higher levels of IAA are more likely to remain positive on subsequent samples and differentiate patients who go on to develop T1DM from those persistently non-diabetic (8). Higher GAA levels also distinguish those with persistent islet autoantibodies from those transiently positive. In a cohort from Germany and the Bart's Oxford (BOX) study, IA2 titers in the highest 75% had significantly higher risk (79% over 10 years) than the lowest 25% (15). In the same study, the highest IAA quartile had a 10-year risk for T1DM much higher than the lowest three quartiles (77% vs. 37% at 10 years).

Similarly, higher affinity autoantibodies to insulin are associated with development of T1DM. Achenbach et al. have analyzed the affinity of anti-insulin autoantibodies for children followed prospectively (16). Children who went on to develop multiple anti-islet autoantibodies or to progress to diabetes tended to express high-affinity IAA autoantibodies.

Metabolic Abnormalities Prior to the Development of T1DM

Long-term follow-up of families positive for islet-cell antibodies with serial intravenous glucose tolerance tests (IVGTT) suggested a model where β-cell loss is linear (1,17). However, β-cell loss can show considerable variability, where in some ICA-positive individuals it may be so slow that diabetes never develops during their lifetime (18). Researchers have proposed models to further define and predict the natural history of the prediabetic period using both first-phase insulin response (FPIR), as a measure of residual β-cell function measured on IVGTT, and antibody titers. This model found that the time remaining before developing clinically significant hyperglycemia was predictable from the FPIR and IAA level (19).

The type 1 DIPP performed in Finland, where the highest rates of childhood T1DM in the world are found, confirmed that FPIRs on IVGTT were below the fifth percentile of normal in more than 40% of children at the time of seroconversion to ICA positivity (20). Antibodies were measured at maximum intervals of 12 months, and FPIR was measured at a mean time of 0.6 years after the positive result. Those with higher ICA titers had significantly lower FPIR than those with lower ICA titers. Multiregression analysis showed that low FPIR was associated with being positive for multiple autoantibodies and high titers of IAA. Approximately, half of those with a low FPIR went on to develop diabetes at a mean interval of 2.2 years after they converted to positive ICA. Data from the diabetes-prevention trial (DPT) showed similar results with 80% of those in the lowest quartile for FPIR developing T1DM within four years (Fig. 1). Oral glucose tolerance tests (oral GTTs) and IVGTTs together predict diabetes-free survival with greater sensitivity than FPIR alone (21).

The Diabetes Prevention Trial Type-1 (DPT-1) provided further data on the prediabetic period. In both the oral and parenteral insulin intervention arms (22,23), oral GTTs were performed at six-month intervals until a diagnosis of T1DM

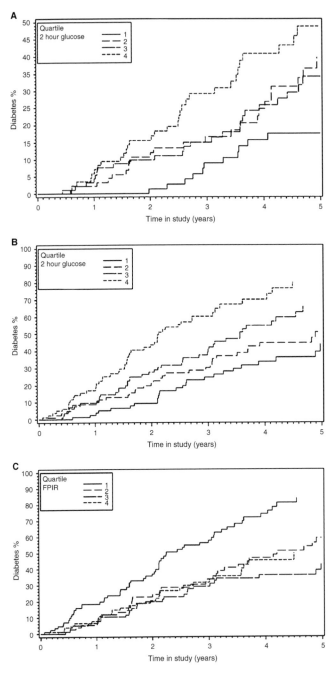

FIGURE 1 **(A)** Time to diabetes by quartile of two-hour glucose on oral glucose tolerance testing in the oral insulin prevention trial. *Subjects in the highest quartile of 2-hour glucose had a shorter diabetes-free survival time compared with subjects in the lowest quartile.* **(B)** Time to diabetes by quartile of two-hour glucose on oral glucose-tolerance testing in the parenteral insulin-prevention trial. **(C)** Time to diabetes by quartile of FPIR on intravenous glucose tolerance testing in the parenteral insulin-prevention trial. *Abbreviation*: FPIR, first-phase insulin response. *Source*: From Ref. 21.

was made. Inclusion criteria for this trial are described elsewhere (see later in this chapter), but briefly, participants were relatives of people with T1DM positive for ICA with a high five-year risk for developing diabetes. Available oral GTT data collected every six months were used to describe the metabolic prodrome in the 30-month period prior to a diagnosis of T1DM (24). Forty-five percent of those in the parenteral arm had impaired fasting glycemia (IFG-fasting BGL 100–126 mg/dL) or impaired glucose tolerance (IGT-2 hour BGL 140–199 mg/dL) 30 months prior to diagnosis of T1DM. Nearly one quarter of those in the oral insulin arm also had either IFG or IGT 30 months out from a diagnosis of T1DM. This collective incidence of IFG or IGT increased to >80% of all patients six months prior to diagnosis. There was a slight but steady decline in stimulated C-peptide levels up until six months before diagnosis, but fasting C-peptide levels did not change. This slight deviation away from normal glycemia significantly accelerates in the last six months before diagnosis with increased glucose area under the curve (AUC) on oral GTT. Importantly, and reflecting β-cell failure, post-challenge C-peptide:glucose ratios decline markedly in the last six months. In other words, β-cell response (insulin production) to a given change in blood glucose declines much more steeply in the last six months before diagnosis when compared with that two to three years prior. Interestingly, fasting C-peptide levels were not found to change significantly, and in fact were increased at diagnosis compared with six months prior to diagnosis. This observation may reflect insulin resistance at the time of diagnosis.

Thus, it appears that the glycemic progression to T1DM can occur gradually over years and is characterized by a steady decline in insulin response to a glucose load that is measurable in many patients at least two years prior to diagnosis, with relative preservation of fasting C-peptide. Within six months of diagnosis, there appears to be a steep increase in glycemia and steep decline in β-cell function, most illuminatingly documented by increases in stimulated C-peptide:glucose ratios. It is important to note that in some individuals, such as those diagnosed with T1DM prior to 12 months of age, the progression to β-cell failure may be very rapid.

FPIR and ΔC-peptide:Δglucose ratios are measures of β-cell function. A reliable measure of β-cell mass may also be useful clinically in following the natural history of the prediabetic and early post-diagnosis period. Imaging with magnetic resonance imaging (MRI) and/or isotope scans that directly image and thus quantify islet-cell mass is not yet in routine clinical practice, and clinical trials of their utility and accuracy in children are complicated by the ethical dilemmas associated with introducing a procedure or dose of radiation to a child. Studies like these are more likely to be successfully approved in adults, and at this time imaging is not routinely used to follow β-cell mass. More sensitive assays for HbA1c may also provide utility in following the natural history of the prediabetic period. It has been shown, for example, that in ICA-positive nondiabetic individuals, mean HbA1c is higher (within the normal range) than ICA-negative subjects. Results such as this suggest that a highly sensitive HbA1c may be useful before the onset of overt diabetes and may be able to detect early changes in glucose metabolism such as those described above.

It must be said, too, that the diagnosis of diabetes is a clinically important but essentially arbitrary point along the pathway of autoimmune β-cell destruction. Actual timing of overt diabetes may vary according to insulin requirements at a given time of life. For example, at times of physiologically exaggerated insulin resistance, a given reduction in insulin secretory capacity may produce symptoms when at a more insulin-sensitive period of life it would not. Insulin response to glucose increases with age (18), and so an attenuation or loss of this increase with age, without symptoms of hyperglycemia, probably, in fact, represents β-cell loss.

Additionally, autoimmune β-cell loss continues after the diagnosis of diabetes. Many patients will experience a temporary remission from insulin dependency, or a reduction in required insulin dose—the so-called "honeymoon period," which may be attributed to β-cell rest from insulin therapy with slowing of loss of measurable C-peptide. Intensive insulin therapy slows this loss further (25). More rapid loss of C-peptide is known to occur in those presenting at a young age of onset (e.g., 12 months of age), in those with higher ICA titers and in those in diabetic ketoacidosis (DKA) at diagnosis (26).

Studies documenting individuals with confirmed positive islet autoantibodies, mentioned above, who show disappearance of antibodies, suggest progression to diabetes may not be completely predictable, and perhaps islet-cell destruction occurs along a variety of paradigms with some individuals able to "switch off" the process at a certain point in time along the pathway and achieve remission. This model shows overlap with the model of other autoimmune diseases, some of which have an increased risk in the same patients affected by T1DM, such as autoimmune thyroid disease. The alternative interpretation might be, however, that there is a subset of individuals in whom detectable T1DM antibodies are not associated with islet autoimmunity.

PREVENTION OF TYPE 1 DIABETES

A thorough understanding of the natural history of type 1 diabetes provides a framework for the treatment strategies that are currently under development and/ or investigation. As subjects pass through the different stages of the natural history of T1DM, our ability to identify them as at risk increases. On the other hand, our ability to identify subjects depends on measuring markers of the autoimmune process such as autoantibodies and T-cell assays against β-cell proteins. Therefore, subjects that we are able to identify are already experiencing an autoimmune process that may be firmly established and difficult to alter. Interventions targeted early in the disease process, by necessity, will treat some people that were never going to develop diabetes. Interventions targeted late in the diagnosis may be less likely to be effective. Therefore, the paradox of prevention/treatment strategies is that the subjects most likely to benefit from these strategies are also at a relatively low risk for T1DM (Fig. 2) (27,28). This observation has major implications for study design. In early stages, large numbers of subjects are needed to adequately power the studies and the treatments must be very safe. Additionally, T1DM is a disease of childhood with a natural history of autoimmunity for many years. Therefore, earlier interventions will on average be targeted at younger children, requiring special consideration of physiological and ethical implications.

The diabetes control and complications trial (DCCT) (29) and its follow-up study (The Epidemiology of Diabetes Interventions and Complications [EDIC]) (30) have clearly shown the benefit of excellent glycemic control for the prevention of diabetes-related complications. Additionally, subjects participating in these studies had a lower incidence of complications in the presence of evidence for endogenous insulin secretion as measured by C-peptide (31). Despite the unequivocal findings of the DCCT, achieving tight glycemic control is not easily achieved, nor without complication, and requires a large commitment on the part of the patient, family,

The Treatment Dilemma

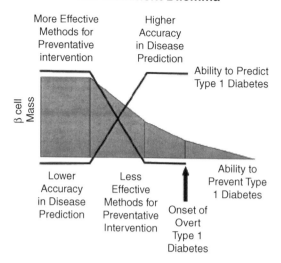

FIGURE 2 The treatment dilemma in type 1 diabetes prevention. *Source*: From Ref. 27 (reprinted with permission from the American Diabetes Association).

and health-care team. Physiologic states such as puberty and pregnancy can further complicate the ability to achieve targets of diabetes therapy. Therefore, goals of diabetes research in the decades to come include both the prevention of T1DM as well as treatment of established patients to preserve C-peptide production.

Treatment strategies employed have generally evolved from animal data in which many different methods are available to prevent the development of T1DM (32). Strategies have been classified as antigen specific (targeting the β cell) and antigen nonspecific (affecting the immune system in general) (28). With these issues in mind, we will discuss strategies paralleling the natural history of type 1 diabetes. Table 1 outlines characteristics of interventions proposed at different stages in terms of outcome monitored, safety, and targeted mechanisms.

GENETIC SUSCEPTIBILITY

We are now able to identify groups of subjects on the basis of family history and HLA genotyping that have risk for the development of diabetes-related auto-immunity and T1DM greater than 50% (33,34). Prevention strategies that work in this very high genetic risk group may be eventually applied to groups at a relatively lower risk, for example children from the general population with the high-risk HLA genotypes. In general, these studies test very safe interventions with the outcome of measurable diabetes-related autoantibodies (27,28).

TRIGR (Trial to Reduce IDDM in the Genetically at Risk)

There is conflicting evidence for cow's milk as an environmental antigen associated with T1DM (35,36). Despite this controversy, a prevention study has begun to test the hypothesis that avoidance of cow's milk within the first nine months of life will decrease β-cell autoimmunity in young children at high genetic risk for T1DM.

TABLE 1 ' General Scheme for Diabetes Prevention

Stage	Subject identifiers	Mechanism	Outcome	Examples
Genetic risk	Family history, HLA genotypes	Prevent autoimmunity Promote a toleragenic response	Diabetes-related autoimmunity	TRIGR NIP-diabetes POINT
Autoimmunity	IAA, GAD, ICA/ IA2 family history	Alter immune response	Diabetes	DPT-1 ENDIT TrialNet oral insulin trial
Metabolic abnormalities	IGT Decreased FPIR	Alter immune response Promote β-cell expansion	Diabetes	DPT-1 parenteral insulin trial
New-onset diabetes	Diagnosis of diabetes	Alter immune response Promote β-cell expansion	C-peptide	See Table 2

Abbreviations: DPT, diabetes prevention trial; ENDIT, European nicotinamide diabetes intervention trial; FPIR, first-phase insulin response; GAD, glutamic acid decarboxylase; IAA, antibodies to insulin; IGT, impaired glucose tolerance; NIP-diabetes, nutritional intervention to prevent diabetes; POINT, primary oral/intranasal insulin trial; TRIGR, trial to reduce IDDM in the genetically at risk.

Children participating in this study are high risk on the basis of family history of T1DM and the presence of HLA genes that are associated with diabetes. All mothers of children participating in this study are encouraged to breast-feed their children and are randomized to receive cow's milk formula or a hydrolyzed casein formula when formula is introduced. The study is enrolling children from multiple centers throughout the world. A pilot study has shown that the intervention is safe and feasible and suggested that infants given the hydrolyzed casein formula may be at a decreased risk for diabetes-related autoantibodies (37).

NUTRITIONAL INTERVENTION TO PREVENT DIABETES

Administration of cod-liver oil during pregnancy and the first year of life has been associated with a decreased risk for T1DM (38). Cod-liver oil contains both vitamin D and docosahexanoic acid (DHA), a 22:6 n-3 fatty acid. Laboratory studies have suggested that DHA may be associated with a decrease in inflammation (39). Studies of the natural history of T1DM have suggested that children who develop diabetes have higher levels of inflammatory markers prior to the diagnosis of diabetes compared with those who have not developed diabetes (40). Nutritional intervention to prevent diabetes (NIP-diabetes) is a multicenter randomized clinical trial to test the hypothesis that the administration of DHA in pregnancy and early infancy in high genetic risk subjects will delay the development of diabetes-related autoimmunity. Pregnant women and infants less than five months of age will be enrolled into the study, with infants continued in the study if they carry a high-risk HLA genotype. Participants will be randomized to DHA or placebo and followed for the development of two or more diabetes-related autoantibodies. The initial study is a pilot and progression to a full study will be dependent on the ability to demonstrate an increased level of DHA in treated subjects, the ability to identify a change in an inflammatory cytokine (IL-1B) and compliance with the treatment protocol. This protocol is administered through TrialNet and has begun enrollment.

POINT (Primary Oral/Intranasal Insulin Trial)

A large amount of animal and human data implicates insulin as a primary auto-antigen for T1DM. The NOD mouse model of T1DM expresses autoantibodies to insulin (41). T cells reactive to insulin have been identified in these mice and in humans (42). Mucosal insulin delays the onset of diabetes in mice (43) and has been tested in humans and found to be safe (23,44). This result has prompted inves-tigators to propose the use of mucosal insulin (intranasal insulin) as a prevention strategy. The initial stage will be a pilot to investigate the safety, feasibility, and immune efficacy of mucosal insulin. It is a multicenter randomized placebo-controlled dose escalation study called Pre-POINT. Progression to the larger, randomized controlled trial, POINT, will be dependent on the establishment of a safe dose that induces an immune response to insulin.

Studies such as these are pushing forward with a new approach to diabetes prevention. Previously performed studies have targeted subjects after the devel-opment of diabetes-related autoimmunity when the autoimmune process has begun. Investigators carrying out studies in pregnant women, babies, and young children who express no autoimmunity carry the burden to prove that the inter-vention is safe. Only very safe treatments will be feasible to evaluate for efficacy. If these treatments are found to be safe and efficacious in these high-risk populations, there is the potential to extend them to the general population, providing a ratio-nale for widespread HLA genotype screening.

DIABETES-RELATED AUTOIMMUNITY

The majority of prevention studies have focused on subjects already expressing diabetes-related autoimmunity. To date, no study has shown a clear decrease in the incidence of diabetes in the treated group compared with control. However, as this group has a risk for diabetes from 20–80% within 5–10 years, they continue to be enrolled in studies of diabetes prevention.

Insulin: Parenteral, Oral, and Intranasal

The DPT-1 tested the related hypotheses that parenteral (22) or oral insulin (23) would delay the onset of T1DM in subjects at high risk compared with placebo. First-degree and young second-degree relatives of subjects with T1DM were invited to be screened. Subjects identified with a 50–75% risk for T1DM were offered enrollment in the parenteral insulin trial and randomized to parenteral insulin or observation. Subjects with a 25–50% five-year risk for T1DM were offered enrollment in the oral insulin trial and randomized to oral insulin or placebo. The overall study showed no difference in the incidence of diabetes in the treatment versus control groups, and neither showed a delay in the onset of T1DM. However, a subgroup of subjects in the oral insulin trial with the highest insulin autoanti-bodies appeared to have a delay in diabetes development of approximately four years that approached statistical significance. Therefore, a repeat trial of oral insulin is planned in TrialNet.

Intranasal insulin has been tested in a phase I trial and shown to not accel-erate the destruction of pancreatic β cells (44). Additionally, immune changes observed were consistent with mucosal tolerance to insulin. Therefore, a larger trial powered to detect a delay in diabetes development has begun enrollment as intra-nasal insulin trial II (INIT II). This response is also being tested in young children with diabetes-related antibodies through the DIPP study.

European Nicotinamide Diabetes Intervention Trial

Nicotinamide is a vitamin B3 derivative. Studies in patients with newly diagnosed T1DM suggested that treatment with nicotinamide was associated with preservation of C-peptide. Therefore, a large clinical trial of relatives of subjects with T1DM who were ICA positive was performed to determine if the administration of nicotinamide could delay the onset of diabetes in this high-risk cohort. Almost 30,000 first-degree relatives were screened and 552 were randomized to nicotinamide versus placebo. No delay in diabetes development was detected over five-years of follow-up (45).

Current studies include the TrialNet oral insulin trial, and the INIT and DIPP intranasal insulin trials. Results of these trials will be available within the next decade. Trials testing other agents are also under development and will likely begin enrolling over the several years.

These studies represent a monumental effort over many years. Combined, these studies screened ~130,000 subjects to identify a combined total of 1263 for participation. They represent a major commitment of time and resources within the diabetes research community and family members of subjects with T1DM. Although methods to prevent diabetes were not developed through the DPT-1 or European nicotinamide diabetes intervention trial (ENDIT), the diabetes community has benefited from these studies. First, a network of investigators was established that continues today through TrialNet. This network provides the venue in which to study the natural history of T1DM and trials for its prevention or cure. Secondly, the risk algorithms developed for diabetes, detailed earlier in this chapter, were confirmed by these trials.

NEW-ONSET DIABETES

Advancements in immunology have been pivotal to the development of prevention and treatment trials for T1DM. Specifically, the understanding of the maintenance of self-tolerance as an active process mediated by regulatory T cells has provided the immunologic basis for some of the treatment trials in new-onset T1DM. The autoimmune process is conceptualized as a balance between autoreactive and regulatory T cells; researchers have hypothesized that tipping the balance in favor of tolerance might arrest autoimmunity in newly diagnosed patients allowing for preservation of β-cell function.

Treatment trials in patients newly diagnosed with T1DM are targeted at preservation of endogenous insulin secretion as marked by the presence of detectable stimulated C-peptide (46). This group is easy to identify and often highly motivated to participate in treatment trials. However, the treatments employed include immunosuppressive medications and are not without significant side effects. Table 2 summarizes the planned and ongoing studies in this group. To date, no method has been shown to permanently reverse the autoimmune attack against the β cell. Both antigen-specific and non-antigen-specific methods have been used in this group.

Anti-CD3

Perhaps the most promising data regarding treatment in early-onset T1DM has been generated with the use of monoclonal antibodies against CD3 (47,48). These antibodies have been modified to decrease complement binding and cytokine release.

TABLE 2 Current Studies to Preserve C-peptide Production in Newly Diagnosed Patients with T1DM

Agent	Status	Results	References
NBI-6024 (altered peptide ligand of insulin)	Phase I	Change in T-cell phenotype	51
Insulin B chain plus incomplete Freund's adjuvant	Phase I, completed		http://www.immunetolerance .org/research/autoimmune/ trials/orban1.html
DiaPep277	Phase II, completed	Reports preservation of c-peptide in adults; no results in children	52
Proinsulin peptide vaccine	Phase I	Await results	http://www.dvdc.org/au
GAD65	Phase I in LADA		53
	Phase II in children with T1DM		http://www.diamyd.com
Proinsulin-based DNA vaccine	Phase I Planned		www.bayhilltherapeutics.com
Interferon-gamma	Phase I	Small pilot; possible effect	54
Anti-CD3 monoclonal AB Single course	Phase I/II completed Phase II/III planned	Remission out to 18 months	48,55
Anti-CD3 monoclonal AB Two courses one-year apart	Phase II	Ongoing	
Anti-CD20 MoAb	Phase II	Ongoing	http://diabetestrialnet.org
Anti-thymocyte globulin	Phase I Phase II	Ongoing Planned	http://diabetestrialnet.org http://www.immunetolerance.org
Anti-CD52	Phase I	Planned	
Autologous umbilical cord blood cell	Phase I	Ongoing	
Autologous gene-engineered dendritic cells	Phase I	Planned	www.chp.edu/research/ 03_diabetes_research_stud .php#safestudy

Abbreviations: GAD, glutamic acid decarboxylase; T1DM, type 1 diabetes mellitus.
Source: Adapted from Ref. 28 (reprinted with permission, Blackwell Publishing).

Despite this modification, treated subjects experienced a significant decline in T-cell number and side effects consistent with cytokine release. Subjects randomized to treatment versus observation were shown to have preservation of C-peptide production that lasted for approximately 12 to 18 months, after which time, C-peptide levels declined at a rate that appeared to parallel levels in untreated subjects (49). Therefore, trials of repeat administration of anti-CD3 are underway.

Additional therapies have been employed in this population with little effect. Please see extensive reviews for details (28).

The classic wisdom that β cells do not replicate has recently been challenged by tantalizing data such as the identification of β-cell replication in an elderly patient recently diagnosed with T1DM (50). The suggestion that β cells may be present in subjects with long-standing diabetes and may be able to divide, given the correct stimuli, provides the basis for trials using exenatide. This represents a paradigm shift in the development of trials to treat and/or prevent T1DM. In the future, combination strategies will likely be employed. These combinations may include an antigen-specific agent (such as insulin or GAD65), an agent active in the immune system and an agent to stimulate β-cell regeneration or replication (28).

CONCLUSION

Over the last two decades, as a result of the recognition of T1DM as an autoimmune disease, the ability to predict the development of T1DM has reached a level of considerable sophistication. Using antibody markers, researchers have come to understand more of the natural history of glucose metabolism in the prediabetic period; marked in many cases by years of mildly declining β-cell function followed by rapid deterioration in the ability of the β cell to respond to a rise in blood glucose in the immediate months before diagnosis.

Yet most importantly, for the future of the field, our patients living with T1DM, and those yet to be diagnosed, a more sophisticated understanding of this process allows studies to be designed and undertaken that target patients at highest risk. The ultimate dual aims of prevention of β-cell loss and preservation of residual β-cell function remain tantalizingly on the horizon.

REFERENCES

1. Eisenbarth GS. Type I diabetes mellitus. A chronic autoimmune disease [review]. N Engl J Med 1986; 314(21):1360–1368.
2. Yu L, Eisenbarth GS. Humoral autoimmunity. In: Eisenbarth GS, ed. Type 1 Diabetes: Molecular, Cellular and Clinical Immunology. 2007. Online edition 2.5.
3. Bottazzo GF, Florin-Christensen A, Doniach D. Islet-cell antibodies in diabetes mellitus with autoimmune polyendocrine deficiencies. Lancet 1974; 2(7892):1279–1283.
4. Palmer JP, Asplin CM, Clemons P, et al. Insulin antibodies in insulin-dependent diabetics before insulin treatment. Science 1983; 222(4630):1337–1339.
5. Ziegler AG, Vardi P, Gross DJ, et al. Production of insulin antibodies by mice rejecting insulin transfected cells. J Autoimmun 1989; 2(3):219–227.
6. Payton MA, Hawkes CJ, Christie MR. Relationship of the 37,000- and 40,000-M(r) tryptic fragments of islet antigens in insulin-dependent diabetes to the protein tyrosine phosphatase-like molecule IA-2 (ICA512). J Clin Invest 1995; 96(3):1506–1511.
7. Verge CF, Gianani R, Kawasaki E, et al. Prediction of type I diabetes in first-degree relatives using a combination of insulin, GAD, and ICA512bdc/IA-2 autoantibodies. Diabetes 1996; 45(7):926–933.
8. Barker JM, Barriga KJ, Yu L, et al. Prediction of autoantibody positivity and progression to type 1 diabetes: diabetes autoimmunity study in the young (DAISY). J Clin Endocrinol Metab 2004; 89(8):3896–3902.
9. Verge CF, Gianani R, Kawasaki E, et al. Number of autoantibodies (against insulin, GAD, or ICA512/IA2) rather than particular autoantibody specificities determines risk of type I diabetes. J Autoimmun 1996; 9(3):379–383.
10. Ziegler AG, Hummel M, Schenker M, et al. Autoantibody appearance and risk for development of childhood diabetes in offspring of parents with type 1 diabetes: the 2-year analysis of the German BABYDIAB Study. Diabetes 1999; 48(3):460–468.
11. Nejentsev S, Sjoroos M, Soukka T, et al. Population-based genetic screening for the estimation of Type 1 diabetes mellitus risk in Finland: selective genotyping of markers in the HLA-DQB1, HLA-DQA1 and HLA-DRB1 loci. Diabet Med 1999; 16(12):985–992.
12. Kimpimaki T, Kulmala P, Savola K, et al. Natural history of beta-cell autoimmunity in young children with increased genetic susceptibility to type 1 diabetes recruited from the general population. J Clin Endocrinol Metab 2002; 87(10):4572–4579.

13. Kimpimaki T, Kupila A, Hamalainen AM, et al. The first signs of beta-cell autoimmunity appear in infancy in genetically susceptible children from the general population: the Finnish type 1 diabetes prediction and prevention study. J Clin Endocrinol Metab 2001; 86(10):4782–4788.
14. Yu L, Rewers M, Gianani R, et al. Antiislet autoantibodies usually develop sequentially rather than simultaneously. J Clin Endocrinol Metab 1996; 81(12):4264–4267.
15. Achenbach P, Warncke K, Reiter J, et al. Stratification of type 1 diabetes risk on the basis of islet autoantibody characteristics. Diabetes 2004; 53(2):384–392; [erratum appears in Diabetes 2004; 53(4):1175–1176].
16. Achenbach P, Koczwara K, Knopff A, et al. Mature high-affinity immune responses to (pro)insulin anticipate the autoimmune cascade that leads to type 1 diabetes. J Clin Invest 2004; 114(4):589–597.
17. Srikanta S, Ganda OP, Jackson RA, et al. Type I diabetes mellitus in monozygotic twins: chronic progressive beta cell dysfunction. Ann Intern Med 1983; 99(3):320–326.
18. Eisenbarth GS. Prediction of type 1A diabetes: the natural history of the prediabetic period. In: Eisenbarth GS, ed. Type 1 Diabetes: Molecular, Cellular and Clinical Immunology. 2007. Online edition 2.5.
19. Eisenbarth GS, Gianani R, Yu L, et al. Dual-parameter model for prediction of type I diabetes mellitus. Proc Assoc Am Physicians 1998; 110(2):126–135.
20. Keskinen P, Korhonen S, Kupila A, et al. First-phase insulin response in young healthy children at genetic and immunological risk for Type I diabetes. Diabetologia 2002; 45 (12):1639–1648.
21. Barker JM, McFann K, Harrison LC, et al. Pre-type 1 diabetes dysmetabolism: maximal sensitivity achieved with both oral and intravenous glucose tolerance testing. J Pediatr 2007; 150(1):31–36. e6.
22. Diabetes PT. Effects of insulin in relatives of patients with type 1 diabetes mellitus [see comment]. N Engl J Med 2002; 346(22):1685–1691.
23. Skyler JS, Krischer JP, Wolfsdorf J, et al. Effects of oral insulin in relatives of patients with type 1 diabetes: the diabetes prevention trial—Type 1. Diabetes Care 2005; 28(5):1068–1076.
24. Sosenko JM, Palmer JP, Greenbaum CJ, et al. Patterns of metabolic progression to type 1 diabetes in the Diabetes Prevention Trial-Type 1. Diabetes Care 2006; 29(3):643–649.
25. Sherry NA, Tsai EB, Herold KC. Natural history of beta-cell function in type 1 diabetes [review]. Diabetes 2005; 54(suppl 2):S32–S39.
26. Schiffrin A, Suissa S, Weitzner G, et al. Factors predicting course of beta-cell function in IDDM. Diabetes Care 1992; 15(8):997–1001.
27. Atkinson MA. ADA Outstanding Scientific Achievement Lecture 2004. Thirty years of investigating the autoimmune basis for type 1 diabetes: why can't we prevent or reverse this disease? Diabetes 2005; 54(5):1253–1263.
28. Staeva-Vieira T, Peakman M, von Herrath M. Translational mini-review series on Type 1 diabetes: Immune-based therapeutic approaches for type 1 diabetes. Clin Exp Immunol 2007; 148(1):17–31.
29. The effect of intensive treatment of diabetes on the development and progression of long-term complications in insulin-dependent diabetes mellitus. The Diabetes Control and Complications Trial Research Group [see comment]. N Engl J Med 1993; 329(14):977–986.
30. Writing Team for the Diabetes Control and Complications Trial/Epidemiology of Diabetes Interventions and Complications Research Group. Sustained effect of intensive treatment of type 1 diabetes mellitus on development and progression of diabetic nephropathy: the Epidemiology of Diabetes Interventions and Complications (EDIC) study. JAMA 2003; 290(16):2159–2167.
31. Effect of intensive therapy on residual beta-cell function in patients with type 1 diabetes in the diabetes control and complications trial. A randomized, controlled trial. The Diabetes Control and Complications Trial Research Group [see comment]. Ann Intern Med 1998; 128(7):517–523.
32. Shoda LK, Young DL, Ramanujan S, et al. A comprehensive review of interventions in the NOD mouse and implications for translation [review]. Immunity 2005; 23(2): 115–126.
33. Aly TA, Ide A, Jahromi MM, et al. Extreme genetic risk for type 1A diabetes. Proc Natl Acad Sci U S A 2006; 103(38):14074–14079.

34. Bonifacio E, Hummel M, Walter M, et al. IDDM1 and multiple family history of type 1 diabetes combine to identify neonates at high risk for type 1 diabetes. Diabetes Care 2004; 27(11):2695–2700.
35. Gerstein HC, VanderMeulen J. The relationship between cow's milk exposure and type 1 diabetes [review]. Diabet Med 1996; 13(1):23–29.
36. Norris JM, Beaty B, Klingensmith G, et al. Lack of association between early exposure to cow's milk protein and beta-cell autoimmunity. Diabetes Autoimmunity Study in the Young (DAISY) [see comment]. JAMA 1996; 276(8):609–614.
37. Akerblom HK, Virtanen SM, Ilonen J, et al. Dietary manipulation of beta cell auto-immunity in infants at increased risk of type 1 diabetes: a pilot study. Diabetologia 2005; 48(5):829–837; erratum appears in Diabetologia 2005; 48(8)1676. Note: Riikjarv MA [added]; Ormisson A [added]; Ludvigsson J [added]; Dosch HM [added]; Hakulinen T [added]; Knip M [added].
38. Stene LC, Joner G. Norwegian Childhood Diabetes Study Group. Use of cod liver oil during the first year of life is associated with lower risk of childhood-onset type 1 diabetes: a large, population-based, case-control study [see comment]. Am J Clin Nutr 2003; 78(6):1128–1134.
39. Endres S, Ghorbani R, Kelley VE, et al. The effect of dietary supplementation with n-3 polyunsaturated fatty acids on the synthesis of interleukin-1 and tumor necrosis factor by mononuclear cells [see comment]. N Engl J Med 1989; 320(5):265–271.
40. Chase HP, Cooper S, Osberg I, et al. Elevated C-reactive protein levels in the development of type 1 diabetes. Diabetes 2004; 53(10):2569–2573.
41. Yu L, Robles DT, Abiru N, et al. Early expression of antiinsulin autoantibodies of humans and the NOD mouse: evidence for early determination of subsequent diabetes. Proc Natl Acad Sci U S A 2000; 97(4):1701–1706.
42. Kent SC, Chen Y, Bregoli L, et al. Expanded T cells from pancreatic lymph nodes of type 1 diabetic subjects recognize an insulin epitope [see comment]. Nature 2005; 435 (7039):224–228.
43. Maron R, Melican NS, Weiner HL. Regulatory Th2-type T cell lines against insulin and GAD peptides derived from orally- and nasally-treated NOD mice suppress diabetes. J Autoimmun 1999; 12(4):251–258.
44. Harrison LC, Honeyman MC, Steele CE, et al. Pancreatic beta-cell function and immune responses to insulin after administration of intranasal insulin to humans at risk for type 1 diabetes. Diabetes Care 2004; 27(10):2348–2355.
45. Gale EA, Bingley PJ, Emmett CL, et al. and European Nicotinamide Diabetes Intervention Trial (ENDIT) Group. European Nicotinamide Diabetes Intervention Trial (ENDIT): a randomised controlled trial of intervention before the onset of type 1 diabetes [see comment]. Lancet 2004; 363(9413):925931.
46. Schatz D, Cuthbertson D, Atkinson M, et al. Preservation of C-peptide secretion in subjects at high risk of developing type 1 diabetes mellitus—a new surrogate measure of non-progression? Pediatr Diabetes 2004; 5(2):72–79.
47. Keymeulen B, Vandemeulebroucke E, Ziegler AG, et al. Insulin needs after CD3-antibody therapy in new-onset type 1 diabetes [see comment]. N Engl J Med 2005; 352 (25):2598–2608.
48. Herold KC, Hagopian W, Auger JA, et al. Anti-CD3 monoclonal antibody in new-onset type 1 diabetes mellitus [see comment]. N Engl J Med 2002; 346(22):1692–1698.
49. Herold KC, Gitelman SE, Masharani U, et al. A single course of anti-CD3 monoclonal antibody hOKT3gamma1(Ala–Ala) results in improvement in C-peptide responses and clinical parameters for at least 2 years after onset of type 1 diabetes. Diabetes 2005; 54 (6):1763–1769.
50. Meier JJ, Lin JC, Butler AE, et al. Direct evidence of attempted beta cell regeneration in an 89-year-old patient with recent-onset type 1 diabetes. Diabetologia 2006; 49(8): 1838–1844.
51. Alleva DG, Maki RA, Putnam AL, et al. Immunomodulation in type 1 diabetes by NBI-6024, an altered peptide ligand of the insulin B epitope. Scand J Immunol 2006; 63(1): 59–69.

52. Raz I, Elias D, Avron A, et al. Beta-cell function in new-onset type 1 diabetes and immunomodulation with a heat-shock protein peptide (DiaPep277): a randomised, double-blind, phase II trial [see comment]. Lancet 2001; 358(9295):1749–1753.
53. Agardh CD, Cilio CM, Lethagen A, et al. Clinical evidence for the safety of GAD65 immunomodulation in adult-onset autoimmune diabetes. J Diabetes Complications 1919; (4):238–246.
54. Brod SA, Atkinson M, Lavis VR, et al. Ingested IFN-alpha preserves residual beta cell function in type 1 diabetes. J Interferon Cytokine Res 2001; 21(12):1021–1030.
55. Keymeulen B, Vandemeulebroucke E, Ziegler AG, et al. Insulin needs after CD3-antibody therapy in new-onset type 1 diabetes [see comment]. N Engl J Med 2005; 352 (25):2598–2608.

13 Prevention and Screening for Type 2 Diabetes in Youth

Phil Zeitler
Department of Pediatrics, University of Colorado at Denver and Health Sciences Center, Denver, Colorado, U.S.A.

Orit Pinhas-Hamiel
Pediatric Endocrinology and Diabetes, Sheba Medical Center, Ramat-Gan, Israel

PREVENTION

Prevention can occur at multiple stages in the development of the disease. Primordial prevention refers to efforts to prevent the development of risk factors for the disease, while primary prevention refers to efforts to prevent the development of the disease in the presence of risk factors. Secondary prevention aims to identify existing but undiagnosed cases in an attempt to alter the early natural history of the clinical condition. Finally, tertiary prevention refers to efforts focused on prevention and control of complications once the disease is present.

Type 2 diabetes (T2DM) should itself be considered a complication of obesity in susceptible children. Therefore, primordial prevention of T2DM entails the prevention of obesity in children and adolescents in general, as well as in those patients who are most at risk for development of T2DM and its associated disorders. Primary prevention efforts focus on the prevention of the development of diabetes once obesity is established. Secondary prevention includes screening for T2DM in order to modify the clinical course of diabetes. Tertiary intervention would involve efforts to prevent and control complications of T2DM in affected children and will not be discussed further.

Primordial Prevention—Prevention of Obesity

The available modes of treatment for obesity (secondary intervention) include diet, exercise, behavior modification, drugs, and surgery. However, as discussed below, the effectiveness of obesity treatment is limited once obesity is established, and there is considerable weight regain. Furthermore, secondary interventions, particularly those relying on medications and surgery, are not necessarily benign. Therefore, the greatest emphasis must be directed at prevention of obesity in at-risk populations of children.

Risk Factors

Genetic factors clearly influence the susceptibility of an individual to gain weight and there is evidence for many genes linked or associated with predisposition to adiposity (1). In addition, a small number of single-gene mutations that cause severe, early-onset obesity in childhood have been identified. However, these are rare and of limited clinical relevance. Furthermore, it is obvious that changes in genetic background cannot be responsible for the secular changes in prevalence of obesity in our children and youth (2). Instead, we must look for changes in the environment that, in combination with genetic predisposition, have resulted in the development of obesity in susceptible individuals.

While some of the details remain to be identified, there is widespread consensus that expanding waistlines reflect the simple functioning of the laws of thermodynamics in an environment with too many calories ingested and too few expended (3). This imbalance is not the consequence of a single factor, but rather, arises from the accumulation of many small changes that have been occurring progressively over the last 30 years. Food has became progressively cheaper and more calorie dense, portion sizes have expanded, snacking, restaurant, and fast food have become routine, and calorie-containing beverages are now a standard part of daily intake (4). Meanwhile, the need to expend energy on a regular basis has diminished and, for many people, it is now necessary to pay for the privilege of exercising. Essentially, calorie burning has become a hobby rather than a fact of daily life.

These changes affected children later than adults. Well into the 1970s and 1980s, children were more likely than adults to walk and run, to spend time outdoors, and to have their eating restricted to the home or school. In addition, schools continued to provide routine physical activity in the form of gym class and recess, and lunch rooms rarely provided prepared foods or calorie-containing beverages. However, in the 1980s, the environment for children began to change. Schools became a contributor to the trend with the appearance of fast food and calorie-containing beverages in the lunchroom and cutbacks in physical education requirements. Opportunities for activity outside of school also decreased and children were more likely to be told to remain indoors until a parent came home from work. Organized team participation has grown, but this is an expensive option, and opportunities for nonathletic children are limited. At the same time, the explosion of sedentary offerings, such as multichannel TV, video games, and computers meant that children were happy to stay indoors and routine daily activity by adolescents decreased steadily (5). Indeed, a number of studies have demonstrated that TV viewing is associated with an increase in new cases of obesity (6,7).

Families began to rely more on convenient foods and restaurant meals rather than family dinner, and caloric intake within the home increased. Unfortunately, the increasing prevalence of adult obesity compounds the deleterious environmental effects on children and adolescents, since parental obesity and eating patterns have a strong influence of pediatric obesity. Thus, the presence of parental obesity more than doubles the risk of later obesity in both obese and non-obese children, and maternal weight strongly predicts weight gain in preschool and school-age children (8–10).

In summary, social and cultural changes over the last 20 years in the West, and increasingly in the developing world, have lead to an environment in which children and adolescents are exposed to an obesitogenic environment in which there is an accumulated imbalance of caloric intake and expenditure.

While the causes of increased weight gain are reasonably well understood, it has been harder to figure out how to reverse it. Attempts to prevent obesity in children and adolescents (primary intervention) have, therefore, focused on reversing these environmental risks through interventions delivered in the community, school, or clinic, either individually or in groups. Epstein et al., among others, have been able to promote sustained weight loss with family-based behaviorally oriented interventions among selected young patients in a research setting (11,12). However, adaptation of these approaches to a broader less-motivated population remains of unproven efficacy. Similarly, experience with clinic-based interventions have been inconsistent, with few systematic studies available. Finally, campaigns to change the environment such as the removal of soda from some school systems and reconfiguring neighborhoods, while necessary in the long run, are painstaking, labor intensive, and slow.

Designing an intervention to be delivered through the schools, where children spend a large part of their day, is an obvious approach. Summerbell et al. (13) performed a systematic review of randomized controlled trials of obesity interventions from 1990 to 2005 with a minimum duration of 12 weeks. They were able to identify 22 studies that met the criteria of being randomized by group or individual and had a nonintervention control group. There were no restrictions on types of intervention, intervention personnel or setting, though nearly all the studies were school based. The authors identified 10 long-term studies (>1 year) and 12 short term studies (3–11 months). Overall, the analysis indicates that the interventions have little or no sustained impact on weight status of the children participating. Even the largest, most comprehensive, multifactorial behavior change intervention conducted over three years has been unable to demonstrate a change in weight status, though this study, like others, has been able to demonstrate an effect on process variables, such as knowledge, reported intake, and reported physical activity (14).

Thus, at a time of increasing public awareness of the need for interventions to reduce the development of obesity, there is little scientific evidence on which to base the design of behavioral intervention programs, except that interventions will need to be multifactorial, intensive, and sustained, in order to be effective.

Primary Prevention

In the setting of risk for diabetes, interventions focus on prevention of development of overt diabetes in at-risk obese youth. These can be divided into interventions to reduce obesity and other risk factors, either through behavioral or pharmacologic intervention, and those designed specifically to prevent the onset of diabetes.

Behavioral Interventions to Treat Obesity

Summerbell et al. (15) reviewed trials of lifestyle intervention to treat obesity in children from 1985 to 2001. Studies were included if they were randomized, controlled, and had a duration of at least six months. The authors identified 18 studies that met these criteria. Most of the studies were from North America and included children aged 7 to 12 years, and 7 of the 18 were reported by the same research group. Overall, the results suggest that there may be some benefit to interventions where the parent is given responsibility for behavior change, rather than the child. None of the trials exploring the effect of changing levels of physical activity or sedentary behavior were large enough to draw conclusions, though there is some support for reduction in sedentary behavior as an efficacious intervention (16).

One consideration in the assessment of behavioral intervention in the at-risk children is the choice of outcome. Thus, there may be a reduction in health risks of obesity and/or reduction in the rate of progression to diabetes in the absence of significant change in overall weight status. However, evaluation of metabolic outcomes requires a more intensive research paradigm, with greater burden on the participants. A number of groups have succeeded in demonstrating that measurement of such outcomes is feasible. Rosenbaum et al. in the El Camino Diabetes Prevention Project report the results of a school-based intervention in a predominately Dominican middle school in New York City (17). The investigators examined a relatively standard three-month intervention consisting of weekly didactics and an aerobic exercise. However, the novelty of this study was that all participants were assessed prior to and following the intervention with fasting blood draw, anthropometrics, including body fat by bioimpedance, and a brief IV glucose tolerance test. The investigators were able to demonstrate changes in body fat and insulin sensitivity that may be more important than changes in body weight or BMI. More importantly, they demonstrated the feasibility of obtaining robust physiologic measures in the school setting. Similarly, Reinehr et al. (18) demonstrated changes in laboratory measures of cardiovascular risk, though not diabetes risk, in 203 children who participated in a one-year after-school, lifestyle change intervention. These studies point out the importance of distinguishing between failure of an intervention to promote a meaningful change in health risk and the failure to demonstrate that change through insufficiently sensitive outcome measures.

Pharmacologic Interventions to Treat Obesity
The use of medications to promote weight loss in children and adolescents has been limited, and there are few published clinical trials. Berkowitz et al. (19) studied the serotonin and norepinephrine reuptake inhibitor, sibutramine, which has been shown to facilitate weight loss and maintenance in adults and is approved by the FDA for that indication. In an initial six-month randomized double-blind trial with 82 adolescents aged 13 to 17 years comparing behavior therapy with and without the addition of sibutramine, the group receiving sibutramine lost 7.8 kg compared to 3.2 kg in the control group, with a similar reduction in BMI. In a subsequent one-year multicenter trial of similar design with 498 adolescents aged 12 to 16 years, weight loss at 12 months was greater in the sibutramine group (6.5 kg vs. 1.9 kg), with similar changes in BMI and BMI z-score. Weight loss and change in BMI plateaued around eight months with no further loss. However, side effects, including tachycardia, dry mouth, and hypertension, were more common with placebo, and overall completion rates for the full one year were somewhat disappointing (20).

Orlistat is an inhibitor of gastrointestinal lipases and, therefore, prevents the absorption of dietary fat. It promotes weight loss in adults with obesity and has been associated with improvements in measures of comorbidity, such as lipid and glucose abnormalities. The drug is not absorbed and the primary side effects relate to fecal fat loss (21). There have been two trials in adolescents. The first trial was a one-year multicenter randomized, double-blind comparison of orlistat and placebo in 539 adolescent subjects who were also given a mildly hypocaloric diet, exercise, and behavior therapy (22). This trial demonstrated a decrease in BMI in both treatments for 12 weeks. Subsequently, patients on placebo gained weight, while the patients on orlistat stabilized. However, decrease in BMI was minimal in the orlistat group (0.55) and only 26% attained a change in BMI of >5%. A second shorter (6 months) and smaller randomized controlled study of 40 adolescents failed to show any difference in change in BMI or weight between orlistat and placebo (23).

Prevention of Diabetes in High-Risk Patients

A number of controlled randomized clinical trials have demonstrated that moderate interventions designed to modify lifestyle risk factors, such as weight, diet, and physical activity, can lead to substantial delay or reduction in progression to T2DM in high-risk adults. Two early studies, the Malmo Feasibility study (24) and the Da Qing Impaired Glucose Tolerance and Diabetes Study (25) demonstrated the potential success of this concept by showing that lifestyle change in subjects with impaired glucose tolerance (IGT) can reduce the incidence of progression to overt diabetes.

The Diabetes Prevention Program (26,27) was a three-year, three-arm randomized controlled study that explored the efficacy of a moderate lifestyle change intervention, or metformin (500 mg, twice a day) in reducing progression from IGT to diabetes among adults. This study demonstrated that a lifestyle program designed to promote intake of a low-fat diet, moderate physical activity of 150 min/week, and target weight loss of 5–7% of initial body weight reduced the conversion to diabetes by 58% compared with no lifestyle intervention. Furthermore, only 38% of the participants achieved 7% long-term weight loss, while 58% achieved long-term physical activity goals, suggesting an effect of weight loss and physical activity on progression to diabetes at relatively modest levels of change. Weight loss, however, was the best predictor of reduction in diabetes incidence, while physical activity predicted maintenance of weight loss (28). Remarkably, similar effects of lifestyle intervention on the progression of IGT to diabetes among adults were also reported from the Finnish Diabetes Prevention Study (29).

Metformin was also successful at reducing risk by 38%. Unfortunately, while the effect of lifestyle change persisted beyond the end of the intervention, the effect of metformin was relatively short lived, with a substantial number of participants developing diabetes by oral glucose tolerance test (OGTT) criteria within few weeks of discontinuation (26). Of interest to this discussion of prevention in adolescents, achievement of weight loss and activity goals increased with age in the cohort (30), and this was reflected in the observation that lifestyle change was substantially more efficacious than metformin among older participants. On the other hand, lifestyle changes and metformin were of equivalent efficacy in young adults aged 25 to 35 years, and the younger patients were less likely to achieve their goals.

Medications other than metformin have also been studied as possible pharmacologic approaches to reduction of progression to diabetes in at-risk adults with IGT. In STOP-NIDDM, a randomized placebo-controlled trial of acarbose, active drug was associated with a 32% decrease in conversion to diabetes and increased reversion to normal glucose tolerance (31). Similarly, in TRIPOD, troglitazone, a member of the thiazolidinedione family, subsequently removed from the market due to hepatic toxicity, was associated with a 56% decrease in conversion to diabetes among Hispanic women with prior gestational diabetes compared with placebo (32). Initial follow-up studies suggest that this reduced risk of progression to diabetes persists for one to two years following discontinuation of the medication. Orlistat has also been shown to reduce progression to diabetes among obese adults when used in conjunction with lifestyle change (33).

There have been no studies to date specifically examining approaches to reducing the progression of high-risk adolescents to overt diabetes. The numbers of children with IGT remains limited, and available data suggest that the progression to diabetes in these children over the short periods of time characteristic of clinical trials is relatively low, making the design and execution of such studies challenging.

The use of metformin has been examined in small randomized six-month trials of high-risk (positive family history, insulin resistance) adolescents and has been associated with modest improvements in BMI, fasting glucose, and glucose tolerance. However, these studies were not designed or powered to demonstrate prevention of progression to diabetes (34,35).

Clearly, additional research will be necessary to clarify the potential benefits of lifestyle and/or pharmacologic intervention in this population. These studies will need to identify the risk factors that are most predictive of progression and be of sufficient size and adequate duration to rigorously test intervention strategies appropriate for a group, that while at high-risk of eventual development of diabetes, have relatively low disease prevalence and short-term progression rates. Until that time, behavioral approaches to weight loss and moderate lifestyle change interventions that have no substantial risk to the patient must remain the preferred prevention strategies in children and adolescents.

SCREENING

The microvascular complications of T2DM, such as hypertension, nephropathy, and retinopathy, are frequently identified at the time of diagnosis of T2DM in children and adolescents (36). The presence of complications at diagnosis implies the existence of long-standing hyperglycemia and suggests that the diagnosis of T2DM could have been made earlier, allowing for earlier intervention. In addition to the presence of complications at diagnosis, adolescents with T2DM may have acute diabetes presentations, including hyperglycemic hyperosmolar state (HHS) (37) and malignant hyperthermia-like syndrome with rhabdomyolysis (38). These conditions are associated with high rates of morbidity and mortality that might be preventable if diagnosis were made earlier in the course of disease development. Therefore, there has been great interest in the development of screening strategies aimed at identifying early diabetes in children at risk in order to avoid life-threatening presentations and the development of chronic complications that are associated with significant patient and economic burden. In this section, we briefly review screening strategies in adults, current recommendations for screening of at-risk children, and the outcomes of those studies done to date based on these recommendations.

Screening for T2DM in Adults

T2DM in adults has a long preclinical period and approximately one-third to half of all people with diabetes remains undiagnosed for many years (39). Therefore, screening for T2DM in order to identify and start treating patients at an early stage might prevent or delay the development of complications. For example, tight glycemic control, along with aggressive control of hypertension, lipid-lowering therapy, and aspirin use reduce cardiovascular events. Nevertheless, screening for T2DM among adults remains controversial.

Results from the U.K. Prospective Diabetes Study (40), showing better outcomes for patients identified with lower initial fasting glucose and hemoglobin A1c, support the presumption that screening and intervention programs are likely to reduce mortality and lead to considerable economic savings. Consequently, routine screening for T2DM is increasingly recommended (41). However, in a recent systematic review performed by the U.S. Preventive Services Task Force (42) of the effectiveness of screening and earlier treatment in reducing morbidity and mortality associated with diabetes, it was concluded that the additional benefit of starting treatment of diabetes in the preclinical phase, following detection by screening, is uncertain. In addition, little is known about the direct cost-effectiveness of screening (42), and data regarding risks and side effects of screening (e.g., physical, psychological, and social harm, as well as economic cost, due to falsely positive screening tests) are lacking.

Screening for T2DM in Children and Adolescents

According to the Centers for Disease Control and Prevention, one in three children born in 2000 in the United States will become diabetic over their lifetime. The odds are higher for African-American and Hispanic children, as nearly 50% of them will develop diabetes. However, despite the increasing prevalence of T2DM among adolescents, it remains a relatively rare disorder and, therefore, random screening is not cost-effective in identifying children at risk for early-onset T2DM. Therefore, there is a need for carefully designed and evidence-based screening strategies to guide the development of appropriate diagnostic and intervention efforts.

Prevalence of Abnormal Glucose Metabolism in Children and Adolescents

The design of screening strategies requires an understanding of the underlying prevalence and incidence of a disorder, since these characteristics will have a profound effect on the positive and negative predictive values of a test outcome. There are, however, limited data regarding population prevalence of T2DM and glucose abnormalities among obese adolescents. Fagot-Campagna et al. (43) have reviewed the limited epidemiology available from U.S. case reports, while we have previously presented the data on prevalence available from the international literature (44).

There are some data on prevalence available from population-based studies. The prevalence of impaired fasting glucose (IFG) in a nationally representative sample of 915 U.S. adolescents aged 12 to 19 years was examined in the 1999–2000 National Health and Nutrition Examination Survey (NHANES). Participants were classified as overweight (BMI > 95th percentile) or at risk for overweight (BMI between the 85th and 95th percentiles). The prevalence of IFG in U.S. adolescents was 7.0% and was higher in boys than in girls (10.0% vs. 4.0%). Prevalence of IFG was higher in overweight adolescents (17.8%), but was similar in those with normal weight and those who were at risk for overweight (5.4% vs. 2.8%). The prevalence of IFG was significantly different across racial/ethnic groups (13.0%, 4.2%, and 7% in Mexican-Americans, non-Hispanic black individuals, and non-Hispanic white individuals, respectively). These data, representing 27 million U.S. adolescents, reveal a very high prevalence of IFG (1 in 10 boys and 1 in 25 girls) among adolescents, with the condition affecting one in every six overweight adolescents (45).

The SEARCH for Diabetes in Youth Study is a six-center population-based ascertainment of physician-diagnosed diabetes in youth <20 years of age in the United States, according to age, gender, race/ethnicity, and diabetes type. Among older youth, the proportion of T2DM ranged from 6% (0.19 cases per 1000 youth for non-Hispanic white youth) to 76% (1.74 cases per 1000 youth for American-Indian youth) (46).

In a study at 12 middle schools around the United States, 1740 eighth graders, of whom 49% had BMI greater than the 85th percentile, underwent fasting and two hour postload glucose determinations. IFG was present in 40.5%, and diabetes by fasting criteria (glucose > 126 mg/dL) was identified in only 0.4%. Following a glucose load, only 2% had IGT and 0.1% had diabetes (47). Thus, despite a sample that was otherwise high in risk factors for insulin resistance and diabetes, the prevalence of IGT and T2DM was low. On the other hand, IFG was surprisingly prevalent, as noted in the NHANES study discussed above. Of note, the presence of IFG was not a strong predictor of diabetes by OGTT in this sample.

In a cross-sectional survey of schoolchildren aged 4 to 19 years during 1996 to 1997 in the remote northern Ojibwa-Cree community of St. Theresa Point First Nation, 717 out of 873 children registered at the school had standing height, weight, fasting serum glucose, and insulin measured (48). Among these 717 children, 19 (2.7%) had IFG. Six new cases of diabetes were identified, all of whom were obese, female, symptom-free, unrelated, and aged 8 to 17 years. The total prevalence of diabetes among children aged 4 to 19 years was 1.1%, with a female/male ratio of 8. Only one child was younger than 10 years and, thus, for girls aged 10 to 19 years, the prevalence of diabetes was 3.6.

Current ADA Recommendations

In 2000, the American Diabetes Association (ADA) issued recommendations for T2DM screening among children. These recommendations were based on clinical reports, showing that affected children were obese, pubertal, had a family history of T2DM, and other clinical signs of insulin resistance. The guidelines from 2007 are presented in Table 1.

However, several studies have reported that these ADA screening guidelines are inconsistently applied, with both under- and overscreening described. The medical records for 997 patients (96% Hispanic), 10 to 18 years of age, who were seen for health maintenance visits in an urban pediatric clinic in Chicago, Illinois were reviewed. Forty-eight percent ($n = 477$) of the patients had a BMI greater than the 85th percentile (including 26% with a BMI greater than or equal to the 95th percentile). Of these 477 subjects, 100% were in high-risk racial/ethnic groups, about one-third had a family history of diabetes, and one-fifth demonstrated

TABLE 1 Testing for T2DM in Children—ADA Recommendations

Criteria:

- Overweight (BMI > 85th percentile for age and sex, weight for height > 85th percentile, or weight > 120% of ideal for height)

Plus any two of the following risk factors:

- Family history of T2DM in first- or second-degree relative
- Race/ethnicity (Native American, African-American, Latino, Asian-American, Pacific Islander)
- Signs of insulin resistance or conditions associated with insulin resistance (acanthosis nigricans, hypertension, dyslipidemia, or PCOS)
- Maternal history of diabetes or GDM

Age of initiation: age 10 yr or at onset of puberty, if puberty occurs at a younger age
Frequency: every 2 yr
Test: FPG preferred

Abbreviations: T2DM, type 2 diabetes; ADA, American Diabetes Association; PCOS, polycystic ovary syndrome; GDM, gestational diabetes mellitus; FPG, fasting plasma glucose.

evidence of insulin resistance. In all, 194 (41%) met the criteria for screening. Of those who met the criteria, only 38% ($n = 73$) had screening ordered and only 65 of those subjects (89%) completed screening. Three of the screened subjects exhibited IGT and none had overt T2DM (49).

In a study of attitudes, barriers, and practices related to T2DM screening among 62 pediatricians, pediatric nurse practitioners, and physician assistants in a multispecialty group practice in Eastern Massachusetts, 21% of respondents reported ADA-consistent screening practice, 39% were also screening low-risk patients, and 35% were screening only very high-risk patients. Furthermore, many clinicians ordered screening tests other than those recommended by the ADA (50).

Similarly, the rates of diabetes screening and the prevalence of screening abnormalities in overweight and non overweight individuals in an urban primary care clinic were studied in a retrospective chart review conducted in a hospital-based urban primary care setting in Boston, Massachusetts. A total of 7710 patients aged 10 to 19 years met the study criteria. Patients were 73.0% black or Hispanic and 47.0% female; 42.0% of children exceeded normal weight, with 18.2% at risk for overweight and 23.8% overweight. On the basis of BMI, family history, and race, 8.7% of patients ($n = 671$) met ADA criteria for T2DM screening. However, 2452 screening tests were performed for 1642 patients. Screening rates were significantly higher (45.4% vs. 19.0%) for patients who met the ADA criteria; however, less than one-half of adolescents who should have been screened by these guidelines were, in fact, screened, while a large number of children who did not meet the criteria had laboratory testing. The strongest predictor of likelihood of having screening blood drawn was increasing BMI percentile. The low prevalence of abnormalities in this population overall was reflected in the observation that abnormal glucose metabolism was demonstrated in only 9.2% of patients screened (51).

Given that the current consensus ADA criteria have not met with general acceptance and do not reliably identify a group of patients at high risk, and with the benefit of increased information about diabetes epidemiology among adolescents, it would be helpful to generate criteria that select obese children at higher than average risk for further testing. We will review the information regarding possible criteria studied to date.

Obesity

The risk of T2DM is greatly increased by excess weight. Several studies have evaluated the prevalence of T2DM and IGT in obese children and adolescents. In a multiethnic cohort of 167 obese children and adolescents, IGT was detected in 25% of the 55 obese children (aged 4 to 10 years) and 21% of the 112 obese adolescents (aged 11 to 18 years). Silent T2DM was identified in 4% of the obese adolescents (52). Similarly, an OGTT was done in 427 asymptomatic obese Argentinean children with a mean age of just under 11 years and mean BMI of 30 ± 5.3 kg/m^2. IGT was seen in 30 patients (7%) and T2DM in 7 (1.6%). The patients with diabetes were older than the others (53). On the other hand, in a group of 150 overweight Latino children with a family history of T2DM in Los Angeles, IGT was present in 28% of children, while no cases of diabetes were identified (54).

In a cross-sectional study from Europe, a cohort of 491 subjects was screened for the presence of two signs of insulin resistance. From this selected high-risk subgroup ($n = 102$) of obese pediatric subjects, 6 patients (5.9%) with T2DM and 37 (36.3%) patients with IGT were identified (55). In another study from Denmark, screening of adolescents at risk was done using random capillary blood glucose (RCBG). All ninth grade pupils ($n = 589$) who were overweight and/or had a family history of T2DM were invited to have RCBG measured. Of the 384 who participated, one had diagnosed T2DM. Two others had elevated RCBG values, one of whom was identified with undiagnosed T2DM upon further testing (56).

Among 117 obese children and adolescents of Greek origin aged 12.1 ± 2.7 years old who underwent an OGTT, a total of 17 patients (14.5%) had IGT, and none had T2DM. IGT was present in 9% of prepubertal subjects compared with 18% of pubertal subjects (57). Among 196 obese Turkish children aged 7 to 18 years, 15 (6.6%) had IFG, 35 (18%) had IGT, and 6 (3%) were diagnosed with T2DM (58).

The prevalence of T2DM and impaired glucose regulation was also studied in a large group of obese Caucasian children and adolescents in Germany. The cohort included a total of 520 subjects (237 boys, 283 girls) [mean age: 14.0 ± 2.0 years (range 8.9–20.4 years) with body mass index standard deviation score (BMI-SDS): 2.7 ± 0.5 (range 1.9–4.6)], who were consecutively admitted to an in-patient obesity unit, T2DM was present in 1.5% ($n = 8$) of the patients, two of whom were known to have diabetes at admission, and six were identified with undiagnosed diabetes during the admission. IFG was detected in 3.7% ($n = 19$) and IGT in 2.1% ($n = 11$) of the patients (59).

Family History

Various case series have suggested that a positive family history of T2DM is common among adolescents with T2DM (43), and this observation is reflected in the ADA guidelines. However, studies directly exploring the prevalence of family history among adolescents with T2DM compared with adolescents without T2DM are limited. The influence of family history and obesity on glucose intolerance was studied in 105 children and adolescents aged 10 to 18 years in Turkey. All children and adolescents were divided into three groups according to positive family history of T2DM and obesity, and an OGTT was performed in all. The prevalence of prediabetes (IGT and/or IFG) was 15.2% in the whole group, while 25.5% in obese children who also had a positive family history of T2DM (60).

Age

The risk of T2DM increases steeply with age throughout the lifespan. Accordingly, the cost effectiveness of screening will be lower at younger ages, while the prevalence of diabetes is greater in puberty and young adulthood. In the Greek cohort discussed above, the incidence of impaired glucose metabolism among the prepubertal subjects was 9%, whereas it was 18% in the pubertal population (57). Similarly, in the cross-sectional survey of schoolchildren in the northern Ojibwa-Cree community of St. Theresa Point First Nation, only one of six children diagnosed with T2DM was younger than 10 years (48). The proportion of new onset cases of diabetes at a large urban diabetes center that are T2DM increases with age, becoming substantial only at pubertal ages in both males and females (61).

Ethnicity

T2DM has been reported to disproportionately affect ethnic minority groups in the United States, Europe, Canada, and New Zealand (43,44). About two-third of adolescents with T2DM in reported series are African-American or Mexican-American, respectively, the rest being Caucasian (44). Thus, T2DM appears to be more prevalent in some ethnic groups than others. These groups are the same as those with a higher prevalence of T2DM in adulthood. Published reports indicate, however, that overall pediatric patients with T2DM belong to all ethnic groups— Hispanics, blacks, Caucasians, Japanese, First Nation children of Canada, and Ashkenazi or Sephardic Jews. Ethnicity is, therefore, not a useful predictive factor in an individual case (44), and guidelines that rely heavily on ethnicity will be of limited use outside the United States and risk missing substantial numbers of at-risk Caucasian adolescents.

Gestational Diabetes Mellitus (GDM)
The prevalence of IGT and obesity in otherwise low-risk offspring of mothers whose pregnancies were complicated by GDM was studied in 89 children (mean age 9.1 years, 93% Caucasian) recruited through a follow-up study of women previously involved in a randomized controlled trial of minimal intervention (control group) versus tight glycemic control (treatment group) for GDM. Of those offspring, 6.9% had abnormal glucose metabolism, four children had IGT, and one had T2DM. Of the four children with IGT, three were male, three had normal BMI, and three had a family history of T2DM. Thus, the incidence of impaired glucose metabolism and T2DM appears to be increased in school-age children of mothers with GDM, even when they are otherwise at low risk (62). Similarly, IGT was found to be more prevalent in Latino children exposed to GDM, particularly children in later stages of puberty (54).

Screening Approaches
There are several tests that could be used in a screening program for IGT and T2DM in adolescents. These include urine glucose, casual (nonfasting) blood glucose, fasting glucose, formal glucose tolerance tests, and hemoglobin A1c. In general, urine testing, though convenient and amenable to wide-spread screening that does not require a blood draw (63), has been considered too insensitive for identification of cases of diabetes in high-risk patients. Similarly, hemoglobin A1c has not proven to be a useful substitute for measurement of blood glucose directly in adolescents with glucose abnormalities (64). Thus, most proposals have focused on screening approaches based on measurement of blood glucose.

Determining the accuracy and reliability of screening tests for diabetes is complicated by uncertainty about the most appropriate reference standard. Among adults, two diagnostic criteria are in general use: one based on the two-hour postload plasma glucose concentration and the other based on the fasting plasma glucose (FPG) (65). Both tests require a second independent confirmation in the absence of frank diabetes symptoms, i.e., in the screening scenario. To complicate matters further, it is unclear whether the ADA guidelines for diagnosis of diabetes, which are based on increased risk for microvascular complications in adults, are appropriate for use in children and adolescents, in whom normal glucose concentrations are generally lower. However, no studies to date have identified more appropriate threshold values for the pediatric population. Therefore, these adult values are in general use and form the basis of all screening studies to date.

A fasting glucose determination has been recommended as the screening method of choice for T2DM because of its practical advantage relative to the OGTT. The ADA and the American Academy of Pediatrics (AAP) endorsed a statement in 2000 recommending screening of children and adolescents at high risk for diabetes with a fasting glucose in every two years. However, studies have suggested that many high-risk patients with normal fasting glucose may have diabetes by OGTT criteria (66,67).

There are similar concerns about the use of fasting glucose in screening programs for adolescents. In a study of 112 obese adolescents (aged 11–18 years), 21% had IGT and 4% had diabetes diagnosed following OGTT (52). However, the fasting glucose was normal in all of these patients and did not predict the presence of IGT or T2DM. Similarly, the glycemic status assessed by OGTT was studied in a 21 (three male, 18 female) Australian children and adolescents at risk, with a mean age of 14.2 ± 1.6 years and BMI 38.8 ± 7.0 kg/m^2. T2DM was diagnosed in one patient, IGT in four patients, and impaired fasting glycemia (IFG) in one patient. The patients with IGT and T2DM had normal fasting glucose measurements (68).

Therefore, screening with a fasting glucose alone may not identify patients with IGT or T2DM. Yet, in clinical practice, performing a two-hour OGTT on all adolescents with risk factors for the development of T2DM may be impractical, given the numbers of obese patients potentially in need of evaluation. Furthermore, undertaking glucose tolerance testing on a wide spread basis would create significant economic burdens that are poorly justified by the relatively small numbers of patients identified (47). Thus, the identification of relatively simple screening methods that effectively identify those adolescents in whom an OGTT will be most useful would facilitate appropriate evaluation of obese adolescents.

In a study of 258 overweight nondiabetic volunteers exploring this question, the fasting plasma triglyceride concentration, the triglyceride/HDL ratio, and fasting serum insulin concentration were the most useful metabolic markers at identifying insulin-resistant individuals (69). Subsequently, a study of normoglycemic men aged 26 to 45 years showed elevated fasting triglycerides >150 mg/ dL (1.69 mmol/L) to be associated with increased risk of development of T2DM over a six-year follow-up period. This association persisted across all categories of fasting glucose but was most pronounced in subjects with high-normal fasting glucose of 91 to 99 mg/dL (5.05–5.50 mmol/L) (70). In a recent study of 84 obese, insulin-resistant, predominantly Hispanic adolescents, 7 (8%) had IGT alone, 7 (8%) had IFG alone, and 3 (4%) had both IFG and IGT. No subject had confirmed diabetes by OGTT criteria (71). Overall, 34 subjects (40%) had fasting triglycerides ≥ 150 mg/dL. However, all 10 (100%) subjects with IGT had fasting triglycerides ≥ 150 mg/dL. In univariate logistic regression, the best predictors for IGT were fasting glucose ($p = 0.023$) and fasting triglycerides ($p = 0.035$). The likelihood ratio for IGT with fasting triglycerides ≥ 150 was 3.1, while that for fasting glucose >100 was 3.3. However, the negative predictive value for a normal fasting triglyceride was 100% in this cohort, while that for a normal glucose was 91%. These results suggest that a combination of fasting glucose and fasting triglyceride determination may be useful in identifying patients who should have formal glucose tolerance testing, since normal fasting glucose and normal triglycerides in combination have a very strong negative predictive value and can exclude most patients from further testing.

SUMMARY

Despite the rising prevalence of T2DM in adolescents and the significant implication that this has for future health and healthcare, T2DM and more mild forms of impairment in glucose metabolism remain relatively uncommon in the general pediatric population, and there is no evidence that widespread screening for glucose abnormalities is cost-effective. Even among children presumed to be at high risk due to medical or family history, ethnicity, or associated comorbidities, the low prevalence of unrecognized T2DM in children and adolescents does not support extensive screening efforts of unselected patients. Furthermore, both clinicians and clinical investigators need to address the economic and ethical implications of identifying number of children with impaired glucose metabolism that far exceed those with frank diabetes. Until we have evidence for prevention of progression to diabetes and related comorbidities through early intervention in these children, the value of identifying them is uncertain. Rather, studies reviewed here suggest that screening for T2DM in the pediatric population should be clinically focused and take into account not only those risk factors identified in the ADA guidelines, but also the clinical context, pubertal status, and the results of simple screening measures such as fasting glucose and triglycerides. The aim of such screening should be the identification of overt T2DM early enough to minimize risk for acute and chronic complications. More outcome-based research is required before general screening to identify children and adolescents with prediabetes or insulin-resistance can be recommended.

REFERENCES

1. Rankinen T, Zuberi A, Changon YC, et al. The human obesity gene map: the 2005 update. Obesity 2006; 14:529–644.
2. Ogden CL, Carroll MD, Curtin LR, et al. Prevalence of overweight and obesity in the United States, 1999–2004. JAMA 2006; 295:1549–1555.
3. Hill JO. Understanding and addressing the epidemic of obesity: an energy balance perspective. Endocr Rev 2006; 27:750–761.
4. Kant AK, Graubard BI. Secular trends in patterns of self-reported food consumption of adult Americans: NHANES 1971–1975 to NHANES 1999–2002. Am J Clin Nutr 2006; 84:1215–1226.
5. Janssen I, Katzmarzyk PT, Boyce WF, et al. Comparison of overweight and obesity prevalence in school-aged youth from 34 countries and their relationships with physical activity and dietary patterns. Obes Rev 2005; 6:123–132.
6. Robinson TN. Television viewing and childhood obesity. Pediatr Clin North Am 2001; 48:1017–1025.
7. Proctor MH, Moore LL, Gao D, et al. Television viewing and change in body fat from preschool to early adolescence: The Framingham Children's Study. Int J Obes Relat Metab Disord 2003; 27:827–833.
8. Whitaker RC, Wright JA, Pepe MS, et al. Predicting obesity in young adulthood from childhood and parental obesity. N Engl J Med 1997; 337:869–873.
9. Hood MY, Moore LL, Sundarajan-Ramamutri A et al. Parental attitudes and the development of obesity in children: the Framingham Children's Study. Int J Obes Relat Metab Disord 2000; 24:1319–1325.
10. Klesges RC, Caotes TJ, Brown G, et al. Parental influences on children's eating behaviors and relative weight. J Appl Behav Anal 1983; 16:371–378.
11. Goldfield GS, Raynor HA, Epstein LH. Treatment of pediatric obesity. In: Stunkard AJ, Wadden TA, eds. Obesity: Theory and Therapy. New York: Guilford Press, 2002:532–555.
12. Epstein LH, Valoski A, Wing RR, et al. Ten-year follow-up of behavioral family-based treatment for obese children. JAMA 1990; 264:2519–2523.
13. Summerbell CD, Waters E, Edmunds LD, et al. Interventions for preventing obesity in children. Cochrane Database Syst Rev, 2005, CD001871.
14. Caballero B, Clay T, Davis SM, et al. Pathways: a school-based, randomized controlled trial for the prevention of obesity in American Indian Schoolchildren. Am J Clin Nutr 2003; 78:1030–1038.

15. Summerbell CD, Ashton V, Campbell KJ, et al. Interventions for treating obesity in children. Cochrane Database Syst Rev 2003, CD001872.

16. Epstein LH, Valoski AM, Vara LS, et al. Effects of decreasing sedentary behavior and increasing activity on weight change in obese children. Health Psychol 1995; 14:109–115.

17. Rosenbaum M, Nonas C, Weil R, et al. School-based intervention acutely improves insulin sensitivity and decreases inflammatory markers and body fatness in junior high school students. J Clin Endocrinol Metab 2006; 92:504–508.

18. Reinehr T, deSousa G, Toschke AM, et al. Long-term followup of cardiovascular disease risk factors in children after an obesity intervention. Am J Clin Nutr 2006; 84:490–496.

19. Berkowitz RJ, Wadden TA, Tershakovec AM, et al. Behavior therapy and sibutramine for the treatment of adolescent obesity: a randomized controlled trial. JAMA 2003; 289:1805–1812.

20. Berkowitz RJ, Fujioka K, Daniels SR, et al. Effects of sibutramine treatment in obese adolescents: a randomized trial. Ann Intern Med 2006; 145:81–90.

21. Henness S. Perry CM. Orlistat: a review of its use in the management of obesity. Drugs 2006; 66:1625–1656.

22. Chanoine JP, Hampl S, Jensen C, et al. Effect of orlistat on weight and body composition in obese adolescents: a randomized controlled trial. JAMA 2005; 293:2873–2883.

23. Maahs D, deSerna DG, Kolotkin RL, et al. Randomized, double-blind, placebo-controlled trial of orlistat for weight loss in adolescents. Endocr Pract 2006; 12:18–28.

24. Eriksson KF, Lindgarde F. Prevention of type 2 (non-insulin-dependent) diabetes mellitus by diet and physical exercise: the 6-year Malmo Feasibility Study. Diabetologia 1991; 34:891–898.

25. Pan XR, Li GW, Hu YH, et al. Effects of diet and exercise in preventing NIDDM in people with impaired glucose tolerance. The Da Qing IGT and Diabetes Study. Diabetes Care 1997; 20:537–544.

26. Diabetes Prevention Program Research Group. Effects of withdrawal from metformin on the development of diabetes in the Diabetes Prevention Program. Diabetes Care 2003; 26:977–980.

27. Diabetes Prevention Program Research Group. Reduction in the incidence of type 2 diabetes with lifestyle intervention or metformin. New Engl J Med 2002; 346:393–403.

28. Hamman RF, Wing RR, Edelstein SL, et al. Effect of weight loss with lifestyle intervention on risk of diabetes. Diabetes Care 2006; 29:2102–2107.

29. Tuomilehto J, Lindstrom J, Eriksson JG, et al. Prevention of type 2 diabetes mellitus by changes in lifestyle among subjects with impaired glucose tolerance. N Engl J Med 2001; 344:1343–1350.

30. Wing RR, Hamman RF, Bray GA, et al. Achieving weight and activity goals among diabetes prevention program lifestyle participants. Obes Res 2004; 12:1426–1434.

31. Chiasson JL, Josse RG, Gomis R, et al. Acarbose for prevention of T2DM diabetes mellitus: the STOP-NIDDM randomised trial. Lancet 2002; 359:2072–2077.

32. Buchanan T, Xiang AH, Peters RK, et al. Preservation of pancreatic beta-cell function and prevention of type 2 diabetes by pharmacologic treatment of insulin resistance in high-risk Hispanic women. Diabetes 2002; 51:2796–2803.

33. Torgerson JS, Hauptman J, Boldrin MN, et al. A randomized study of orlistat as an adjunct to lifestyle changes for the prevention of type 2 diabetes in obese patients. Diabetes Care 2004; 27:155–161.

34. Freemark M, Bursey D. The effects of metformin on body mass index and glucose tolerance in obese adolescents with fasting hyperinsulinemia and a family history of T2DM diabetes. Pediatrics 2001; 107:E55.

35. Love-Osborn K, Sheeder J, Zeitler P. The addition of metformin to a lifestyle intervention in obese insulin-resistant adolescents. J Pediatr 2007 (in press).

36. Pinhas-Hamiel O, Zeitler P. Acute and chronic complications of type 2 diabetes mellitus in children and adolescents. Lancet 2007; 369:1823–1831.

37. Fourtner SH, Weinzimer SA, Levitt Katz LE. Hyperglycemic hyperosmolar non-ketotic asyndrome in children with type 2 diabetes. Pediatr Diabetes 2005; 6:129–135.

38. Hollander AS, Olney RC, Blackett PR, et al. Fatal malignant hyperthermia-like syndrome with rhabdomyolysis complicating the presentation of diabetes mellitus in adolescent males. Pediatrics 2003; 111:1447–1452.

39. Harris M. Undiagnosed NIDDM: clinical and public health issues. Diabetes Care 1993; 16:643–652.

40. Colagiuri S, Cull CA, Holman RR. Are lower fasting plasma glucose levels at diagnosis of type 2 diabetes associated with improved outcomes? UK Prospective Diabetes Study 61. Diabetes Care 2002; 25:1410–1417.

41. Mogensen CE, Borch-Johnsen K, Wenzel H, et al. Is screening and intervention for microalbuminuria worthwhile in patients with insulin dependent diabetes? BMJ 1993; 306:1722–1725.

42. Harris R, Donahue K, Rathore SS, et al. Screening adults for type 2 diabetes: a review of the evidence for the US Preventive Services Task Force. Ann Int Med 2003; 138:215–229.

43. Fagot-Campagna A, Pettitt DJ, Engelgau MM, et al. Type 2 diabetes among north American children and adolescents: an epidemiological review and public health perspective. J Pediatr 2000; 136:664–672.

44. Pinhas-Hamiel O, Zeitler P. The global spread of type 2 diabetes in children and adolescents. J Pediatr 2005; 145:693–700.

45. Williams DE, Cadwell BL, Cheng YJ, et al. Prevalence of impaired fasting glucose and its relationship with cardiovascular disease risk factors in US adolescents, 1999–2000. Pediatrics 2005; 116:1122–1126.

46. SEARCH for Diabetes in Youth Study Group. Liese AD, D'Agostino R Jr., et al. The burden of diabetes mellitus among US youth: prevalence estimates from the SEARCH for Diabetes in Youth Study. Pediatrics 2006; 118:1510–1518.

47. Baranowski T, Cooper DM, Harrell J, et al. Presence of diabetes risk factors in a large U.S. eighth-grade cohort. Diabetes Care 2006; 29:212–217.

48. Dean HJ, Young TK, Flett B, et al. Screening for type-2 diabetes in aboriginal children in northern Canada. Lancet 1998; 352:1523–1524.

49. Drobac S, Brickman W, Smith T, et al. Evaluation of a type 2 diabetes screening protocol in an urban pediatric clinic. Pediatrics 2004; 114:141–148.

50. Rhodes ET, Finkelstein JA, Marshall R, et al. Screening for type 2 diabetes mellitus in children and adolescents: attitudes, barriers, and practices among pediatric clinicians. Ambul Pediatr 2006; 6:110–114.

51. Anand SG, Mehta SD, Adams WG. Diabetes mellitus screening in pediatric primary care. Pediatrics 2006; 118:1888–1895.

52. Sinha R, Fisch G, Teague B, et al. Prevalence of impaired glucose tolerance among children and adolescents with marked obesity. N Engl J Med 2002; 346:802–810.

53. Mazza CS, Ozuna B, Krochik AG, et al. Prevalence of type 2 diabetes mellitus and impaired glucose tolerance in obese Argentinean children and adolescents. J Pediatr Endocrinol Metab 2005; 18:491–498.

54. Goran MI, Bergman RN, Avila Q, et al. Impaired glucose tolerance and reduced β-cell function in overweight Latino children with a positive family history for type 2 diabetes. J Clin Endocrinol Metab 2004; 89:207–212.

55. Wiegand S, Dannemann A, Krude H, et al. Impaired glucose tolerance and type 2 diabetes mellitus: a new field for pediatrics in Europe. Int J Obes (Lond) 2005; 29(suppl l2):S136–S142.

56. Pearson S, Brolos EJ, Herner EB, et al. Screening Copenhagen school children at risk of type 2 diabetes mellitus using random capillary blood glucose. Acta Paediatr 2007; 96:885–889.

57. Xekouki P, Nikolakopoulou NM, Papageorgiou A, et al. Glucose dysregulation in obese children: predictive, risk, and potential protective factors. Obesity (Silver Spring) 2007; 15:860–869.

58. Atabek ME, Pirgon O, Kurtoglu S. Assessment of abnormal glucose homeostasis and insulin resistance in Turkish obese children and adolescents. Diabetes Obes Metab 2007; 9:304–310.

59. Wabitsch M, Hauner H, Hertrampf M, et al. Type II diabetes mellitus and impaired glucose regulation in Caucasian children and adolescents with obesity living in Germany. Int J Obes Relat Metab Disord 2004; 28:307–313.

60. Babaoglu K, Hatun S, Arslanoglu I, et al. Evaluation of glucose intolerance in adolescents relative to adults with type 2 diabetes mellitus. J Pediatr Endocrinol Metab 2006; 19:1319–1326.
61. Wang J, Miao D, Babu S, et al. Prevalence of autoantibody-negative diabetes is not rare at all ages and increases with older age and obesity. J Clin Endocrinol Metab 2007; 92:88–92.
62. Malcolm JC, Lawson ML, Gaboury I, et al. Glucose intolerance of offspring of mothers with gestational diabetes in a low-risk population. Diabet Med 2006; 23:565–570.
63. Urakami T, Morimoto S, Nitadori Y, et al. Urine glucose screening program at schools in Japan to detect children with diabetes and its outcome-incidence and clinical characteristics of childhood type 2 diabetes in Japan. Pediatr Res 2007; 61:141–145.
64. Shultis WA, Leary SD, Ness AR, et al. Haemoglobin A1c is not a surrogate for glucose and insulin measures for investigating the early life and childhood determinants of insulin resistance and Type 2 diabetes in healthy children. An analysis from the Avon Longitudinal Study of Parents and Children (ALSPAC). Diabet Med 2006; 23:1357–1363.
65. American Diabetes Assocation. Diagnosis and classification of diabetes. Diabetes Care 2005; 28:S37–S42.
66. Melchionda N, Forlani G, Marchesini G, et al. WHO and ADA criteria for the diagnosis of diabetes mellitus in relation to body mass index. Insulin sensitivity and secretion in resulting subcategories of glucose tolerance. Int J Obes Relat Metab Disord 2002; 26:90–96.
67. Shaw JE, deCourten M, Boyko EJ, et al. Impact of new diagnostic criteria for diabetes on different populations. Diabetes Care 1999; 22:762–766.
68. Conwell LS, Batch JA. Oral glucose tolerance test in children and adolescents: positives and pitfalls. J Paediatr Child Health 2004; 40:620–626.
69. McLaughlin T, Abbasi F, Cheal K, et al. Use of metabolic markers to identify overweight individuals who are insulin resistant. Ann Intern Med 2003; 139:802–809.
70. Tirosh A, Shai I, Tekes-Manova D, et al. Normal fasting plasma glucose levels and type 2 diabetes in young men. New Engl J Med 2005; 353:1454–1462.
71. Love-Osborn K, Butler N, Gao D, et al. Elevated fasting triglycerides predict impaired glucose tolerance in adolescents at risk for type 2 diabetes. Pediatr Diabetes 2006; 7:205–210.

Chronic Complications of Childhood Diabetes

Kim C. Donaghue
Institute of Endocrinology and Diabetes, The Children's Hospital at Westmead, University of Sydney, Westmead, Australia

Fauzia Mohsin
Department of Pediatrics, BIRDEM and Ibrahim Medical College, Dhaka, Bangladesh

Monique L. Stone
Department of Pediatric Endocrinology and Diabetes, Royal North Shore Hospital, The University of Sydney, St. Leonards, Australia

MICROVASCULAR COMPLICATIONS

The microvascular complications of diabetes, retinopathy, nephropathy, and neuropathy cause significant morbidity and mortality in childhood onset diabetes. In the 1980s, interventions to reduce the risk of blindness and renal failure due to diabetes were established, specifically laser therapy and antihypertensive therapy. Because these treatments are most successful prior to the onset of symptoms, the advent of screening programs for diabetes complications has occurred. One such comprehensive screening program was introduced for adolescents at the Children's Hospital at Westmead (CHW), Sydney, Australia, in 1990.

Considerable new insights have been gained into the natural history of microvascular complications, and the interplay between risk factors such as hyperglycemia, high blood pressure, lipid abnormalities, and smoking. Attention to these factors has occurred during a time when there has been a decrease in retinopathy and nephropathy.

The diabetes control and complications trial (DCCT) established the causative role of hyperglycemia and showed that complications could be reduced by intensive diabetes management, including in adolescents cohorts (1). The United Kingdom Prospective Diabetes Study (UKPDS) group showed the same for adults with type 2 diabetes mellitus (T2DM) (2). To date there are only few reports of T2DM complications in adolescents, but studies comparing complications in type 1 diabetes mellitus (T1DM) and T2DM diabetes are emerging (Fig. 1).

During this time, however, there has been a general population increase in obesity, which includes adolescents with T1DM (3). Higher body mass index (BMI) increases the risk for microvascular complications (4). Many of the accompanying conditions of the metabolic syndrome are risk factors for T1DM and contribute to the risk for microvascular complications in T2DM. Furthermore, shared familial factors of T2DM place the proband with T1DM at greater risk, especially for nephropathy and retinopathy (5).

Microalbuminuria, hyperlipidemia, and hypertension are part of the "metabolic syndrome" and may be present at diagnosis of T2DM in adolescents (6). In addition, subclinical neuropathy has also been found in adults with prediabetes and obesity (7), prior to the development of diabetes.

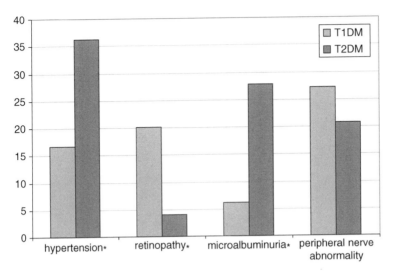

FIGURE 1   Prevalence of diabetes complications in children and adolescents with T1DM versus T2DM between 1996 and 2005. Hypertension was defined as systolic or diastolic blood pressure > 95th percentile, microalbuminuria was defined as AER > 20 μg/min or ACR > 2.5 mg/mmol in two-third urine collections; peripheral nerve abnormalities were assessed by thermal threshold and vibration threshold; * indicates a significant difference ($p < 0.05$) between T1DM and T2DM. *Abbreviations*: ACR, albumin/creatinine ratio; AER, albumin excretion rate; T1DM, type 1 diabetes mellitus; T2DM, type 2 diabetes mellitus. *Source*: Adapted from Ref. 18.

Retinopathy

Retinopathy is the leading cause of blindness among young adults in Western countries. It appears to be generally less common in T2DM than is microalbuminuria. Retinopathy can be diagnosed by ophthalmoscopy or fundal photography. The latter is threefold more sensitive. Fluorescein photography is similarly sensitive, but is generally reserved now as a functional test of blood vessel leakage and is used to stage the timing of laser treatment. The Wisconsin Epidemiology Study of Diabetic Retinopathy (WESDR) was the first large-scale population-based study to use seven-field stereoscopic fundal photography and this technique was also used in the DCCT and at CHW. Fundal photography of two central fields is also used but reduces the sensitivity of peripheral fields. Studies of retinopathy in adolescents are shown in Table 1.

Natural Progression of Retinopathy

The initial abnormalities are increased blood flow with leakage of albumin. There is pericyte loss and endothelial proliferation. Subsequently, hypoxia develops and promotes neovascularization. Larger retinal arteriolar caliber can be measured predating signs of retinopathy in children and adolescents with T1DM independent of conventional risk factors for retinopathy, consistent with increased blood flow (8).

   Background retinopathy can progress to vision-threatening retinopathy, which includes preproliferative retinopathy, proliferative retinopathy, and maculopathy. The earliest features of background retinopathy are microaneurysms and

TABLE 1 Prevalence of Retinopathy in Young People with Diabetes

References	Location	Age (yrs)	Participants	Prevalence	Screening procedures
93	Berlin	17.6 ± 4.0	231 T1	47%	Fluorescein angiography
94	Norway	8–30.3	371 T1	33%	Fundus photography
95	Finland	12.2	194 T1	11%	Fundus photography
96	Australia	11.0–19.8	255 T1	42%	Stereoscopic fundus photography
97	Sweden	12.4–17	557 T1	15%	Stereoscopic fundus photography
98	Denmark	12–26.9	339 T1	60%	40–60° color fundus photography
99	India	26.3 ± 6.9	617 T1	13%	Indirect ophthalmoscopy
100	Sweden	12–30	94 T1	48%	Fundal photography
80	Australia	13.9–17	1,433 T1	20%	Stereoscopic fundus photography
			68 T2	4%	
81	New York	10–35	40 T2	2.5%	Direct and indirect ophthalmoscopy
101	Bangladesh	13 ± 2.3	37 FCPD	2.7%	Direct and indirect ophthalmoscopy

Abbreviation: FCPD, fibrocalculous pancreatopathy.

pre- and intraretinal hemorrhage. Microaneurysms develop because of loss of supporting pericytes around the capillary wall and are often transient, lasting from months to years (9). Later features are soft exudate caused by microinfarcts, hard exudate caused by protein, and lipid leakage and microvascular abnormalities. Background retinopathy is not vision threatening and does not invariably progress to proliferative retinopathy.

Preproliferative retinopathy is characterized by vascular obstruction, progressive intraretinal microvascular abnormalities, and infarctions of the retinal nerve fibers causing "cotton wool spots."

Proliferative retinopathy is characterized by the formation of new blood vessels (neovascularization) in the retina and/or vitreous posterior surface and is vision threatening. The vessels may rupture or bleed into the vitreoretinal space. Encasement in connective tissue results in adhesions, which can cause hemorrhage and retinal detachment. Visual loss may occur depending on location and extent of neovascularization.

In diabetic maculopathy, decreased vascular competence and microaneurysm formation produce exudation and swelling in the central retina that can significantly decrease visual acuity. This characteristic is far more common in T2DM than T1DM.

The WESDR showed an orderly progression of increasing severity from background to proliferative retinopathy in their group with diabetes onset before 30 years (of these, 200 were aged less than 20 years at first assessment in 1980–1982). The prevalence of any retinopathy was 17% in those with less than five years diabetes duration, 50% after five to six years diabetes duration, and rose to 98% after 15 or more years' duration. Proliferative retinopathy was present in 4% after 10 years' duration, 25% after 15 years, and 67% after 35 years (10).

Our population-based study of children diagnosed before 15 years of age documented a 24% prevalence of retinopathy at six years' duration (11). While this rate is very similar to the WESDR, we found a lower rate of retinopathy in a more recent follow-up of young adults with long diabetes duration (73%). That cohort was clinic based and examined initially as adolescents in 1990–1993, at which time 47% had retinopathy. At 12-year follow-up at a median age of 26 years and duration 19 years, severe retinopathy requiring laser treatment was found in 10%, moderately severe retinopathy in 15%, mild retinopathy in 44%, and no retinopathy in 30% (12). At the four-year follow-up of the WESDR, progression of retinopathy had occurred in 41%, retinopathy was unchanged in 55%, and had improved in 4% (13). The predictors of progression to proliferative retinopathy were severity of retinopathy at baseline and glycemic control.

In children and adolescents we found a much higher rate of regression. Between 1990 and 2005 at CHW, retinopathy was assessed longitudinally in 618 adolescents aged 11–20 years, and 50 children less than 11 years (14). In the older group, retinopathy was present in 22% of which only 13% had progressed one to two years later and 36% had regressed. In the younger group, retinopathy was present in 16%, of whom none progressed and 80% regressed one to two years later. Significant increase in the proportion with retinopathy only occurred at two-year follow-up in the older group and at six-year follow-up in the younger group. Progression and persistence of retinopathy were associated with worse glycemic control (HbA1c of 9.1% vs. 8.5%) and longer duration (7.8 years vs. 5.9 years) than those whose retinopathy regressed. In this group, the highest severity of retinopathy was moderate (grade 41). This observation was very reassuring but the authors subsequently became aware of two females in the cohort who rapidly progressed to loss of vision at age 21 and 23 years, after 17 years' duration and persistently poor control (15).

In an earlier follow-up study of 196 adults with prepubertal-onset diabetes, the median duration until the earliest signs of background retinopathy was 9.7 years (16). For the subgroup of children diagnosed before five years of age, the median time till retinopathy was 12.2 years compared with 8.9 years for those diagnosed after five years of age, indicating that the effect of prepubertal diabetes duration is more important the closer to onset of puberty.

Diabetic Nephropathy

Clinically, diabetic nephropathy refers to deterioration in renal function or proteinuria with albumin excretion rate (AER) > 200 µg/min. Earlier studies have led to estimates that 30–40% of patients with T1DM will develop end-stage renal disease (17). Nephropathy is associated with increased risk of mortality, usually as a consequence of cardiovascular disease (18).

Diabetic nephropathy is rare in children with T1DM; however, early signs of renal disease such as microalbuminuria and hypertension are not uncommon. Hyperfiltration and renal hypertrophy precede the development of microalbuminuria in adolescents followed from diagnosis for 10 years (19).

There is a large variation in the reported prevalence of microalbuminuria in children (20–23), which reflects real differences because of racial, genetic, or metabolic factors, but different definitions of microalbuminuria and study methodology must also be considered (Table 2).

Borderline Microalbuminuria

Borderline microalbuminuria has been defined as an AER > 7.5 µg/min as this value is abnormal (above the 95th centile for AER in nondiabetic school children), but not yet at the level generally accepted as significant microalbuminuria. Presence of borderline microalbuminuria at first complication assessment more than doubles the risk of future development of persistent microalbuminuria (24,25).

TABLE 2 Prevalence or Incidence of Nephropathy and Microalbuminuria: Longitudinal Studies

References	Location	Age at diagnosis (Dx); follow-up (yrs)	Participants	Prevalence or incidence	Outcome
25	Australia	Dx < 18; follow-up: 6	991 T1	4.6 per 1000 patient years	AER > 20 µg/min for > 12 months
77	Japan	Dx 10–19; follow-up, 30	25 T1	6.4 per 1000 patient years	Proteinuria > 300 mg/dL
			37 T2	13.1 per 1000 patient years	
100	Sweden	Dx 15–34; follow-up, 9	426 T1	5.6%	AER > 20 µg/min or elevated high albumin/creatinine ratio
			43 T2	16.2%	
20	Oxford	Dx < 16; follow-up, 11	514 T1	Persistent in 4.8%	ACR > 3.5 mg/mmol (males); 4.0 mg/mmol (females)
102	Arizona	Dx < 20; follow-up, 20	96 T2	25.0 cases per 1000 patient years	End-stage renal disease

Abbreviations: ACR, albumin/creatinine ratio; AER, albumin excretion rate.

Our population-based study of childhood diabetes at six years diabetes duration found AER > 7.5 in 18%, which is slightly lower than the prevalence of retinopathy (24%). Only 2% had microalbuminuria (based on 2 of 3 albumin excretion rate > 20 µg/min at a single time point in 1996–1998) (11).

Early Elevation of AER
Several longitudinal studies have found an association between early elevation of AER and the development of microalbuminuria (26–28). This association has remained significant when the outcomes were adjusted for age, duration, HbA1c, and blood pressure (25,29,30). A progressive increase in AER before onset of persistent microalbuminuria has been shown (25,31).

Transient Microalbuminuria
A single episode of microalbuminuria is found in 2–18% of children and adolescents with T1DM (22,23,32). This characteristic is transient in 32–49% of cases (20,33). Transient microalbuminuria may arise in the context of intercurrent illness, strenuous exercise, urinary tract infections, glomerulonephritis, menstrual bleeding, vaginal discharge, or hyperglycemia. The significance of transient microalbuminuria is unclear. Regression of microalbuminuria has also been observed in adults with T1DM (34), particularly those with HbA1c < 8%, systolic blood pressure < 115 mmHg, cholesterol < 5.1 mmol/L, triglycerides < 1.64 mmol/L.

Persistent Microalbuminuria
Generally, persistent microalbuminuria refers to an elevated AER of greater than 20 µg/min or alternatively albumin/creatinine (ACR) greater than 2.5 mg/mmol, for greater than six months; however, there is no consistency in the definition used in either clinical practice or research (35).

At CHW, we have followed 972 adolescents between the years 1989–2004 (25). Only six progressed from microalbuminuria to macroalbuminuria at a median duration of 11.5 years. Overall, 124 had an episode of microalbuminuria, which was transient in 60 adolescents. Persistent microalbuminuria developed in 45 adolescents at a median duration of 9.3 years with the earliest at 1.6 years.

Predictors of persistent microalbuminuria from baseline assessment were higher cholesterol and borderline albuminuria, and independent predictors over time using Cox regression were HbA1c, older age at diagnosis, obesity, and higher insulin dose. Higher androgens and lower sex hormone–binding globulin supported a role for hyperandrogenism in its development. The Oxford longitudinal study found microalbuminuria associated with higher growth hormone and androgens (36,37).

In our adult follow-up of those initially assessed in 1990–1993, only 19% had microalbuminuria (elevated albumin/creatinine) and none had renal failure (12). In the prepubertal-onset cohort reexamined at adult age, the median follow-up time until development of microalbuminuria was 21.2 years, while the median follow-up time to AER > 7.5 was 11.1 years (again similar to the survival till "retinopathy") (16). For the subgroup of children diagnosed before five years of age, the median follow-up time to AER > 7.5 was 13.8 years compared with 9.5 years for those diagnosed after five years of age.

Other longitudinal studies have demonstrated that nocturnal hypertension (38), increased ambulatory blood pressure (39–41), impaired diastolic function (42,43), and septal hypertrophy (44) precede the development of microalbuminuria in T1DM. The effect of high blood pressure as a risk factor persists after adjustment for HbA1c (25,26,45).

Hyperlipidemia can occur secondary to poor glycemic control or constitutively (46). An association between hyperlipidemia and diabetic renal disease has been demonstrated in cross-sectional studies (47,48).

Elevations of LDL cholesterol (>3.3 mmol/L) and triglycerides (>1.1 mmol/L), even when corrected for HbA1C, were identified as risk factors for proteinuria in the Pittsburgh Epidemiology of Diabetes Complications Study (49). This was a prospective study of 589 adults with childhood-onset T1DM. Similarly, in the EURODIAB study of 1865 T1DM patients followed for a mean of 7.3 years, fasting triglycerides, HDL, and LDL cholesterol were significant predictors of the development of microalbuminuria even when this association was adjusted for duration, HbA1c, and baseline AER (29).

Diabetic Neuropathy

Neuropathy is a major complication of diabetes that causes considerable morbidity and increased mortality in adults. Both the autonomic and peripheral nervous systems can be affected. Peripheral neuropathy predisposes to foot ulceration and amputation and autonomic neuropathy is associated with an increased risk of sudden death.

Longer duration and worse metabolic control were established as risk factors for clinical neuropathy in Pirart's longitudinal study from 1947 to 1973 (50). Neuropathy developed in 45% of individuals after 20–25 years of T1DM.

The largest prevalence study of neuropathy was the EURODIAB Prospective Complications Study group, which investigated complications in 3250 randomly selected patients with T1DM from 16 countries in 1989–1991 (51). Neuropathy was present in 19% of the group aged 15–29 years. It was defined as two of four abnormal measures: presence of one or more symptoms, absence of two tendon reflexes, high

TABLE 3 Prevalence of Subclinical Peripheral and Autonomic Neuropathy

References	Location	Age (yrs)	Participants	Abnormal	Method
103	Scotland	16–19	71 T1	72%	Nerve conduction
				31%	CVS tests
104	Netherlands	11.3 ± 3.9	55 T1	2%	Vibration threshold
				15%	Thermal threshold
56	Australia	15.0 ± 1.9	181 T1	20%	Thermal threshold
				7%	Vibration threshold
				28%	CVS tests
105	Denmark	15.5 (10–21)	61 T1	20%	Vibration threshold >95th PC
106	Sweden	15.4 ± 3.6	75 T1	57%	Nerve conduction >95th PC
107	Australia	12.8 ± 3.2	130 T1	15%	Spectral analysis of heart rate
53	Finland	13.7 ± 2.0	100 T1	10%	Nerve conduction <1st or >99th PC
108	Spain	8–16	35 T1	43%	Thermal threshold
109	Belgium	15 (5–19)	60 T1	23%	Long QTc
110	Canada	13.7 ± 2.6	73 T1	51%	Vibration nerve
				57%	Conduction
				26%	tactile perception
80	Australia	15.7	1453 T1	27%	Thermal threshold or vibration
		15.3	24 T2	21%	

vibration threshold for age, and abnormal autonomic tests of lying/standing heart rate variation or systolic blood pressure fall on standing. At seven-year follow-up, incident neuropathy had developed in 24% of individuals without neuropathy at baseline (52). Incident neuropathy was associated with longer duration of diabetes, higher HbA1c, triglyceride level and BMI, history of smoking and presence of hypertension at baseline, and increase in HbA1c, all significant in multivariate analysis.

In a recent study of 101 Finnish adolescents, 10% were diagnosed with distal polyneuropathy. While the diagnosis was based on neurophysiological tests (at least 2 abnormal), these adolescents also had less heart rate variation and three had symptoms. An additional nine adolescents had symptoms of tingling or numbness in their feet (53). This represents a clinical diagnosis in 3%. Other studies in adolescents have focused on subclinical testing and reported single abnormalities (Table 3).

Peripheral Neuropathy
Symmetrical distal polyneuropathy is the commonest manifestation of neuropathy. The most commonly reported symptoms are dys-, para-, hypo-, or hyperaesthesia, burning, and superficial or deep pain.

Physical examination typically shows sensory loss in a glove and stocking distribution and loss of deep tendon reflexes. Sensory loss can involve vibration, pressure, pain, and temperature perception. Pressure can be assessed with a monofilament and vibration with a tuning fork. Muscle weakness occurs late in the disease and usually involves the intrinsic foot muscles and ankle dorsiflexors.

Diabetic patients can have acute and disabling pain at any stage of their diabetes. It can occur in a stocking distribution, in the thighs (femoral neuropathy) or in the trunk as a radiculopathy. Pain is usually worse at night. Correlation with physical examination and electrophysiological abnormalities may be poor. The pain is protracted and unremitting, lasting on average 10 months until complete recovery, when return of lost tendon reflexes may occur. Exquisite contact discomfort is characteristic. It is unrelated to other complications of diabetes and can be precipitated by a period of improved glycemic control.

The mechanism of pain may be sprouting, regenerating small nerve fibers because sural nerve biopsies show fiber loss and atrophy of myelinated and unmyelinated fibers as well as regeneration of fibers.

Nerve conduction studies primarily reflect the function of large myelinated motor and sensory nerves. Improvement in velocity and amplitude has been shown with reduction in blood glucose levels after onset of disease and with intensive treatment (54). Axonal loss causes initially reduction in amplitude, and segmental demyelination is reflected by decreased nerve conduction velocity. The earliest sign is reduction in sural nerve amplitude or action potential (55).

Quantitative sensory tests use the method of levels or method of limits to measure ability to detect a stimulus. Small unmyelinated and thinly myelinated fibers are tested by temperature discrimination and large fibers by vibration discrimination.

At CHW, we found heat discrimination was more frequently abnormal than vibration in the foot (12% vs. 5%) (56). During 10-year follow-up, heat discrimination in the foot was the most consistently abnormal test, which increased over time (57). Vibration perception abnormalities did not increase.

Autonomic Neuropathy

The symptoms of autonomic neuropathy include postural hypotension, vomiting, diarrhea, bladder paresis, erectile dysfunction, and sweating abnormalities. Clinical signs are resting tachycardia, gastroparesis, small pupils, and reduced response to light. The autonomic nerves enervate the vasculature systemically.

There is evidence that subclinical and especially neurophysiological abnormalities of autonomic function are present early in the course of the disease (Table 3). The most frequently used tests to evaluate the autonomic system are the cardiovascular and the pupillary tests. While meta-analysis of 15 studies shows an increase in mortality with one and two cardiovascular test abnormalities, abnormal pupillary tests, may also have prognostic significance for subsequent development of complications in adolescents (12,58).

Ewing et al. first described a battery of five cardiovascular autonomic tests (59). They are the heart rate response to deep breathing, the Valsalva maneuver and to standing, and the blood pressure response to standing from a lying position.

At CHW, we found 28% of 181 had at least one abnormal autonomic test: four girls had two and one girl had three abnormal tests (56). Our longitudinal analysis did not show any increase in abnormalities in 150 adolescents followed up to 10 years (57).

Using computerized infrared pupillometry, we found 10% of adolescents had reduced pupillary size and 21% had at least one abnormal pupillary test, using the pupillary response to light (60). The reflex amplitude (difference between maximum and minimum pupil diameter) was smaller and the conduction velocity slower.

Reassessment in 150 adolescents 1.5 years later suggested that pupillometry was a more reliable and sensitive test than standard cardiovascular reflexes (61). There was significant decrease in maximum constriction velocity and resting pupil diameter. At reassessment, pupillary abnormalities increased from 21% to 30% with 17 (54%) of the initial abnormalities persisting. This greater sensitivity persisted over time. Smaller pupillary size was associated with subsequent development of retinopathy and microalbuminuria but no such association was found with cardiovascular autonomic tests (12).

Heart rate variability has also been tested using ECG recordings of longer duration, up to 24 hours. The R–R interval can be analyzed using time domain and frequency domain (or power spectral analysis) and nonlinear methods of maximal entropy (Table 3).

Inheritance of Risk Factors for Complications

There is increasing evidence that factors associated with "insulin resistance" are important in the development of micro (52,62) and macrovascular (63) complications of T1DM. Cross-sectional studies in adults with T1DM have described associations between microalbuminuria and insulin dose (64), family history of T2DM, hypertension, waist circumference, hypercholesterolemia (65), elevated serum triglycerides, endothelial dilatation (66), and insulin sensitivity (64). Prospective studies have identified endothelial dysfunction (67) and impaired glucose uptake (68) to precede the development of microalbuminuria. BMI (25) and waist/hip ratio (29) remain significant predictors of microalbuminuria in T1DM when adjusted for age, duration, initial AER, and HbA1c.

In addition, risk factors for microvascular complications in the proband with T1DM can be identified in first-degree relatives. A familial insulin resistance score comprising hypertension, lipid disorders, T2DM, and obesity was also linked to the development of nephropathy and retinopathy in a prospective, multicenter study of 275 probands with T1DM (5). Obesity and lipid disorders in relatives cosegregated with nephropathy in the proband and obesity and hypertension in relatives cosegregated with retinopathy, even after allowing for nephropathy. Even more interestingly, the probands themselves did not differ for BMI between those with and without the complication. Another family study did not confirm this association of parental hypertension, lipids, and apoproteins A1 and B with microalbuminuria; however, microalbuminuria was associated with paternal nighttime systolic blood pressure, night to day systolic blood pressure, and albumin/creatinine ratio (69).

The DCCT provided the first evidence for familial clustering of proliferative retinopathy and nephropathy, which is independent of metabolic control. There was a threefold increased risk of retinopathy in probands who had a diabetic relative with retinopathy compared with those who had a diabetic relative without retinopathy, and fivefold increased risk for nephropathy in probands with a relative positive for nephropathy compared with a relative negative for nephropathy (70).

Candidate gene association studies have included the aldose reductase gene for retinopathy (71), nephropathy (72), and neuropathy (73,74) in young patients with T1DM. Limited in vivo studies link susceptible polymorphisms with changes in expression of the aldose reductase gene itself (75).

The Changing Epidemiology of Diabetes Complications

Recent studies from Sweden, Denmark, Japan, and US have reported a marked decline in proliferative retinopathy and nephropathy in adults (76–78). This decline has happened during a time when there have been major improvements in diabetes

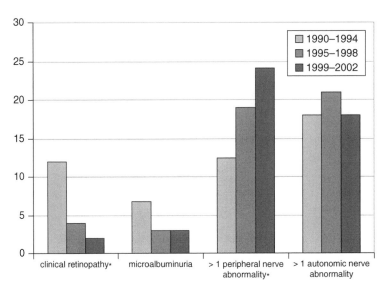

FIGURE 2 Changes in prevalence of complications in T1DM between 1990 and 2002 in Sydney, Australia. Microalbuminuria was defined as AER > 20 μg/min in two-third urine samples; (∗) indicates a statistically significant difference ($p < 0.01$) in the incidence of complications between time periods using χ^2 test. *Abbreviation*: AER, albumin excretion rate. *Source*: Adapted from Ref. 13.

management and better management of hypertension, and the use of angiotensin converting enzyme inhibitors and angiotensin II receptor blockers (79).

At CHW, we have reported a decline in background retinopathy and elevated albumin excretion in adolescents, between 1990 and 2002 (32). Adolescents with median age of 14.6 years and duration of 7.5 years were compared in three assessment periods: 1990–1994, 1995–1998, and 1992–2002. The prevalence of retinopathy declined from 49%, 31%, and 24%, and AER > 7.5 from 38%, 30% to 25%. However, peripheral nerve test abnormalities increased from 12%, 19% to 24%, but cardiovascular autonomic test abnormalities did not change (Fig. 2).

During this time, the mean blood pressure and BMI of the clinic population also increased. There was no significant change in HbA1c; however, more patients were managed with intensive treatment using multiple daily injections (80) (Table 1). Improvements in blood glucose control, in particular postprandial glycemic excursions, which are not detectable using HbA1c are likely to be responsible for this reduction in prevalence of retinopathy and microalbuminuria. Of concern is the relationship of increasing BMI and peripheral nerve abnormalities.

Complications in Adolescents with T2DM

A comparative study of 1433 adolescents with T1DM (duration 6.8 years, HbA1c 8.5%) and age-matched 68 patients with T2DM was performed in Australia 1996–2005 (80). Duration of diabetes was shorter in type 2 (1.3 years vs. 6.8 years) and HbA1c was lower (7.3% vs. 8.5%). No retinopathy was present at diagnosis in the group with T2DM but did develop in 1 of 25 assessed. This prevalence of 4% compares with 20% of those with T1DM. Microalbuminuria and hypertension were more common in T2DM (Fig. 1).

Similarly, in a cohort of 40 African-American and Carribean-Hispanic adolescents with T2DM, retinopathy was rare (2.5%) but microalbuminuria was common (27.3%) (81). In young Pima Indians (less than 20 years at diagnosis) who were followed longitudinally, only three developed retinopathy (by ophthalmoscopy) but nine developed nephropathy after 10 years (82). The adolescents being relatively protected from retinopathy was confirmed in the subgroup aged less than 20 years who underwent stereoscopic fundal photography: only 1 of 31 was diagnosed with early background retinopathy.

Rapid onset of proliferative retinopathy was reported in a subgroup of early-onset type 2 Japanese diabetic patients. This subgroup of patients was characterized by inadequate glycemic control and a high familial prevalence of diabetes supporting the role of gene-environmental interactions in the risk of diabetes vascular complications (83).

Some racial groups, in particular Aboriginal Australians, New Zealand Mauri, and Pacific Islanders, appear to be at increased risk of nephropathy compared with those of European origin (84). In young Japanese patients with T2DM, nephropathy occurs more frequently and progresses more rapidly than in T1DM, particularly in those with poor glycemic control (77).

Like in adults with T2DM, microalbuminuria in youth with T2DM is associated with other risk factors for the metabolic syndrome such as hypertension, obesity, hypercholesterolemia, hypertriglyceridemia.

Microalbuminuria occurs in obese adolescents with insulin resistance (85); however, it is not described in obese individuals with normal glucose tolerance (86). At CHW, peripheral and autonomic nerve-function abnormalities occurred at a similar rate in T2DM and T1DM despite a shorter duration in T2DM. Nerve conduction abnormalities and intrepidemal nerve fiber abnormalities on biopsy have been documented during the time of prediabetes, a metabolic syndrome with normoglycemia (7). Abnormal glucose tolerance tests occur in painful neuropathy (87).

POLYCYSTIC OVARIAN SYNDROME AND DIABETES

Polycystic ovarian syndrome (PCOS) and hyperandrogenism are more common in women with T1DM (88,89). Although the pathophysiology of PCOS in T1DM is unclear, it is thought that the exogenous administration of insulin in relatively high doses and a nonphysiological pattern stimulates the synthesis of androgens by the ovaries.

PCOS is associated with hyperinsulinism and T2DM. However, nonobese women also develop PCOS. Research evaluating glucose and insulin levels in PCOS has suggested that the insulin resistance in PCOS may not be due to obesity (90).

THE LIVER AND DIABETES

The most common chronic liver disease seen in patients with diabetes mellitus is nonalcoholic fatty liver disease (NAFLD), a term encompassing the spectrum hepatic steatosis, nonalcoholic steatohepatitis (NASH), cirrhosis, end-stage liver disease, and hepatocellular carcinoma (HCC). NAFLD is associated with hepatic and peripheral insulin resistance. Those with NASH and diabetes are more likely to develop fibrosis. Conversely, up to 80% of patients with cirrhosis have insulin resistance and 20–63% of these will develop diabetes (91).

Elevated transaminases are frequently found in adolescents with T2DM. In the United States, levels more than double the upper limit of normal were found in 48% of adolescents with short duration and median BMI of 33 kg/m^2 (92). At CHW, we found abnormal liver function tests (above the normal range) in 49% of adolescents who had a comparatively lower BMI (BMI SDS, 1.86) (80).

Fatty liver and elevated transaminases are less commonly observed in T1DM but are well recognized in extremely poorly controlled T1DM (often in association with poor growth as in the Mauriac syndrome).

In T1DM, lower levels of liver glycogen are found—most likely as a consequence of low portal insulin concentrations. This consequence may be a contributing factor to the predisposition to hypoglycemia during exercise.

CONCLUSIONS

The good news is that there has been a decrease in the incidence of retinopathy and nephropathy in T1DM in specialized centers, since the advent of screening and attention to modifiable risk factors. There is no evidence for such a reduction in T2DM complications, nor for neuropathy in T1DM.

The bad news is that the increase in obesity not only increases the risk for T2DM but may also be associated with an increased risk of developing diabetes-related complications, especially neuropathy, in both T1DM and T2DM. Our challenge ahead remains to alter or modify all the risk factors for diabetes-related long-term complications.

REFERENCES

1. DCCT Research Group. The effect of intensive treatment of diabetes on the development and progression of long-term complications in insulin-dependent diabetes mellitus. N Engl J Med 1993; 329:977–986.
2. Intensive blood-glucose control with sulphonylureas or insulin compared with conventional treatment and risk of complications in patients with type 2 diabetes (UKPDS 33). UK Prospective Diabetes Study (UKPDS) Group. Lancet 1998.352(9131). 837–853.
3. Clarke SL, Craig ME, Garnett SP, et al. Increased adiposity at diagnosis in younger children with type 1 diabetes does not persist. Diabetes Care 2006; 29(7):1651–1653.
4. Dorchy H, Claes C, Verougstraete C. Risk factors of developing proliferative retinopathy in type 1 diabetic patients: role of BMI. Diabetes Care 2002; 25(4):798–799.
5. Hadjadj S, Pean F, Gallois Y, et al. Different patterns of insulin resistance in relatives of type 1 diabetic patients with retinopathy or nephropathy: the Genesis France-Belgium Study. Diabetes Care 2004; 27(11):2661–2668.
6. Fagot-Campagna A, Pettitt DJ, Engelgau MM, et al. Type 2 diabetes among North American children and adolescents: an epidemiologic review and a public health perspective. J Pediatr 2000; 136(5):664–672.
7. Vinik A, Ullal J, Parson HK, et al. Diabetic neuropathies: clinical manifestations and current treatment options. Nat Clin Pract Endocrinol Metab 2006; 2(5):269–281.
8. Alibrahim E, Donaghue KC, Rogers S, et al. Retinal vascular caliber and risk of retinopathy in young patients with type 1 diabetes. Ophthalmology 2006; 113(9):1499–1503.
9. Kohner EM, Dollery CT. The rate of formation and disappearance of microaneurysms in diabetic retinopathy. Trans Ophthalmol Soc U K 1970; 90:369–74.
10. Klein R, Klein BE, Moss SE, et al. The Wisconsin epidemiologic study of diabetic retinopathy. II. Prevalence and risk of diabetic retinopathy when age at diagnosis is less than 30 years. Arch Ophthalmol 1984; 102(4):520–526.

11. Donaghue KC, Craig ME, Chan AK, et al. Prevalence of diabetes complications 6 years after diagnosis in an incident cohort of childhood diabetes. Diabet Med 2005; 22(6):711–718.
12. Maguire AM, Craig ME, Craighead A, et al. Autonomic nerve testing predicts the development of complications: a 12-year follow-up study. Diabetes Care 2007; 30(1): 77–82.
13. Klein R, Klein BE, Moss SE, et al. The Wisconsin Epidemiologic Study of Diabetic Retinopathy. IX. Four-year incidence and progression of diabetic retinopathy when age at diagnosis is less than 30 years. Arch Ophthalmol 1989; 107(2):237–243.
14. Maguire A, Chan A, Cusumano J, et al. The case for biennial retinopathy screening in children and adolescents. Diabetes Care 2005; 28(3):509–513.
15. Maguire AM, Chan A, Cusumano JM, et al. Changing attitudes towards retinal screening in type 1 diabetes. Response to Stefanson. Diabetes Care 2006; 29:178–179.
16. Donaghue KC, Fairchild JM, Craig ME, et al. Do all prepubertal years of diabetes duration contribute equally to diabetes complications? Diabetes Care 2003; 26(4): 1224–1229.
17. Brink SJ. Complications of pediatric and adolescent type 1 diabetes mellitus. Curr Diab Rep 2001; 1(1):47–55.
18. Borch-Johnsen K, Kreiner S. Proteinuria: value as predictor of cardiovascular mortality in insulin dependent diabetes mellitus. Br Med J (Clin Res Ed) 1987; 294(6588): 1651–1654.
19. Zerbini G, Bonfanti R, Meschi F, et al. Persistent renal hypertrophy and faster decline of glomerular filtration rate precede the development of microalbuminuria in type 1 diabetes. Diabetes 2006; 55(9):2620–2625.
20. Schultz CJ, Konopelska-Bahu T, Dalton RN et al. Microalbuminuria prevalence varies with age, sex, and puberty in children with type 1 diabetes followed from diagnosis in a longitudinal study. Oxford Regional Prospective Study Group. Diabetes Care 1999; 22(3):495–502.
21. Twyman S, Rowe D, Mansell P, et al. Longitudinal study of urinary albumin excretion in young diabetic patients–Wessex Diabetic Nephropathy Project. Diabet Med 2001; 18 (5): 402–408.
22. Donaghue KC, Fairchild JM, Chan A, et al. Diabetes complication screening in 937 children and adolescents. J Pediatr Endocrinol Metab 1999; 12(2):185–192.
23. Svensson M, Sundkvist G, Arnqvist HJ, et al. Signs of nephropathy may occur early in young adults with diabetes despite modern diabetes management: results from the nationwide population-based Diabetes Incidence Study in Sweden (DISS). Diabetes Care 2003; 26(10):2903–2909.
24. Couper JJ, Clarke CF, Byrne GC, et al. Progression of borderline increases in albuminuria in adolescents with insulin-dependent diabetes mellitus. Diabet Med 1997; 14 (9):766–771.
25. Stone ML, Craig ME, Chan AK, et al. Natural history and risk factors for microalbuminuria in adolescents with type 1 diabetes: a longitudinal study. Diabetes Care 2006; 29(9):2072–2077.
26. Hovind P, Tarnow L, Rossing P, et al. Predictors for the development of microalbuminuria and macroalbuminuria in patients with type 1 diabetes: inception cohort study. BMJ 2004; 328(7448):1105.
27. Rossing P, Hougaard P, Parving HH. Risk factors for development of incipient and overt diabetic nephropathy in type 1 diabetic patients: a 10-year prospective observational study. Diabetes Care 2002; 25(5):859–864.
28. Schultz CJ, Neil HA, Dalton RN, et al. Risk of nephropathy can be detected before the onset of microalbuminuria during the early years after diagnosis of type 1 diabetes. Oxford Regional Prospective Study Group. Diabetes Care 2000; 23(12):1811–1815.
29. Chaturvedi N, Bandinelli S, Mangili R, et al. Microalbuminuria in type 1 diabetes: rates, risk factors and glycemic threshold. Kidney Int 2001; 60(1):219–227.
30. Predictors of the development of microalbuminuria in patients with Type 1 diabetes mellitus: a seven-year prospective study. The Microalbuminuria Collaborative Study Group. Diabet Med 1999; 16(11):918–925.

31. Bach LA, Gilbert RE, Cooper ME, et al. Prediction of persistent microalbuminuria in patients with diabetes mellitus. J Diabetes Complications 1993; 7(2):67–72.
32. Mohsin F, Craig ME, Cusumano J, et al. Discordant trends in microvascular complications in adolescents with type 1 diabetes from 1990 to 2002. Diabetes Care 2005; 28(8):1974–1980.
33. Gorman D, Sochett E, Daneman D. The natural history of microalbuminuria in adolescents with type 1 diabetes. J Pediatr 1999; 134(3):333–337.
34. Perkins BA, Ficociello LH, Silva KH, et al. Regression of microalbuminuria in type 1 diabetes. N Engl J Med 2003; 348(23):2285–2293.
35. Mogensen CE, Keane WF, Bennett PH, et al. Prevention of diabetic renal disease with special reference to microalbuminuria. Lancet 1995; 346(8982):1080–1084.
36. Amin R, Schultz C, Ong K, et al. Low IGF-I and elevated testosterone during puberty in subjects with type 1 diabetes developing microalbuminuria in comparison to normoalbuminuric control subjects: the Oxford Regional Prospective Study. Diabetes Care 2003; 26(5):1456–1461.
37. Amin R, Williams RM, Frystyk J, et al. Increasing urine albumin excretion is associated with growth hormone hypersecretion and reduced clearance of insulin in adolescents and young adults with type 1 diabetes: the Oxford Regional Prospective Study Clin Endocrinol (Oxf) 2005; 62(2):137–144.
38. Lurbe E, Redon J, Kesani A, et al. Increase in nocturnal blood pressure and progression to microalbuminuria in type 1 diabetes. N Engl J Med 2002; 347(11):797–805.
39. Poulsen PL, Hansen KW, Mogensen CE. Ambulatory blood pressure in the transition from normo- to microalbuminuria. A longitudinal study in IDDM patients. Diabetes 1994; 43:1248–1253.
40. Page SR, Manning G, Ingle AR, et al. Raised ambulatory blood pressure in type 1 diabetes with incipient microalbuminuria. Diabet Med 1994; 11(9):877–882.
41. Poulsen PL, Ebbehoj E, Hansen KW, et al. 24-h blood pressure and autonomic function is related to albumin excretion within the normoalbuminuric range in IDDM patients. Diabetologia 1997; 40(6):718–725.
42. Watschinger B, Brunner C, Wagner A, et al. Left ventricular diastolic impairment in type 1 diabetic patients with microalbuminuria. Nephron 1993; 63(2):145–151.
43. Sampson MJ, Chambers JB, Sprigings DC, et al. Abnormal diastolic function in patients with type 1 diabetes and early nephropathy. Br Heart J 1990; 64(4):266–271.
44. Sampson MJ, Chambers J, Sprigings D, et al. Intraventricular septal hypertrophy in type 1 diabetic patients with microalbuminuria or early proteinuria. Diabet Med 1990; 7(2):126–131.
45. Marshall G, Garg SK, Jackson WE, et al. Factors influencing the onset and progression of diabetic retinopathy in subjects with insulin-dependent diabetes mellitus. Ophthalmology 1993; 100(8):1133–1139.
46. Abraha A, Schultz C, Konopelska-Bahu T, et al. Glycaemic control and familial factors determine hyperlipidaemia in early childhood diabetes. Oxford Regional Prospective Study of Childhood Diabetes. Diabet Med 1999; 16(7):598–604.
47. Coonrod BA, Ellis D, Becker DJ, et al. Predictors of microalbuminuria in individuals with IDDM. Pittsburgh Epidemiology of Diabetes Complications Study. Diabetes Care 1993; 16(10):1376–1383.
48. Krolewski AS, Warram JH, Christlieb AR. Hypercholesterolemia—a determinant of renal function loss and deaths in IDDM patients with nephropathy. Kidney Int Suppl 1994; 45:S125–S131.
49. Orchard TJ, Forrest KY, Kuller LH, et al. Lipid and blood pressure treatment goals for type 1 diabetes: 10-year incidence data from the Pittsburgh Epidemiology of Diabetes Complications Study. Diabetes Care 2001; 24(6):1053–1059.
50. Pirart J. Diabetes mellitus and its degenerative complications: a prospective study of 4,400 patients observed between 1947 and 1973. Diabete Metab 1977; 3(3):173–182.
51. Tesfaye S, Stevens LK, Stephenson JM, et al. Prevalence of diabetic peripheral neuropathy and its relation to glycaemic control and potential risk factors: the EURODIAB IDDM Complications Study. Diabetologia 1996; 39(11):1377–1384.
52. Tesfaye S, Chaturvedi N, Eaton SE, et al. Vascular risk factors and diabetic neuropathy. N Engl J Med 2005; 352(4):341–350.

53. Riihimaa PH, Suominen K, Tolonen U, et al. Peripheral nerve function is increasingly impaired during puberty in adolescents with type 1 diabetes. Diabetes Care 2001; 24 (6):1087–1092.

54. DCCT Research Group. Effect of intensive diabetes treatment on nerve conduction in the Diabetes Control and Complications Trial. Ann Neurol 1995; 38(6):869–880.

55. Vinik A. Neuropathies in children and adolescents with diabetes: the tip of the iceberg. Pediatr Diabetes 2006; 7(6):301–304.

56. Donaghue KC, Bonney M, Simpson JM, et al. Autonomic and peripheral nerve function in adolescents with and without diabetes. Diabet Med 1993; 10(7):664–671.

57. Donaghue KC, Al-Jasser A, Maguire AM. Diabetic Autonomic and Peripheral Neuropathy. Pediatr Adolesc Med 2005; 10:259–278.

58. Lafferty AR, Werther GA, Clarke CF. Ambulatory blood pressure, microalbuminuria, and autonomic neuropathy in adolescents with type 1 diabetes. Diabetes Care 2000; 23 (4):533–538.

59. Ewing DJ, Campbell IW, Clarke BF. The natural history of diabetic autonomic neuropathy. Q J Med 1980; 49:95–108.

60. Schwingshandl J, Simpson JM, Donaghue K, et al. Pupillary abnormalities in type I diabetes occurring during adolescence. Comparisons with cardiovascular reflexes. Diabetes Care 1993; 16(4):630–633.

61. Pena MM, Donaghue KC, Fung AT, et al. The prospective assessment of autonomic nerve function by pupillometry in adolescents with type 1 diabetes mellitus. Diabet Med 1995; 12(10):868–873.

62. Chaturvedi N, Sjoelie AK, Porta M, et al. Markers of insulin resistance are strong risk factors for retinopathy incidence in type 1 diabetes. Diabetes Care 2001; 24(2): 284–289.

63. Orchard TJ, Olson JC, Erbey JR, et al. Insulin resistance-related factors, but not glycemia, predict coronary artery disease in type 1 diabetes: 10-year follow-up data from the Pittsburgh Epidemiology of Diabetes Complications Study. Diabetes Care 2003; 26 (5):1374–1379.

64. Yip J, Mattock MB, Morocutti A, et al. Insulin resistance in insulin-dependent diabetic patients with microalbuminuria. Lancet 1993; 342(8876):883–887.

65. Orchard TJ, Chang YF, Ferrell RE, et al. Nephropathy in type 1 diabetes: a manifestation of insulin resistance and multiple genetic susceptibilities? Further evidence from the Pittsburgh Epidemiology of Diabetes Complication Study. Kidney Int 2002; 62 (3):963–970.

66. Zenere BM, Arcaro G, Saggiani F, et al. Noninvasive detection of functional alterations of the arterial wall in IDDM patients with and without microalbuminuria. Diabetes Care 1995; 18(7):975–982.

67. Stehouwer CD, Fischer HR, van Kuijk AW, et al. Endothelial dysfunction precedes development of microalbuminuria in IDDM. Diabetes 1995; 44(5):561–564.

68. Ekstrand AV, Groop PH, Gronhagen-Riska C. Insulin resistance precedes microalbuminuria in patients with insulin-dependent diabetes mellitus. Nephrol Dial Transplant 1998; 13(12):3079–3083.

69. Schultz CJ, Dalton RN, Selwood M, et al. Paternal phenotype is associated with microalbuminuria in young adults with Type 1 diabetes mellitus of short duration. Diabet Med 2004; 21(3):246–251.

70. Clustering of long-term complications in families with diabetes in the diabetes control and complications trial. The Diabetes Control and Complications Trial Research Group. Diabetes 1997; 46(11):1829–39.

71. Kao YL, Donaghue K, Chan A, et al. An aldose reductase intragenic polymorphism associated with diabetic retinopathy. Diabetes Res Clin Pract 1999; 46(2):155–160.

72. Heesom AE, Hibberd ML, Millward A, et al. Polymorphism in the 5′-end of the aldose reductase gene is strongly associated with the development of diabetic nephropathy in type I diabetes. Diabetes 1997; 46(2):287–291.

73. Thamotharampillai K, Chan AK, Bennetts B, et al. Decline in neurophysiological function after 7 years in an adolescent diabetic cohort and the role of aldose reductase gene polymorphisms. Diabetes Care 2006; 29(9):2053–2057.

74. Donaghue KC, Margan SH, Chan AK, et al. The association of aldose reductase gene (AKR1B1) polymorphisms with diabetic neuropathy in adolescents. Diabet Med 2005; 22(10):1315–1320.
75. Hodgkinson AD, Sondergaard KL, Yang B, et al. Aldose reductase expression is induced by hyperglycemia in diabetic nephropathy. Kidney Int 2001; 60(1):211–218.
76. Bojestig M, Arnqvist HJ, Hermansson G, et al. Declining incidence of nephropathy in insulin-dependent diabetes mellitus. N Engl J Med 1994; 330(1):15–18.
77. Yokoyama H, Okudaira M, Otani T, et al. Higher incidence of diabetic nephropathy in type 2 than in type 1 diabetes in early-onset diabetes in Japan. Kidney Int 2000; 58 (1):302–311.
78. Harvey JN, Rizvi K, Craney L, et al. Population-based survey and analysis of trends in the prevalence of diabetic nephropathy in Type 1 diabetes. Diabet Med 2001; 18(12): 998–1002.
79. Ruggenenti P, Remuzzi G. How should patients with, or at risk of, cardiovascular disease be screened for chronic kidney disease? Nat Clin Pract Nephrol 2007; 3(3): 126–127.
80. Eppens MC, Craig ME, Cusumano J, et al. Prevalence of diabetes complications in adolescents with type 2 compared with type 1 diabetes. Diabetes Care 2006; 29(6): 1300–1306.
81. Farah SE, Wals KT, Friedman IB, et al. Prevalence of retinopathy and microalbuminuria in pediatric type 2 diabetes mellitus. J Pediatr Endocrinol Metab 2006; 19(7):937–942.
82. Krakoff J, Lindsay RS, Looker HC, et al. Incidence of retinopathy and nephropathy in youth-onset compared with adult-onset type 2 diabetes. Diabetes Care 2003; 26 (1):76–81.
83. Yokoyama H, Okudaira M, Otani T, et al. Existence of early-onset NIDDM Japanese demonstrating severe diabetic complications. Diabetes Care 1997; 20(5):844–847.
84. Scott A, Toomath R, Bouchier D, et al. First national audit of the outcomes of care in young people with diabetes in New Zealand: high prevalence of nephropathy in Maori and Pacific Islanders. NZ Med J 2006; 119(1235):U2015.
85. Csernus K, Lanyi E, Erhardt E, et al. Effect of childhood obesity and obesity-related cardiovascular risk factors on glomerular and tubular protein excretion. Eur J Pediatr 2005; 164(1):44–49.
86. Hoffmann IS, Jimenez E, Cubeddu LX. Urinary albumin excretion in lean, overweight and obese glucose tolerant individuals: its relationship with dyslipidaemia, hyper-insulinaemia and blood pressure. J Hum Hypertens 2001; 15(6):407–412.
87. Singleton JR, Smith AG, Bromberg MB. Increased prevalence of impaired glucose tolerance in patients with painful sensory neuropathy. Diabetes Care 2001; 24(8): 1448–1453.
88. Codner E, Soto N, Lopez P, et al. Diagnostic criteria for polycystic ovary syndrome and ovarian morphology in women with type 1 diabetes mellitus. J Clin Endocrinol Metab 2006; 91(6):2250–2256.
89. Escobar-Morreale HF, Roldan B, Barrio R, et al. High prevalence of the polycystic ovary syndrome and hirsutism in women with type 1 diabetes mellitus. J Clin Endocrinol Metab 2000; 85(11):4182–4187.
90. Dunaif A, Segal KR, Futterweit W, et al. Profound peripheral insulin resistance, inde-pendent of obesity, in polycystic ovary syndrome. Diabetes 1989; 38(9):1165–1174.
91. El Serag HB, Hampel H, Javadi F. The association between diabetes and hepatocellular carcinoma: a systematic review of epidemiologic evidence. Clin Gastroenterol Hepatol 2006; 4(3):369–380.
92. Nadeau KJ, Klingensmith G, Zeitler P. Type 2 diabetes in children is frequently associated with elevated alanine aminotransferase. J Pediatr Gastroenterol Nutr 2005; 41(1):94–98.
93. Burger W, Hovener G, Dusterhus R, et al. Prevalence and development of retinopathy in children and adolescents with type 1 (insulin-dependent) diabetes mellitus. A lon-gitudinal study. Diabetologia 1986; 29(1):17–22.
94. Joner G, Brinchmann-Hansen O, Torres CG, et al. A nationwide cross-sectional study of retinopathy and microalbuminuria in young Norwegian type 1 (insulin-dependent) diabetic patients. Diabetologia 1992; 35(11):1049–1054.

95. Flack AA, Kaar ML, Laatikainen LT. Prevalence and risk factors of retinopathy in children with diabetes. A population-based study on Finnish children. Acta Ophthalmol (Copenh) 1993; 71(6):801–809.

96. Fairchild JM, Hing SJ, Donaghue KC, et al. Prevalence and risk factors for retinopathy in adolescents with type 1 diabetes. Med J Aust 1994; 160(12):757–762.

97. Kernell A, Dedorsson I, Johansson B, et al. Prevalence of diabetic retinopathy in children and adolescents with IDDM. A population-based multicentre study. Diabetologia 1997; 40(3):307–310.

98. Olsen BS, Johannesen J, Sjolie AK et al. Metabolic control and prevalence of microvascular complications in young Danish patients with Type 1 diabetes mellitus. Danish Study Group of Diabetes in Childhood. Diabet Med 1999; 16(1):79–85.

99. Ramachandran A, Snehalatha C, Sasikala R, et al. Vascular complications in young Asian Indian patients with type 1 diabetes mellitus. Diabetes Res Clin Pract 2000; 48 (1):51–56.

100. Svensson M, Eriksson JW, Dahlquist G. Early glycemic control, age at onset, and development of microvascular complications in childhood-onset type 1 diabetes: a population-based study in northern Sweden. Diabetes Care 2004; 27(4):955–962.

101. Mohsin F, Zabeen B, Zinnat R, et al. Clinical profile of diabetes mellitus in children and adolescents under eighteen years of age. Ibrahim Med Coll J 2007; 1:11–15.

102. Pavkov ME, Bennett PH, Knowler WC, et al. Effect of youth-onset type 2 diabetes mellitus on incidence of end-stage renal disease and mortality in young and middle-aged Pima Indians. JAMA 2006; 296(4):421–426.

103. Young RJ, Ewing DJ, Clarke BF. Nerve function and metabolic control in teenage diabetics. Diabetes 1983; 32(2):142–147.

104. Heimans JJ, Bertelsmann FW, de Beaufort CE, et al. Quantitative sensory examination in diabetic children: assessment of thermal discrimination. Diabet Med 1987; 4(3):251–253.

105. Olsen BS, Nir M, Kjaer I, et al. Elevated vibration perception threshold in young patients with type 1 diabetes in comparison to non-diabetic children and adolescents. Diabet Med 1994; 11(9):888–892.

106. Hyllienmark L, Brismar T, Ludvigsson J. Subclinical nerve dysfunction in children and adolescents with IDDM. Diabetologia 1995; 38(6):685–692.

107. Wawryk AM, Bates DJ, Couper JJ. Power spectral analysis of heart rate variability in children and adolescents with IDDM. Diabetes Care 1997; 20(9):1416–1421.

108. Abad F, Diaz-Gomez NM, Rodriguez I, et al. Subclinical pain and thermal sensory dysfunction in children and adolescents with Type 1 diabetes mellitus. Diabet Med 2002; 19(10):827–831.

109. Suys BE, Huybrechts SJ, De Wolf D, et al. QTc interval prolongation and QTc dispersion in children and adolescents with type 1 diabetes. J Pediatr 2002; 141(1):59–63.

110. Nelson D, Mah JK, Adams C, et al. Comparison of conventional and non-invasive techniques for the early identification of diabetic neuropathy in children and adolescents with type 1 diabetes. Pediatr Diabetes 2006; 7(6):305–310.

15 Cardiovascular Disease Risk Factors

R. Paul Wadwa
Barbara Davis Center for Childhood Diabetes, University of Colorado at Denver and Health Sciences Center, Aurora, Colorado, U.S.A.

Elaine M. Urbina
Department of Pediatrics, Division of Cardiology, Cincinnati Children's Hospital Medical Center, University of Cincinnati, Cincinnati, Ohio, U.S.A.

Stephen R. Daniels
Department of Pediatrics, The Children's Hospital, University of Colorado School of Medicine, Denver, Colorado, U.S.A.

INTRODUCTION

Coronary artery disease and stroke are the most common causes of morbidity and mortality in developed countries. In the past, atherosclerosis has been viewed as a problem of adults and not a focus in the pediatric age range. This is because clinical manifestations of atherosclerosis are often not observed until middle age. However, there is increasing evidence that the process of atherosclerosis begins in childhood and is progressive throughout life.

Diabetes is a known risk factor for cardiovascular disease (CVD). Studies have documented the risk for CVD in adults with diabetes mellitus to be 3 to 10 times that in the general population. Hyperglycemia increases risk for CVD compared with the general population, but there may be other factors related to diabetes leading to increased risk in this population. Youth with diabetes are at increased risk for developing CVD as adults and risk factors present in childhood and adolescence may contribute to this disease later in life.

The prevention of CVD in adults with diabetes begins with the diagnosis and treatment of cardiovascular risk factors in childhood and adolescence. This chapter focuses on the available data for CVD risk factors for youth with type 1 diabetes (T1DM) and type 2 diabetes (T2DM).

Differences Between Type 1 and Type 2 Diabetes

Although T1DM and T2DM both contribute to an increase in risk for CVD, there are significant differences in the features of each. The average age of onset of type 1 diabetes is 11 years. Many young adults with type 1 diabetes will have had diabetes for over 10 years and the effects of hyperglycemia that come with it. The degree of glucose variability and potentially the level of inflammation that accompany the insulin deficiency of type 1 diabetes likely contribute to the CVD risk in a patient with type 1 diabetes.

While insulin resistance is not restricted to T2DM patients, it is more consistently observed in this group. The onset of type 2 diabetes, even in adolescents, can be more subtle than the typical onset of type 1 diabetes. Adolescents with type 2 diabetes may have untreated insulin resistance and even mild hyperglycemia for months to years prior to presenting for medical care. Features of the insulin resistance syndrome, including low HDL cholesterol, elevated triglycerides, and hypertension may be present prior to diagnosis of type 2 diabetes. The period of insulin resistance may begin to set the stage for increased CVD risk prior to the onset of type 2 diabetes. In the absences of insulin resistance, these features are not as common in youth with type 1 diabetes. Given these differences, CVD risk for youth with diabetes will be discussed separately in this chapter for type 1 diabetes and for type 2 diabetes. These sections are followed by a section describing noninvasive tools for assessment of cardiovascular risk in youth.

TYPE 1 DIABETES

Traditional CVD Risk Factors
While the risk for CVD in adults with T1DM has not been as well documented as the risk in adults with T2DM, there have been several large studies documenting traditional factors such as glycemic control, blood pressure, and lipids.

Glycemic Control
The relationship between glycemic control and microvascular complications has been well documented, most notably from the Diabetes Control and Complications Trial (DCCT) (1). Findings from the Epidemiology of Diabetes Interventions and Complications (EDIC) study have shown that glycemic control is also an important factor for the risk of CVD events in adults (2,3). In EDIC, the group that received conventional diabetes therapy and had a higher mean hemoglobin A1c (HbA1c) during the DCCT had a significantly increased risk of CVD events compared with the group on intensive therapy with a lower mean HbA1c. In addition to highlighting the importance of good glycemic control to reduce CVD risk, this study raises the issue of glycemic control during adolescence effecting risk for CVD events in adulthood. Further studies will be necessary to determine the long-term effects of glycemic control during childhood and adolescence.

Evidence from the Coronary Artery Calcification in Type 1 Diabetes (CACTI) study also suggests a link between better blood sugar control and lower risk of coronary disease (4). This study examined progression of coronary artery calcification (CAC), a marker of subclinical coronary atherosclerosis in young adults with T1DM as well as a similar group of nondiabetic control subjects. In an analysis of 109 adults with T1DM, the odds of having progression of coronary calcification were seven times higher for subjects with HbA1c over 7.5% compared with subjects with HbA1c less than 7.5% (odds ratio 7.11 in multivariate logistic regression model).

A meta-analysis of randomized, controlled comparison studies including 1800 T1DM and 4472 T2DM adults identified a reduction in macrovascular events with improvements in glycemic control for both T1DM and T2DM patients (5). The report suggests a larger reduction in macrovascular risk in T1DM and a smaller reduction of risk in T2DM with improved glycemic control.

Pediatric studies using surrogate markers of vascular disease have not identified similar associations of glycemic control with carotid intimal medial thickness (IMT) or arterial stiffness (6–8). These studies were smaller than the previously mentioned adult studies and glycemic control was not a primary focus. This discrepancy suggests that the effects of glycemic control may take several years before vascular changes are detectable with currently available instruments.

In 2005, goals for glycemic control in youth with T1DM were updated by the American Diabetes Association (ADA) (9). The updated goals are based on evidence from DCCT/EDIC that suggests long-term benefits related to the risk for microvascular and macrovascular disease balanced with the potential effects of hypoglycemia in children. In the 2005 ADA guidelines, HbA1c targets are less than 7.5% for adolescents aged 13 to 18 years, less than 8% for children aged 6 to 12 years; and 7.5–8.5% for children under 6 years. As the technology to care for diabetes improves and more patients are able to attain these goals, there is potential for decreased microvascular and macrovascular diabetes complications.

Blood Pressure

Hypertension is known to be an important factor for CVD risk and management of blood pressure has been shown to reduce CVD risk in adults (10,11). Screening for hypertension in youth with diabetes is essential in decreasing risk for both microvascular and macrovascular disease later in life (9).

Several studies have found that hypertension in persons with diabetes is underdiagnosed and undertreated. Saydah et al reported less than 36% of diabetic adults over 20 years old participating in NHANES III (1988–1994) or NHANES 1999–2000 achieved systolic blood pressure less than 130 mmHg and diastolic blood pressure less than 80 mmHg (12). In the CACTI study, blood pressure data for 652 young adults with T1DM (mean age 37 years) and 764 nondiabetic control subjects (mean age 39 years) were analyzed. While T1DM subjects were more likely to have hypertension (43% in T1DM vs. 15% in nondiabetic subjects, $p < 0.001$), they were more aggressively treated with medications (87% of T1DM subjects with hypertension vs. 47% in nondiabetic controls with hypertension, $p < 0.0001$) (13). Rodriguez et al. reported on the prevalence of hypertension in 3- to 19-year-old youth with diabetes enrolled in the SEARCH for Diabetes in Youth Study (14). Hypertension was defined as systolic or diastolic blood pressure over the 90th percentile for age, sex, and height (15) or use of medication for high blood pressure. In 2096 youth with diabetes, 573 (27%) had hypertension. While 22% of the 1376 youth with confirmed type 1a diabetes had hypertension, 73% of the 63 youth with type 2 diabetes had hypertension. No significant difference in the presence of hypertension was seen by sex (26% of females vs. 29% of males). Schwab et al. reported lower rates of hypertension (8.1% systolic hypertension, 2.5% diastolic hypertension) in a large cohort of over 27,000 T1DM subjects in Germany and Austria under age 26 years but similar rates of treatment with medication (2.1% of cohort) (16). In this cohort, significantly more males than females were found to be hypertensive ($p < 0.001$). Most subjects on antihypertensive medications were treated with angiotensin-converting enzyme (ACE) inhibitors (83%).

The ADA guidelines recommend determination of a child's blood pressure at each diabetes care visit for detection of hypertension and also to look for upward trends in blood pressure that may merit further investigation. The family history should also be reviewed (9). Using data from several epidemiological studies, including 1999–2000 NHANES data, blood pressure tables with 50th, 90th, 95th, and 99th percentiles by age, sex, and height are available (15). A child is considered to have hypertension if systolic or diastolic blood pressure is ≥95th percentile on repeated measurements. Levels between the 90th and 95th percentile are considered "prehypertensive" (15).

If hypertension is documented, evaluation of the child should include updating parental history for hypertension, laboratory examination of renal function (urinalysis, serum creatinine, and blood urea nitrogen), and urinary albumin excretion. Patients with type 1 or type 2 diabetes and hypertension should have an echocardiogram to evaluate for left ventricular hypertrophy. The recommended treatment for hypertension in youth with diabetes initially is elimination of added salt in the diet, diet to achieve ideal body weight, and encouragement to exercise if the child is sedentary (9). If lifestyle intervention does not lead to adequate blood pressure improvement in three to six months in children with blood pressure consistently over the 95th percentile, pharmacological therapy is indicated. Pharmacologic treatment of hypertension is also indicated if there is evidence of target organ abnormalities, such as left ventricular hypertrophy on echocardiogram. The goal for treatment is blood pressure at or below the 90th percentile for youth with T1DM and less than the 95th percentile for youth with T2DM unless they have two or more comorbidities, in which case it would also be 90th percentile or less (17). There is evidence supporting the use of ACE inhibitors for treatment of hypertension to decrease CVD risk in adults (18,19). There is also data to support the use of ACE inhibitors in the presence of albuminuria to slow the rate of decline in renal function and decrease progression of retinopathy in diabetic adults (20,21). ACE inhibitors have been proven to be safe in children and are recommended with the diagnosis of hypertension or albuminuria in youth with diabetes. Because ACE inhibitors are contraindicated in pregnancy, this factor must be considered in the care of postpuberty females. Angiotensin receptor blockers have been used in adults with diabetes (22); however, no data are available for the use of these agents in children with diabetes at this time. Dosing information for antihypertensive medications that have been used in children may be found in the Fourth Report on High Blood Pressure in Children (15).

Ambulatory blood pressure monitoring (ABPM) has been used to detect hypertension in diabetic and nondiabetic youth and protocols for pediatric use have been published (23,24). ABPM may be more closely correlated with target organ disease than casual office blood pressure measurement. ABPM is also quite useful to rule out "white coat hypertension." However, the National High Blood Pressure Education Program Working Group on high blood pressure in children and adolescents recommends clinical use of ABPM only by hypertension experts with experience in the use and interpretation of ABPM (25).

Lipids

Dyslipidemia is a major risk factor for atherosclerosis and CVD. Although lipid levels in patients with T1DM have been found to be comparable to or better than in nondiabetic adults (26), adults with T1DM are known to be at higher risk for atherosclerotic disease compared with the general population (27). Some data suggest that lipids in those with diabetes may be more atherogenic. Possible mechanisms for this include differences in lipoprotein particle size, LDL oxidation, and increased transvascular LDL transport in patients with type 1 diabetes (28–30).

Lipid levels in childhood may also have a significant impact on CVD risk in adulthood. In the Bogalusa Heart Study and Young Finns Study, childhood LDL levels were significantly associated with carotid IMT in nondiabetic young adults ($p < 0.001$ and $p = 0.001$, respectively) (31,32).

TABLE 1 American Diabetes Association Recommendations for Lipid Screening and Management in Children and Adolescents with Diabetes

	Type 1 Diabetes	Type 2 Diabetes
Initial screening	>2 yr at diagnosis if other CVD risk factors; otherwise at 12 yr (puberty)	At diagnosis regardless of age
Re-screening if lipid profile is normal	5 yr	2 yr
Initial management of dyslipidemia	Glycemic control, diet, physical activity	
LDL-C concentration for pharmacologic treatment if initial management fails (age 10+ yr)	LDL-C > 160 mg/dL: begin medication LDL-C 130–159 mg/dL "consider" medication based on other adult risk factors: ■ Smoking ■ Hypertension ■ Obesity (>95th percentile for age and sex) ■ Parental TC > 240 mg/dL or family history of cardiovascular event in a parent before 55 yr of age ■ HDL-C < 35 mg/dL	
Optimal concentration	LDL-C < 100 mg/dL HDL-C > 35 mg/dL Triglyceride < 150 mg/dL	

Abbreviations: CVD, cardiovascular disease; LDL-C, low-density lipoprotein cholesterol; HDL-C, high-density lipoprotein cholesterol.
Source: From Ref. 35 with permission from Elsevier Science.

There is evidence that abnormal lipid levels are present in youth with diabetes. In the cohort from Germany and Austria, dyslipidemia (defined as total cholesterol > 200 mg/dL, LDL > 130 mg/dL, or HDL < 35 mg/dL) was detected in 28.6% of T1DM subjects under 26 years old, with a larger percentage (34.2%) in the 17- to 26-year age group. Only 0.4% of all subjects were on lipid lowering medications with 0.8% of 17- to 26-year-olds on lipid-lowering medications (33). A retrospective analysis from Denver, Colorado, revealed 28% of 682 youth (under 21 years old) with T1DM had at least one non-HDL level above 130 mg/dL, 15% had total cholesterol over 200 mg/dL, and 3% with HDL less than 35 mg/dL (34). LDL levels were not examined as fasting status could not be verified in this retrospective analysis. In the SEARCH for Diabetes in Youth study, fasting lipids were examined in 2165 youth with T1DM and 283 youth with T2DM at six centers in the United States. Of the T1DM youth, 3% had LDL levels greater than 160 mg/dL, 14% had greater than 130 mg/dL, and almost half (48%) had LDL levels over the threshold for recommended LDL of 100 mg/dL (35). Of the 1680 youth with T1DM over 10 years old, 242 had LDL levels over 130 mg/dL and only 23 were on lipid-lowering medications at the time of the study. Findings from the American studies indicate that current clinical screening and treatment of lipid abnormalities in T1DM youth in the United States are below recommended ADA standards (Table 1).

The ADA recommends screening of lipid levels in youth with T1DM at 12 years of age and every 5 years thereafter (9,36). In youth with a positive or unknown family history of dyslipidemia or CVD, screening should begin after two years of age (once glycemic control is obtained). In youth with T2DM, screening of lipids is recommended at diagnosis once glycemic control is obtained and every two years if initial values are normal (36). Treatment options should begin with decreasing saturated and total fat in the diet, maximizing glycemic control, and weight reduction when indicated. Thresholds for use of lipid lowering medications have been based on extrapolation from adult data and expert opinion based on epidemiological studies of nondiabetic children (37–39). Treatment with medication is recommended for children over age 10 years for LDL > 160 mg/dL or LDL > 130 mg/dL if not improved with lifestyle changes and significant CVD risk is present. While bile acid sequestrants or "resins" have been considered first-line therapy, compliance with this class of medications is known to be low, and HMG-CoA reductase inhibitors or "statins" are more commonly used. Importantly, statins are contraindicated in pregnancy. Ezetimibe is a relatively new medication that offers the option of using a class of medication with a different mechanism and site of action for LDL lowering (40). While the safety and efficacy of statins has been documented in studies in youth with familial hypercholesteremia (41), studies in youth with diabetes for the efficacy of statins and ezetimibe are lacking at this time. For lowering of triglycerides, diet and glycemic control are recommended unless triglycerides are over 1000 mg/dL, in which case the child is at increased risk for pancreatitis, and fibric acid derivatives should be considered (36). While the most recent dietary guidelines from the American Heart Association mention the benefits of fish oils in the diet and the use of plant stanols/sterols (42), there are no current guidelines for diabetic youth from the ADA regarding these options that have gained recent popularity.

Inflammation

Inflammation is now known to be a key component for the development of atheroma. In the last few years, mechanisms related to immune system involvement in atherosclerosis have become more clear (43,44). Proinflammatory markers C-reactive protein (CRP) and interleukin-6 are associated with worse prognosis in adults who present with unstable angina and myocardial infarction (45–47). More data on markers including adiponectin, E-selectin, and soluble IL-2 receptor in diabetic individuals have become available from clinical research studies associating these markers with clinical and subclinical coronary disease (48–50). Studies in T1DM youth have not shown a significant difference in CRP, IL-6, and metalloproteinase-9 compared with nondiabetic youth (7,51). As the role of inflammation in the atherosclerotic process continues to be clarified, potential opportunities for screening of markers for inflammation and possible interventions may emerge in the future. At this time, however, there is no current role for measuring markers of inflammation in the clinical evaluation of children with diabetes for assessing cardiovascular risk.

TYPE 2 DIABETES

While the increased risk of death from CVD in adults with T2DM compared with the general population has been well documented (52–54), data on CVD risk for youth with T2DM remains relatively sparse.

Recent studies have documented a higher prevalence of CVD risk factors in youth with T2DM compared with youth with T1DM. Data from the SEARCH study have documented abnormalities of blood pressure, lipids, albuminuria, and arterial stiffness that point to an even higher risk for CVD in youth with T2DM compared with those with T1DM (8,14,35,55). Similarly, Eppens et al. reported an increased rate of hypertension and albuminuria in adolescents with T2DM compared with similar aged youth with T1DM despite shorter duration of diabetes and lower HbA1c (56).

In addition to the presence of documented risk factors after diagnosis of T2DM, these youth may have risk factors related to obesity and insulin resistance prior to the development of T2DM. With preexisting risk factors, atherogenesis may begin years prior to diagnosis of diabetes in this population. Given the potential for preexisting comorbidities, screening for hypertension, dyslipidemia, albuminuria, and sleep apnea are recommended soon after the diagnosis of T2DM in youth (36,57).

Studies of youth with T2DM and those at risk for developing T2DM are now shedding more light on the pathophysiology of CVD in this population (58,59). Further work from multicenter studies including larger numbers of youth with T2DM such as SEARCH, STOPP-T2D, and TODAY may also help to clarify the mechanisms leading to increased risk for CVD in this population.

SURROGATE MEASURES OF CVD RISK

Studies to assess CVD in adults have examined risk factors associated with CVD events. The low incidence of overt cardiac disease in youth makes testing any preventive intervention difficult. Therefore, developing and validating noninvasive measures of subclinical atherosclerosis in youth is essential to advance the science of primary prevention in diabetes. Several methods of assessing changes in the heart and vasculature to measure abnormalities in cardiovascular profile are now available and are gaining popularity in clinical research in young individuals with type 1 and type 2 diabetes.

Ultrasound methodology has been utilized to evaluate the presence of atherosclerosis (Fig. 1). In adults, carotid artery IMT has gained acceptance as a useful

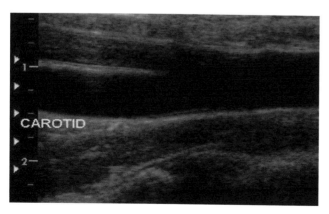

FIGURE 1 Ultrasound of the carotid artery to measure carotid IMT. *Abbreviation*: IMT, intimal medial thickness.

Pulse Wave Velocity

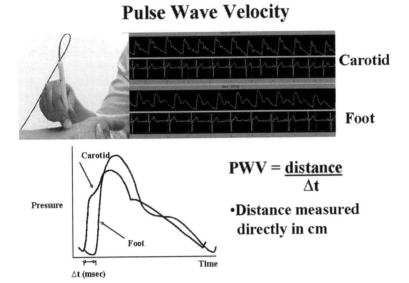

Carotid

Foot

$$PWV = \frac{\text{distance}}{\Delta t}$$

•Distance measured directly in cm

FIGURE 2 Assessment of PWV using arterial tonometry. *Abbreviation*: PWV, pulse wave velocity.

method in epidemiologic studies to evaluate atherosclerosis, and it has been showed that increased carotid IMT is associated with incident myocardial infarction and stroke. Fewer studies have used ultrasound to evaluate carotid IMT in children and adolescents. In nondiabetic studies, associations have been seen with increased childhood cholesterol levels and elevated carotid IMT in adulthood in the Muscatine study and in the Young Finns study (31,60). In youth with diabetes, Krantz et al. found increased carotid IMT in 142 adolescents and young adults with T1DM (age, 16.0 ± 2.6 years) compared with 87 slightly older nondiabetic controls (age, 18.8 ± 3.1 years) (6). Carotid IMT was negatively correlated with HDL and positively correlated with LDL/HDL ratio specifically in male subjects with diabetes, suggesting a gender difference beginning in adolescence. Jarvisalo et al. also found increased carotid IMT in T1DM subjects compared with nondiabetics in a younger group (age, 11 ± 2 years). The 45 T1DM subjects had increased carotid IMT compared with the 30 nondiabetic control subjects and also had decreased brachial flow–mediated dilation (FMD) (61). These findings suggest a link between endothelial dysfunction and carotid atherosclerosis starting at a young age in T1DM.

Arterial stiffness represents a process of vascular damage distinct from the development of atherosclerosis measured by carotid IMT. Arterial stiffness has been measured by several different techniques in the past (62). Pulse wave velocity (PWV), an established measure of arterial stiffness, calculates the speed for the pressure wave generated by cardiac ejection to reach the periphery (Fig. 2). Atherosclerosis results in stiffer vessels and increased PWV. Adults with type 2 diabetes have increased PWV compared with nondiabetic controls. Additional analyses correlated PWV in diabetic patients with higher fasting glucose (63), higher fasting insulin (64), and longer duration of disease (65). PWV was also found to be a powerful predictor of mortality both in type 1 and type 2 diabetic populations as well as those only exhibiting abnormal carbohydrate metabolism (66). Few studies have examined PWV in children (67). In the SEARCH study, PWV was found to be higher in youth with type 2 diabetes compared with those with type 1 diabetes and was associated with longer duration of diabetes in analyses, after adjustment for age and gender (8).

Radial artery tonometry has also been useful in estimating central aortic pressure wave characteristics, i.e., Augmentation Index (AI) (68). This pressure wave augmentation generally occurs in diastole in younger, healthy compliant vessels and produces higher levels of coronary blood flow during diastole. However, in stiffer vessels, the rate of return of the reflected wave is more rapid and augmentation occurs during systole. This augmentation not only decreases coronary blood flow during diastole, but also increases cardiac afterload leading to increased myocardial oxygen demand (69). In adults, increasing AI is correlated with structural arterial changes, such as increased carotid IMT (70). In adults with type 1 diabetes, AI was found to be increased compared with controls (71,72). Similar abnormalities in AI were seen in adults with type 2 diabetes (73) and the increase in arterial stiffness was associated with carotid IMT indicating more extensive atherosclerosis (74). In one study, it was also related to metabolic variables such as higher fasting blood glucose and glycosylated hemoglobin levels (75). While data are largely lacking in children, one study did find increased AI in children (age, 10–18 years) with type 1 diabetes compared with nondiabetic control subjects (76).

Brachial artery distensibility is a method that has been used to measure vascular disease in adults and adolescents without diabetes. The technique provides a measure of arterial stiffness proven to be associated with atherosclerosis at a different site than pulse wave analysis. In the Bogalusa Heart Study, decreased distensibility of the brachial artery has been associated with greater adiposity, high blood pressure, and lipid levels in adults (77,78). Decreased brachial distensibility was also found in nondiabetic adult subjects with a greater coronary artery calcium load (79). Few data are available in children, although one study found that brachial distensibility correlated inversely with cholesterol levels (80), and Whincup et al. found that decreased distensibility in healthy adolescents related to greater adiposity, diastolic blood pressure, inflammation, and insulin resistance (81). A recent report demonstrated decreased brachial distensibility in adolescents and young adults with obesity and further decline with the addition of hyperinsulinemia (82).

In addition to abnormalities in arterial stiffness, endothelial dysfunction has also been documented in diabetic youth. Singh et al. found reduced brachial FMD in adolescents with type 1 diabetes as compared with healthy controls even though they had a mean duration of disease of only 6.8 years (83). Later studies have found the abnormality in FMD in youth with type 1 diabetes to be associated with a concomitant increase in carotid IMT (61) and microalbuminuria (84), other manifestations of vascular disease. Although few data are available in children with type 2 diabetes, similar endothelial dysfunction has been documented in obese children (85) suggesting that these patients are also at increased risk for vascular disease.

In adults, computed tomography (CT) scanning has been used to detect the presence of calcium in the coronary arteries. The presence of calcium deposits has been associated with increased risk for adverse cardiovascular outcomes (86). Studies in adults have demonstrated increased rates of coronary calcium in patients with type 1 diabetes compared with similar age nondiabetic adults (87). An association with glycemic control in adults with type 1 diabetes has also been observed (4).

While CAC appears to be a promising surrogate endpoint in studies of T1DM patients older than 30 years, CAC is unlikely to be a useful surrogate marker of CAD in T1DM adolescents (51,88) given the relatively low likelihood of CAC in this age group. While the CACTI study demonstrated the presence of CAC in 25% of male and 12% of female T1DM patients aged 20 to 29 years, respectively, Starkman et al. detected CAC in only 7% of female and 18% of male T1DM patients aged 17 to 28 years (89).

Magnetic resonance imaging (MRI) may also be used to evaluate the atherosclerotic process. It has been used to evaluate the presence of atherosclerotic plaque and supravalvular aortic stenosis in young patients with homozygous familial hypercholesterolemia (90). Studies in adults have also demonstrated that high resolution multicontrast MRI can be used to evaluate whether arterial plaque is unstable and subject to rupture (91). This is important as other noninvasive methods have been unable to characterize this progression of atherosclerosis. This method allows the fibrous cap to be distinguished from the lipid core. It is not currently known if MRI will be useful in following the evolutions of fatty streaks to fibrous plaques, the process most likely occurring in the pediatric age patient.

Similar to the assessment of inflammatory markers, surrogate measures of cardiovascular health such as carotid IMT, arterial stiffness, coronary calcium, and MRI studies have a role in research, but clinical use of such measures to guide the care of youth is not recommended at this time. As technology continues to evolve and more data on levels in healthy children become available, there may be a role in the future for noninvasive measures of vascular function in the outpatient clinical setting. However, at this time, the assessment of CVD risk should continue to focus on known factors with clinical evidence and guidelines for evaluation and treatment in youth.

CONCLUSION

CVD is the leading cause of mortality in adults with diabetes over the age of 30 years. Adults with diabetes are at significantly higher risk for CVD compared with nondiabetics. Data from several studies indicate that atherosclerosis begins in childhood. The most recent studies in youth with diabetes indicate worse subclinical atherosclerosis and vascular changes compared with nondiabetic youth of similar age. Risk factors for CVD include poor glycemic control, hypertension, dyslipidemia, and possibly increased inflammation. Youth with T2DM appear to be at even higher risk for future CVD compared with youth with T1DM. Surrogate measures including carotid IMT, arterial stiffness measures, CT to assess CAC, and MRI to assess plaques have proven to be important tools in research studies of youth with diabetes. Further studies are necessary to clarify the mechanisms leading to higher rates of CVD in individuals with diabetes and potential avenues for primary prevention beginning in childhood to decrease morbidity and mortality related to CVD.

REFERENCES

1. The effect of intensive treatment of diabetes on the development and progression of long-term complications in insulin-dependent diabetes mellitus. The Diabetes Control and Complications Trial Research Group. N Engl J Med 1993; 329:977–986.

2. Nathan DM, Cleary PA, Backlund JY, et al. Intensive diabetes treatment and cardiovascular disease in patients with type 1 diabetes. N Engl J Med 2005; 353:2643–2653.
3. Nathan DM, Lachin J, Cleary P, et al. Intensive diabetes therapy and carotid intima-media thickness in children with type 1 diabetes mellitus. N Engl J Med 2003; 348:2294–2303.
4. Snell-Bergeon JK, Hokanson JE, Jensen L, et al. Progression of coronary artery calcification in type 1 diabetes: the importance of glycemic control. Diabetes Care 2003; 26:2923–2928.
5. Stettler C, Allemann S, Juni P, et al. Glycemic control and macrovascular disease in types 1 and 2 diabetes mellitus: meta-analysis of randomized trials. Am Heart J 2006; 152:27–38.
6. Krantz JS, Mack WJ, Hodis HN, et al. Early onset of subclinical atherosclerosis in young persons with type 1 diabetes. J Pediatr 2004; 145:452–457.
7. Haller MJ, Samyn M, Nichols WW, et al. Radial artery tonometry demonstrates arterial stiffness in children with type 1 diabetes. Diabetes Care 2004; 27:2911–2917.
8. Wadwa RP, Urbina EM, Dabelea D, et al. Diabetes type and duration are associated with increased arterial stiffness in the SEARCH for Diabetes in Youth study. Diabetes 2006; 55:A2.
9. Silverstein J, Klingensmith G, Copeland K, et al. Care of children and adolescents with type 1 diabetes: a statement of the American Diabetes Association. Diabetes Care 2005; 28:186–212.
10. Hansson L, Zanchetti A, Carruthers SG, et al. Effects of intensive blood-pressure lowering and low-dose aspirin in patients with hypertension: principal results of the Hypertension Optimal Treatment (HOT) randomised trial. HOT Study Group. Lancet 1998; 351:1755–1762.
11. UK Prospective Diabetes Study Group. Tight blood pressure control and risk of macrovascular and microvascular complications in type 2 diabetes: UKPDS 38. BMJ 1998; 317:703–713.
12. Saydah SH, Fradkin J, Cowie CC. Poor control of risk factors for vascular disease among adults with previously diagnosed diabetes. JAMA 2004; 291:335–342.
13. Maahs DM, Kinney GL, Wadwa P, et al. Hypertension prevalence, awareness, treatment, and control in an adult type 1 diabetes population and a comparable general population. Diabetes Care 2005; 28:301–306.
14. Rodriguez BL, Fujimoto WY, Mayer-Davis EJ, et al. Prevalence of cardiovascular disease risk factors in U.S. children and adolescents with diabetes: the SEARCH for diabetes in youth study. Diabetes Care 2006; 29:1891–1896.
15. National High Blood Pressure Education Program Working Group on High Blood Pressure in Children and Adolescents. The fourth report on the diagnosis, evaluation, and treatment of high blood pressure in children and adolescents. Pediatrics 2004; 114:555–576.
16. Schwab KO, Doerfer J, Hecker W, et al. Spectrum and prevalence of atherogenic risk factors in 27,358 children, adolescents, and young adults with type 1 diabetes: cross-sectional data from the German diabetes documentation and quality management system (DPV). Diabetes Care 2006; 29:218–225.
17. Kavey RE, Allada V, Daniels SR, et al. Cardiovascular risk reduction in high-risk pediatric patients: a scientific statement from the American Heart Association Expert Panel on Population and Prevention Science; the Councils on Cardiovascular Disease in the Young, Epidemiology and Prevention, Nutrition, Physical Activity and Metabolism, High Blood Pressure Research, Cardiovascular Nursing, and the Kidney in Heart Disease; and the Interdisciplinary Working Group on Quality of Care and Outcomes Research: endorsed by the American Academy of Pediatrics. Circulation 2006; 114:2710–2738.
18. Hansson L, Zanchetti A, Carruthers SG, et al. Effects of intensive blood-pressure lowering and low-dose aspirin in patients with hypertension: principal results of the Hypertension Optimal Treatment (HOT) randomised trial. HOT Study Group. Lancet 1998; 351:1755–1762.
19. UK Prospective Diabetes Study Group. Tight blood pressure control and risk of macrovascular and microvascular complications in type 2 diabetes: UKPDS 38. BMJ 1998; 317:703–713.

20. Captopril reduces the risk of nephropathy in IDDM patients with microalbuminuria. The Microalbuminuria Captopril Study Group. Diabetologia 1996; 39:587–593.
21. Chaturvedi N, Sjolie AK, Stephenson JM, et al. Effect of lisinopril on progression of retinopathy in normotensive people with type 1 diabetes. The EUCLID Study Group. EURODIAB Controlled Trial of Lisinopril in Insulin-Dependent Diabetes Mellitus. Lancet 1998; 351:28–31.
22. Arauz-Pacheco C, Parrott MA, Raskin P. The treatment of hypertension in adult patients with diabetes. Diabetes Care 2002; 25:134–147.
23. Garg SK, Chase HP, Icaza G, et al. 24-hour ambulatory blood pressure and renal disease in young subjects with type I diabetes. J Diabetes Complications 1997; 11:263–267.
24. Lurbe E, Sorof JM, Daniels SR. Clinical and research aspects of ambulatory blood pressure monitoring in children. J Pediatr 2004; 144:7–16.
25. National High Blood Pressure Education Program Working Group on High Blood Pressure in Children and Adolescents, the fourth report on the diagnosis, evaluation, and treatment of high blood pressure in children and adolescents. Pediatrics 2004; 114:555–576.
26. Wadwa RP, Kinney GL, Maahs DM, et al. Awareness and treatment of dyslipidemia in young adults with type 1 diabetes. Diabetes Care 2005; 28:1051–1056.
27. Weis U, Turner B, Gibney J, et al. Long-term predictors of coronary artery disease and mortality in type 1 diabetes. QJM 2001; 94:623–630.
28. Colhoun HM, Otvos JD, Rubens MB, Taskinen et al. Lipoprotein subclasses and particle sizes and their relationship with coronary artery calcification in men and women with and without type 1 diabetes. Diabetes 2002; 51:1949–1956.
29. Orchard TJ, Virella G, Forrest KY, et al. Antibodies to oxidized LDL predict coronary artery disease in type 1 diabetes: a nested case-control study from the Pittsburgh Epidemiology of Diabetes Complications Study. Diabetes 1999; 48:1454–1458.
30. Kornerup K, Nordestgaard BG, Feldt-Rasmussen B, et al. Increased transvascular low density lipoprotein transport in insulin dependent diabetes: a mechanistic model for development of atherosclerosis. Atherosclerosis 2003; 170:163–168.
31. Raitakari OT, Juonala M, Kahonen M, et al. Cardiovascular risk factors in childhood and carotid artery intima-media thickness in adulthood: the Cardiovascular Risk in Young Finns Study. JAMA 2003; 290:2277–2283.
32. Li S, Chen W, Srinivasan SR, Bond MG, et al. Childhood cardiovascular risk factors and carotid vascular changes in adulthood: the Bogalusa Heart Study. JAMA 2003; 290: 2271–2276.
33. Schwab KO, Doerfer J, Hecker W, et al. Spectrum and prevalence of atherogenic risk factors in 27,358 children, adolescents, and young adults with type 1 diabetes: cross-sectional data from the German diabetes documentation and quality management system (DPV). Diabetes Care 2006; 29:218–225.
34. Maahs DM, Maniatis AK, Nadeau K, et al. Total cholesterol and high-density lipoprotein levels in pediatric subjects with type 1 diabetes mellitus. J Pediatr 2005; 147:544–546.
35. Kershnar AK, Daniels SR, Imperatore G, et al. Lipid abnormalities are prevalent in youth with type 1 and type 2 diabetes: the SEARCH for Diabetes in Youth Study. J Pediatr 2006; 149:314–319.
36. American Diabetes Association. Management of dyslipidemia in children and adolescents with diabetes. Diabetes Care 2003; 26:2194–2197.
37. Freedman DS, Bowman BA, Srinivasan SR, et al. Distribution and correlates of high-density lipoprotein subclasses among children and adolescents. Metabolism 2001; 50:370–376.
38. Srinivasan SR, Myers L, Berenson GS. Distribution and correlates of non-high-density lipoprotein cholesterol in children: the Bogalusa Heart Study. Pediatrics 2002; 110:e29.
39. Lauer RM, Clarke WR. Use of cholesterol measurements in childhood for the prediction of adult hypercholesterolemia. The Muscatine Study. JAMA 1990; 264:3034–3038.
40. Rodenburg J, Vissers MN, Daniels SR, et al. Lipid-lowering medications. Pediatr Endocrinol Rev 2004;2(suppl 1):171–180.

41. de Jongh S, Ose L, Szamosi T, et al. Efficacy and safety of statin therapy in children with familial hypercholesterolemia: a randomized, double-blind, placebo-controlled trial with simvastatin. Circulation 2002; 106:2231–2237.
42. Lichtenstein AH, Appel LJ, Brands M, et al. Diet and Lifestyle Recommendations Revision 2006: a scientific statement from the American Heart Association Nutrition Committee. Circulation 2006; 114:82–96.
43. Hansson GK. Inflammation, atherosclerosis, and coronary artery disease. N Engl J Med 2005; 352:1685–1695.
44. Libby P, Ridker PM, Maseri A. Inflammation and atherosclerosis. Circulation 2002; 105:1135–1143.
45. Lindahl B, Toss H, Siegbahn A, et al. Markers of myocardial damage and inflammation in relation to long-term mortality in unstable coronary artery disease. The FRISC Study Group. Fragmin during Instability in Coronary Artery Disease. N Engl J Med 2000; 343:1139–1147.
46. Fisman EZ, Benderly M, Esper RJ, et al. Interleukin-6 and the risk of future cardiovascular events in patients with angina pectoris and/or healed myocardial infarction. Am J Cardiol 2006; 98:14–18.
47. Zebrack JS, Anderson JL, Maycock CA, et al. Usefulness of high-sensitivity C-reactive protein in predicting long-term risk of death or acute myocardial infarction in patients with unstable or stable angina pectoris or acute myocardial infarction. Am J Cardiol 2002; 89:145–149.
48. Maahs DM, Ogden LG, Kinney GL, et al. Low plasma adiponectin levels predict progression of coronary artery calcification. Circulation 2005; 111:747–753.
49. Wadwa RP, Kinney GL, Ogden L, et al. Soluble interleukin-2 receptor as a marker for progression of coronary artery calcification in type 1 diabetes. Int J Biochem Cell Biol 2006; 38(5–6):996–1003.
50. Costacou T, Lopes-Virella MF, Zgibor JC, et al. Markers of endothelial dysfunction in the prediction of coronary artery disease in type 1 diabetes. The Pittsburgh Epidemiology of Diabetes Complications Study. J Diabetes Complications 2005; 19:183–193.
51. Gunczler P, Lanes R, Soros A, et al. Coronary artery calcification, serum lipids, lipoproteins, and peripheral inflammatory markers in adolescents and young adults with type 1 diabetes. J Pediatr 2006; 149:320–323.
52. Intensive blood-glucose control with sulphonylureas or insulin compared with conventional treatment and risk of complications in patients with type 2 diabetes (UKPDS 33). UK Prospective Diabetes Study (UKPDS) Group. Lancet 1998; 352:837–853.
53. Battisti WP, Palmisano J, Keane WE. Dyslipidemia in patients with type 2 diabetes; relationships between lipids, kidney disease and cardiovascular disease. Clin Chem Lab Med 2003; 41:1174–1181.
54. Caro JJ, Ward AJ, O'Brien JA. Lifetime costs of complications resulting from type 2 diabetes in the U.S. Diabetes Care 2002; 25:476–481.
55. Dabelea D, Maahs DM, Snively BM, et al. High prevalence of elevated albumin excretion in youth with type 2 diabetes: the SEARCH for Diabetes in Youth Study. Diabetologia 2005; 48:A53–A54.
56. Eppens MC, Craig ME, Cusumano J, et al. Prevalence of diabetes complications in adolescents with type 2 compared with type 1 diabetes. Diabetes Care 2006; 29: 1300–1306.
57. Liu L, Hironaka K, Pihoker C. Type 2 diabetes in youth. Curr Probl Pediatr Adolesc Health Care 2004; 34:254–272.
58. Steinberger J, Daniels SR. Obesity, insulin resistance, diabetes, and cardiovascular risk in children: an American Heart Association scientific statement from the Atherosclerosis, Hypertension, and Obesity in the Young Committee (Council on Cardiovascular Disease in the Young) and the Diabetes Committee (Council on Nutrition, Physical Activity, and Metabolism). Circulation 2003; 107:1448–1453.
59. Goran MI, Ball GDC, Cruz ML. Obesity and risk of type 2 diabetes and cardiovascular disease in children and adolescents. J Clin Endocrinol Metab 2003; 88:1417–1427.
60. Davis PH, Dawson JD, Riley WA, et al. Carotid intimal-medial thickness is related to cardiovascular risk factors measured from childhood through middle age: the Muscatine Study. Circulation 2001; 104:2815–2819.

61. Jarvisalo MJ, Raitakari M, Toikka JO, et al. Endothelial dysfunction and increased arterial intima-media thickness in children with type 1 diabetes. Circulation 2004; 109:1750–1755.
62. O'Rourke MF, Gallagher DE. Pulse wave analysis. J Hypertens Suppl 1996; 14:S147–S157.
63. Tedesco MA, Natale F, Di Salvo G, et al. Effects of coexisting hypertension and type II diabetes mellitus on arterial stiffness. J Hum Hypertens 2004; 18:469–473.
64. Meyer C, Milat F, McGrath BP, et al. Vascular dysfunction and autonomic neuropathy in Type 2 diabetes. Diabet Med 2004; 21:746–751.
65. Taniwaki H, Kawagishi T, Emoto M, et al. Correlation between the intima-media thickness of the carotid artery and aortic pulse-wave velocity in patients with type 2 diabetes. Vessel wall properties in type 2 diabetes. Diabetes Care 1999; 22:1851–1857.
66. Cruickshank K, Riste L, Anderson SG, et al. Aortic pulse-wave velocity and its relationship to mortality in diabetes and glucose intolerance: an integrated index of vascular function? Circulation 2002; 106:2085–2090.
67. Ahimastos AA, Formosa M, Dart AM, et al. Gender differences in large artery stiffness pre- and post puberty. J Clin Endocrinol Metab 2003; 88:5375–5380.
68. Lurbe E, Torro MI, Carvajal E, et al. Birth weight impacts on wave reflections in children and adolescents. Hypertension 2003; 41:646–650.
69. O'Rourke MF, Staessen JA, Vlachopoulos C, et al. Clinical applications of arterial stiffness; definitions and reference values. Am J Hypertens 2002; 15:426–444.
70. Liang YL, Teede H, Kotsopoulos D, et al. Non-invasive measurements of arterial structure and function: repeatability, interrelationships and trial sample size. Clin Sci (Lond) 1998; 95:669–679.
71. Brooks B, Molyneaux L, Yue DK. Augmentation of central arterial pressure in type 1 diabetes. Diabetes Care 1999; 22:1722–1727.
72. Wilkinson IB, MacCallum H, Rooijmans DF, et al. Increased augmentation index and systolic stress in type 1 diabetes mellitus. QJM 2000; 93:441–448.
73. Brooks BA, Molyneaux LM, Yue DK. Augmentation of central arterial pressure in Type 2 diabetes. Diabet Med 2001; 18:374–380.
74. Fukui M, Kitagawa Y, Nakamura N, et al. Augmentation of central arterial pressure as a marker of atherosclerosis in patients with type 2 diabetes. Diabetes Res Clin Pract 2003; 59:153–161.
75. Ravikumar R, Deepa R, Shanthirani C, et al. Comparison of carotid intima-media thickness, arterial stiffness, and brachial artery flow mediated dilatation in diabetic and nondiabetic subjects (The Chennai Urban Population Study [CUPS-9]). Am J Cardiol 2002; 90:702–707.
76. Haller MJ, Samyn M, Nichols WW, et al. Radial artery tonometry demonstrates arterial stiffness in children with type 1 diabetes. Diabetes Care 2004; 27:2911–2917.
77. Urbina EM, Brinton TJ, Elkasabany A, et al. Brachial artery distensibility and relation to cardiovascular risk factors in healthy young adults (The Bogalusa Heart Study). Am J Cardiol 2002; 89:946–951.
78. Urbina EM, Kieltkya L, Tsai J, et al. Impact of multiple cardiovascular risk factors on brachial artery distensibility in young adults: the Bogalusa Heart Study. Am J Hypertens 2005; 18:767–771.
79. Budoff MJ, Flores F, Tsai J, et al. Measures of brachial artery distensibility in relation to coronary calcification. Am J Hypertens 2003; 16:350–355.
80. Leeson CP, Whincup PH, Cook DG, et al. Cholesterol and arterial distensibility in the first decade of life: a population-based study. Circulation 2000; 101:1533–1538.
81. Whincup PH, Gilg JA, Donald AE, et al. Arterial distensibility in adolescents: the influence of adiposity, the metabolic syndrome, and classic risk factors. Circulation 2005; 112:1789–1797.
82. Urbina EM, Bean JA, Daniels SR, et al. Overweight and hyperinsulinemia provide individual contributions to compromises in brachial artery distensibility in healthy adolescents and young adults. J Am Soc Hypertens 2007; 1:200–207.
83. Singh TP, Groehn H, Kazmers A. Vascular function and carotid intimal-medial thickness in children with insulin-dependent diabetes mellitus. J Am Coll Cardiol 2003; 41:661–665.

84. Ladeia AM, Ladeia-Frota C, Pinho L, et al. Endothelial dysfunction is correlated with microalbuminuria in children with short-duration type 1 diabetes. Diabetes Care 2005; 28:2048–2050.
85. Pena AS, Wiltshire E, MacKenzie K, et al. Vascular endothelial and smooth muscle function relates to body mass index and glucose in obese and nonobese children. J Clin Endocrinol Metab 2006; 91:4467–4471.
86. Keelan PC, Bielak LF, Ashai K, et al. Long-term prognostic value of coronary calcification detected by electron-beam computed tomography in patients undergoing coronary angiography. Circulation 2001; 104:412–417.
87. Dabelea D, Kinney G, Snell-Bergeon JK, et al. Effect of type 1 diabetes on the gender difference in coronary artery calcification: a role for insulin resistance? The Coronary Artery Calcification in Type 1 Diabetes (CACTI) Study. Diabetes 2003; 52:2833–2839.
88. Starkman HS, Cable G, Hala V, et al. Delineation of prevalence and risk factors for early coronary artery disease by electron beam computed tomography in young adults with type 1 diabetes. Diabetes Care 2003; 26:433–436.
89. Starkman HS, Cable G, Hala V, et al. Delineation of prevalence and risk factors for early coronary artery disease by electron beam computed tomography in young adults with type 1 diabetes. Diabetes Care 2003; 26:433–436.
90. Summers RM, Andrasko-Bourgeois J, Feuerstein IM, et al. Evaluation of the aortic root by MRI: insights from patients with homozygous familial hypercholesterolemia. Circulation 1998; 98:509–518.
91. Hatsukami TS, Ross R, Polissar NL, et al. Visualization of fibrous cap thickness and rupture in human atherosclerotic carotid plaque in vivo with high-resolution magnetic resonance imaging. Circulation 2000; 102:959–964.

16 | Epidemiology of Acute Complications in Youth: Diabetic Ketoacidosis and Hypoglycemia

Arleta Rewers and Georgeanna J. Klingensmith
Department of Pediatrics, University of Colorado at Denver and Health Sciences Center, Barbara Davis Center for Childhood Diabetes, Aurora, Colorado, U.S.A.

INTRODUCTION

Diabetic ketoacidosis (DKA) and hypoglycemia are the major life-threatening complications of diabetes. While the rates appear to be inching down, 20–30% of patients with type 1 diabetes (T1D) in most developed countries are diagnosed in DKA and the rates are much higher in developing countries. A small group of high-risk patients accounts for most of recurring DKA in long-standing T1D, but the incidence remains high, approximately 1 per 10 patient-years in countries where monitoring systems exist. Severe hypoglycemia, i.e., coma or seizure secondary to diabetes treatment remains high (up to 5/10 patient-years) and has recently increased among patients who aim for lower HbA1c targets without appropriate initial education and ongoing support. All three acute complications are theoretically preventable; unfortunately, they still account for an enormous morbidity, hospitalizations, and mortality among diabetic patients and contribute significantly to the high costs of diabetes care.

DIABETIC KETOACIDOSIS

Pathogenesis

DKA results from very low levels of effective circulating insulin and a concomitant increase in counterregulatory hormones levels, such as glucagon, catecholamines, cortisol, and growth hormone. This combination causes catabolic changes in the metabolism of carbohydrates, fat, and protein. Hyperglycemia develops due to impaired glucose utilization and increased glucose production by the liver and kidneys. Lipolysis leads to increased production of ketones, especially β-hydroxybutyrate (B-OHB), ketonemia, and metabolic acidosis. Most common underlying mechanisms of DKA include progressive β-cell failure in previously undiagnosed patients and omission or inadequate insulin dosing in established patients. Elevation of counterregulatory hormones during infection, gastrointestinal illness, trauma, and stress may also precipitate DKA in the absence of appropriate increases in insulin dosing. The clinical picture of DKA includes polyuria, polydipsia, dehydration, Kussmaul's respiration (rapid, deep, and sighting) and progressive worsening of mental status from somnolence to coma.

Definition

The incidence of DKA varies with the definition; therefore, it is important to standardize criteria for comparative epidemiological studies. The American Diabetes Association (ADA) (1,2), the International Society for Pediatric and Adolescent Diabetes (ISPAD) (3) as well as the European Society for Paediatric Endocrinology

TABLE 1 Classification of DKA Severity: Current Inconsistent Guidelines

Severity of DKA	ADA adults[a]	ADA children[b]	ESPE/LWPES and ISPAD children[c]
Severe	Arterial pH < 7.0 Bicarbonate < 10	Venous pH < 7.1	Venous pH < 7.1 Bicarbonate < 5
Moderate	Arterial pH 7.0 to < 7.25 Bicarbonate 10 to < 15	Venous pH 7.1–7.2	Venous pH < 7.2 Bicarbonate < 10
Mild	Arterial pH 7.25 to 7.30 Bicarbonate 15 to 18	Venous pH 7.2–7.3	Venous pH < 7.3 Bicarbonate < 15

[a]From Ref. 2.
[b]From Ref. 1.
[c]From Refs. 3,4.
Abbreviations: ADA, American Diabetes Association; DKA, diabetic ketoacidosis; ESPE, European Society for Paediatric Endocrinology; LWPES, Lawson Wilkins Pediatric Endocrine Society; ISPAD, International Society for Pediatric and Adolescent Diabetes.

(ESPE) and the Lawson Wilkins Pediatric Endocrine Society (LWPES) (4) jointly agreed to define DKA as:

1. Hyperglycemia, i.e., plasma glucose higher than 250 mg/dL or ~14 mmol/L
2. Venous pH < 7.25 (arterial pH < 7.30) and/or bicarbonate < 15 mmol/L
3. Moderate or large ketones level in urine or blood

Caveats

1. Pediatric experts agree that lower level of hyperglycemia (>200 mg/dL or >11 mmol/L) meets criteria for DKA. Pregnant adolescents, young or partially treated children (5), and those fasting during a period of insulin deficiency (6) may have near-normal glucose levels and ketoacidosis (euglycemic ketoacidosis).
2. DKA is generally categorized by the severity of acidosis. In most laboratories, the normal range for arterial pH is 7.35 to 7.45 and venous pH is 7.32 to 7.42 in adults and children older than two years. Currently recommended severity categories differ between adults and children (Table 1) with little evidence to support these differences.
3. While large or moderate ketonuria is sufficient for confirmation of DKA diagnosis, measurement of B-OHB is more helpful in making treatment decisions (7,8). Whole blood B-OHB levels of > 1.5 mmol/L obtained using the Precision Xtra™ meter (MediSense/Abbott, Diabetes Care, Abbott Park, IL, U.S.) combined with blood glucose > 250 mg/dL (~14 mmol/L) indicate probable DKA. With increasing use of B-OHB in home/outpatient diabetes management, more data are needed to define the role of B-OHB measurement in diagnosing milder cases of DKA, now underdiagnosed and treated at home.

For epidemiological studies in the United States, use of consistent ICD-9 or 10 codes are very helpful. In the ICD-9 system, DKA is usually coded as 250.1x (250.10–250.13). However, the code 250.3 (diabetes with other coma) is used for DKA coma as well as for coma caused by severe hypoglycemia. In the ICD-10, categories for diabetes (E10–E14), subdivision E1x.1 denotes DKA while E1x.0 denotes coma with or without ketoacidosis, hyperosmolar, or hypoglycemic (x digit is used to define type of diabetes).

Prevalence and Predictors of DKA at the Diagnosis of Diabetes
Prevalence of DKA at the Diagnosis of T1D
Examples of reports concerning the prevalence and predictors of DKA at diagnosis around the world are presented in Table 2. The largest population-based study to date, SEARCH for Diabetes in Youth Study in the United States, reported that 29% of patients with T1D, younger than 20 years at diagnosis, presented with DKA(9). This estimate was lower than rates previously reported from hospital series (10,11). In European countries, the prevalence varied from 15–67% (12–17). DKA prevalence at diagnosis is generally higher in populations with lower incidence of T1D (14,18). DKA incidence at the time of diagnosis in Asian and African populations is less clear because of the paucity of metabolic and clinical data. However, 42–85% of T1D children in the Arab countries presented with DKA(19–21).

Studies in the United States and elsewhere suggest that the clinical severity at diagnosis of T1D in youth may be decreasing. In Colorado, the proportion of children with T1D who presented with DKA at the time of diagnosis has significantly decreased, from 38% in 1978–1982 to 29% in 1998–2001 (22,23). Similarly, the prevalence of DKA at onset decreased in Finnish children from 30% in 1982–1991 to 19% in 1992–2002 (17). On the other hand, admission rates for any DKA, at onset or later in the course of disease, have remained unchanged and high (over 20/100,000 per year) in Canadian youth between 1991–1999, but severity seems to be decreasing (24,25).

Predictors of DKA at the Diagnosis of T1D
The prevalence of DKA at the diagnosis is significantly higher among younger children (9,12,26), reaching over 50% in those aged less than two years (27). Lower socioeconomic status—lower family income, parental education, and less favorable health insurance creating barriers in access to care—is a powerful independent risk factor (9,10,15,28). Patients from low-income families have higher rates of DKA, and it is frequently more severe (10). Lack of insurance and less favorable health insurance are also associated with more severe onset of diabetes in youth (28,29). It is unlikely that the risk of DKA differs by race or ethnicity independent of socioeconomic factors and access to care. Low societal awareness of diabetes symptoms, as found in populations with low incidence of T1D, adds to the risk, while programs or centers promoting community awareness may decrease the risk (see section "Prevention"). In addition, high-dose glucocorticoids, atypical antipsychotics, diazoxide and immunosuppresive drugs have been reported to precipitate DKA in individuals not previously diagnosed with diabetes (30,31).

Prevalence of DKA at the Diagnosis of Type 2 Diabetes
Few population-based epidemiologic data exist concerning the prevalence of DKA at the time of presentation of type 2 diabetes (T2D) in youth. The SEARCH for Diabetes in Youth Study, which included youth with T2D from six geographic areas in the United States, found that 10% presented with DKA (9). As many as 19% of Thai children and adolescents had DKA at diagnosis of T2D (32).

Incidence of DKA in Established T1D
The overall incidence of DKA in patients with established T1D varies from 1 to 12 per 100 patient-years (12,33,34) (Table 3). The incidence of DKA increases significantly

TABLE 2 Prevalence of DKA in Youth at Diagnosis of Diabetes

References	Country	Age	N	Completeness of record review	Study period	Definition of DKA	Prevalence of DKA(%)	Predictors
9	U.S.A.	0–19	2824	77% Population based	2002–2004	pH < 7.3 (venous) or pH < 7.25 (arterial) bicarbonate < 15 or ICD-9 250.1 or medical record diagnosis	29% type 1 10% type 2	Younger age, lower family income, under insurance, lower parental education
10	U.S.A.	0–18	139	68% Hospital series	1995–1998	pH < 7.3	38%	Younger age, lack of insurance
11	U.S.A.	0–5	247	Hospital series	1990–1999	pH < 7.3 or bicarbonate < 15	44%	
14	Europe (11 countries)	0–14	1260	91% Varied by center	1989–1994	pH < 7.3	26–67% (42% on average)	Area of low incidence of type 1 diabetes
15	Germany	0–14	2121	97% Population based	1987–1997	pH < 7.3 or bicarbonate < 15	26%	Lower socioeconomic status
17	Finland	0–14	585	Hospital series	1982–2001	pH < 7.3 or bicarbonate ≤ 15	18%	Younger age
48	U.K.	0–15	328	Hospital series	1987–1996	pH ≤ 7.25 (arterial) or bicarbonate ≤ 15	27%	Asian minority, Age less than 5 yr
12	U.K.	0–20	23097	Population based	1985–1986 1990	pH < 7.36 or bicarbonate < 21	26%	Younger age
16	Ireland	0–14	283	72% Population based	1997–1998	pH < 7.3	31%	
21	Kuwait	0–12	103	Hospital series	2000–2003	pH < 7.3	84.5%	

Abbreviation: DKA, diabetic ketoacidosis; N, number of patients.

TABLE 3 Incidence of DKA in Youth with Established Type 1 Diabetes

References	Country	Age group	N	Study design	Length of study	Definition of DKA	Incidence(/100 patient-year)	Predictors
33	U.S.A.	0–19	1243	Prospective cohort	3.5 yr	DKA leading to ED visit or hospital admission	8	Female gender, age, higher HbA1c, higher insulin dose, underinsurance, psychiatric disorders
42	U.S.A.	7–16	300	Prospective cohort	1 yr	DKA leading to ED visit or hospital admission	15	Higher HbA1c
178	U.S.A.	13–17	195	Clinical trial	7.4 yr	BG > 250 mg/mL, ketonuria, pH < 7.3 or bicarbonate < 15	4.7-conventional 2.8-intensiveE	NA
104	Sweden	0–18	139	Prospective cohort	3 yr	Acidosis	1.5	NA
179	U.K.	1–17	135	Retrospective	6 yr	pH < 7.3 or bicarbonate < 18	10	Female gender, family, and school problems
180	Australia	1–19	268	Retrospective	3 mo	pH < 7.2 or bicarbonate < 10	12	NA

Abbreviations: BG, blood glucose; DKA, diabetic ketoacidosis; ED, emergency department; N, number of patients.

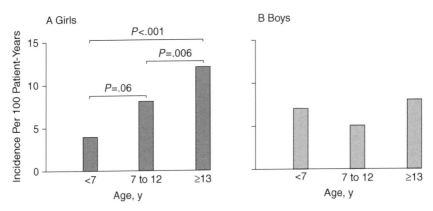

FIGURE 1 Incidence of diabetic ketoacidosis by age and gender, Colorado, 1996–2001.
Source: From Ref. 33.

with age in females (4, 8, and 12 per 100 patient-years in those < 7, 7-12, and ≥ 13 years, respectively), but not in males (7, 5, and 8 per 100 patient-years) (Fig. 1) (33). There are no comparable population-based data for adults.

Most of episodes of DKA beyond diagnosis are associated with insulin omission or treatment error (35,36). Children whose insulin treatment is supervised by a responsible adult rarely have episodes of DKA (34). However, inadequate adjustment of insulin therapy during intercurrent illness may cause DKA (12,34,37). Patients with a history of previous episodes of DKA are at higher risk for recurrent DKA. In one study, 60% of all DKA episodes occurred in 5% of patients with recurrent events (33).

While continuous subcutaneous insulin infusion (CSII) is effective and safe in both adults and adolescents with T1D (38), CSII interruption can lead to DKA (39). The incidence of DKA appears to be unchanged during long-term (4 years) follow-up after introduction of CSII in children and youth (40).

Incidence of DKA in Established T2D
Patients with T2D may develop DKA or of hyperglycemic hyperosmolar syndrome (HHS) and require hospitalization. Hospitalization for other medical or surgical conditions is clearly a risk factor for the development of metabolic deterioration and hospitalization. (41). The number of hospitalizations for any DKA among persons younger than 45 years estimated by the U.S. National Diabetes Surveillance System increased from 37,000 (24/100,000) in 1980 to 87,000 (47/100,000) in 2003, and the number of hospital discharges in the United States with DKA diagnosis almost doubled between 1980 and 2003, from 62,000 discharges in 1980 to 115,000 in 2003. While the rates have nearly doubled, average length of hospital stay in this group has decreased from 6.4 to 3.4 days (http://www.cdc.gov/diabetes/statistics/dkafirst/index.htm, last accessed December 2006).

Risk Factors for Recurrent DKA
The risk of recurrent DKA is higher in patients with poor metabolic control (14,33,42). Lower socioeconomic status and insufficient access to outpatient

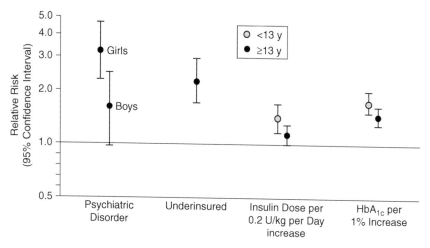

FIGURE 2 Predictors of diabetic ketoacidosis in children with established diabetes, Colorado, 1996–2001. *Source*: From Ref. 33.

diabetes care are often the primary mechanism; however, major psychiatric disorders (depression, bipolar disorder, schizophrenia) also play a significant role (33). Eating disorders, prevalent in adolescent girls, (12) contribute to the highest risk for DKA in this group reaching 12/100 patient-years (33,43,44). This is probably related to issues of body image, as diabetic adolescent girls often omit insulin injections to lose weight (45,46). Girls with recurrent ketoacidosis have also been shown to exhibit more behavioral problems, lower social competence, and higher levels of family conflict (47). The patterns of recurrent DKA vary by age (Fig. 2). In children younger than 13 years of age, the risk increases with higher HbA1c and with higher reported insulin dose. In older children, the risk increases with higher HbA1c, higher reported insulin dose, inadequate insurance, and the presence of psychiatric disorders (33).

The prevalence of DKA at onset (9) and the recurrence of DKA (33) did not differ by race/ethnicity in the United States youth with T1D; however, young Asian children in the United Kingdom were eight times more likely to present with DKA than non-Asian children of the same age (unadjusted risk ratio) (48).

Morbidity and Mortality

DKA is the most common cause of death in children with T1D (49,50). Mortality and morbidity in DKA is mostly due to cerebral edema, which accounts for most hospital deaths in young diabetic children. The incidence of cerebral edema is 0.3–3.0% (51–53). Less frequent causes of mortality related to DKA include hypokalemia, hyperkalemia, thrombosis (54), other neurological complications (55,56), stroke (57,58), sepsis, and other infections such as rhinocerebral mucormycosis (59,60), aspiration pneumonia, and pulmonary edema (61,62).

Cost

Direct medical care charges associated with DKA episodes represent 28% of the direct medical care charges for all patients, and 56% for those with recurrent DKAs (63).

Acute complications in children with T1D also increase directly and indirectly (64) the costs of care.

National Hospital Ambulatory Medical Care Survey has shown that between 1993 and 2003, DKA accounted for ~753,000 visits (95% CI, 610,000–895,000) or an average of 68,000 visits per year. Most DKA visits were evenly distributed among patients aged 10 to 50 years. Most DKA patients (87%) were admitted, with most admissions to a non-ICU setting. The rate of emergency department visits for DKA per 10,000 U.S. population with diabetes was 64 (95% CI 52–76). There was an increase in number of visits for DKA during 1999–2003 compared to 1993–1998 (65).

During 2004, there were approximately 5.2 million of hospitalizations in the United States with diagnostic coding indicative of diabetes (66). Among these, 120,000 admissions were primarily due to DKA, 15,000 due to HHS, and an additional 5,000 were coded as "diabetic coma." On the basis of the Diagnostic Related Group codes in the inpatient records, the total hospital cost for DKA was estimated at $1.4 to 1.8 billion. An independent analysis also arrived to an estimate of the annual hospital cost of DKA in the United States in excess of $1 billion (67). The authors based their estimate on an annual average of over 100,000 hospitalizations for DKA, with an average cost of $13,000 per patient. Newly diagnosed patients may account for approximately 25% of this cost (29).

Prevention

Prevention of DKA should be a major goal of diabetes care and a growing body of evidence suggests that primary prevention of DKA in newly diagnosed children should be possible. In the United States, the Diabetes Autoimmunity Study in the Youth, an observational study following children at genetically high risk for T1D by periodic testing for diabetes autoantibodies, HbA1c, and random blood glucose, demonstrated that the clinical course of diabetes is milder in youth diagnosed without DKA (68). An intensive community intervention to raise awareness of the signs and symptoms of childhood diabetes among school teachers and primary care providers in a region of Italy was found to reduce the prevalence of DKA at diagnosis of type 1 disease from 83% to 13% (69). A follow-up study has shown that the campaign for DKA prevention is still effective in Parma's province eight years later but there is also an indication that the campaign should be periodically renewed (70).

In the diabetes prevention trial (DPT-1), nearly three quarters of the subjects in whom diabetes developed were asymptomatic at the time of diagnosis. Awareness of increased level of risk and close biochemical monitoring increases the likelihood of early diagnosis and prevents DKA (71). Public awareness of signs and symptoms of diabetes also helps earlier diagnosis. If health care providers always consider the possibility of diabetes in ill children and urgently check urine or blood for glucose, early diagnosis will be likely. If confirmation is rapid, and children are promptly referred to an appropriate centre, development of DKA will be less common. Although these strategies are intuitive, programs to decrease DKA at onset need to be designed and evaluated in diverse populations and age groups. These should include approaches that target both the public at large and health care providers.

Studies to date also suggest that most, if not all, episodes of DKA beyond disease diagnosis are preventable. Four studies on the effect of a comprehensive diabetes program and telephone help line reported a reduction in the rates of DKA from 15–60 to 5–6 per 100 patient-years (72–74). In the adolescent cohort of the DCCT, intensive diabetes management was associated with less DKA (conventional and intensive treatment groups: 4.7 and 2.8/100 patient-years, respectively (75). In patients treated with insulin pumps, episodes of DKA can be reduced with introduction of educational algorithms. Therefore, it is likely that most episodes of DKA after diagnosis could be avoided if all children with diabetes received comprehensive diabetes health care and education, and had access to a 24-hour diabetes telephone help line (33,72,76). The extent to which home measurement of B-OHB may assist in the prevention of hospitalization needs to be further assessed (7).

HYPOGLYCEMIA

Pathogenesis
Hypoglycemia is the most common life-threatening complication of diabetes treatment. It is characterized by multiple risk factors and complex pathophysiology (77). Hypoglycemia is more common in young children and adolescents and causes a spectrum of acute complications from mild cognitive impairment to coma, seizure, and sudden death. The brain depends on a continuous supply of glucose for energy, although it can also utilize ketone bodies.

In insulin-treated patients, common causes of hypoglycemia include missed meals, exercise, insulin-dosing errors, and rapid insulin absorption due to intramuscular injection or hot shower/bath shortly after injection. Rarely, secondary-gain ideation or suicidal attempt may lead to insulin overdose. In all these situations, insulin overdose reduces hepatic glucose output in addition to increasing glucose utilization. Physical activity increases glucose utilization and may lead to hypoglycemia if not matched by lowering of the insulin dose and increasing carbohydrate intake. Oral hypoglycemic agents may cause hypoglycemia by either decreasing hepatic glucose output (metformin) or increasing insulin levels (sulfonylureas and metiglinides). In contrast, enhancers of peripheral glucose utilization (thiazolidenediones) do not cause hypoglycemia in patients with residual insulin and glucagon secretion. Release of glucagon—the major counterregulatory response to hypoglycemia in nondiabetic persons—is progressively lost within a few years after diagnosis of T1D. Catecholamine release, the other powerful counterregulatory mechanism, is also impaired in diabetic patients, especially type 1, and in those on β-blocker treatment (78).

Definition
Hypoglycemia is usually defined as a blood glucose level below 2.8 mmol/L (50 mg/dL). In the diabetes control and complications trial (DCCT), severe hypoglycemia was defined as an episode in which the patient required assistance with treatment from another person to recover, blood glucose level had to be documented as <50 mg/dL, and/or the clinical manifestations had to be reversed by oral carbohydrate, subcutaneous glucagon, or intravenous glucose (79). This definition is not very practical in children, particularly the youngest, because they require assistance from others even for mild episodes of hypoglycemia. Other studies have limited the definition of severe hypoglycemia in children to episodes leading to unconsciousness or seizure (80,81). We have previously proposed (33) the following categories:

Severe hypoglycemia: Loss of consciousness or seizure; definite, if confirmed by blood glucose level below 2.8 mmol/L (50 mg/dL), or probable, if such a confirmation is lacking.

Moderate hypoglycemia: Episode associated with typical signs and symptoms requiring assistance of another person (including administration of glucagon or intravenous glucose) but not leading to complete loss of consciousness or seizure; definite, if confirmed by blood glucose level below 3.3 mmol/L (60 mg/dL), or probable, if such a confirmation is lacking.

Mild hypoglycemia: Episode associated with typical signs and symptoms that objectively do not require assistance of another person (beyond simply making oral fluids or food available to the patient) and not leading to loss of consciousness or seizure; definite, if confirmed by blood glucose level below 3.9 mmol/L (70 mg/dL), or probable, if such a confirmation is lacking.

In addition, "asymptomatic hypoglycemia (biochemical)" is defined as a blood glucose level of 50 mg/dL or less without any recognizable symptoms.

In the ICD-9, hypoglycemic coma secondary to diabetes treatment is coded 250.3; however, this code is also used for coma with DKA. Other forms of diabetic hypoglycemia are coded 250.8. Additional E code is recommended to identify the drugs that induced hypoglycemia. In the ICD-10, E1x.0 denotes coma with or without ketoacidosis, hyperosmolarity, or hypoglycemia (x digit is used to define type of diabetes), while E16.0 denotes diabetic drug-induced hypoglycemia without coma.

Incidence in Type 1 Diabetic Patients

The true incidence of moderate or mild hypoglycemia is difficult to ascertain; therefore, this review is limited to studies of severe hypoglycemia, unless noted otherwise. Studies completed before the DCCT (82–86) reported rates of severe hypoglycemia ranging from 3 to 86 per 100 patient-years. The studies differed in event definition, patients' age, duration of diabetes, and treatment modalities.

In the DCCT, intensive insulin treatment increased the incidence of hypoglycemia three times compared with that observed with conventional therapy; for hypoglycemia requiring assistance 61 versus 19 per 100 patient-years; for coma or seizure 16 versus 5 per 100 patient-years, respectively (79). Most (55%) of the episodes occurred during sleep. Of the episodes that occurred while subjects were awake, 36% were not accompanied by warning symptoms (87). Among 195 adolescent participants, the incidence of hypoglycemia requiring assistance was 86/100 patient-years in the intensively treated group and 28/100 patient-years in those conventionally treated (75). The incidence of coma or seizure in the adolescents was 27 and 10/100 patient-years, respectively.

Post-DCCT studies of severe hypoglycemia and its predictors in children are summarized in Table 4. Few used a prospective design or were population based. A cohort study of 1243 type 1 diabetic children, aged 0 to 19 years, residing in the six-county Denver Metropolitan Area between 1996 and 2000 reported incidence of severe hypoglycemia of 19/100 patient-years (33). The rates decreased significantly with age in females, but not in males (Fig. 3).

A Joslin Clinic study used a similar definition in a cohort of older children, aged 7 to 16 years, and found a lower rate of 8/100 patient-years (42). However, high-risk children with documented psychiatric disorders and unstable living conditions were excluded. The rates were comparable in Europe and Australia,

TABLE 4 Incidence of Severe Hypoglycemia in Youth in the Post-DCCT Era

References	Country	Age group	N	Study design	Length of study	Definition of hypoglycemia	Incidence/100 patient-year	Predictors
33	U.S.A.	0–19	1243	Prospective cohort	3.5 yr	Coma, seizure, or admission	19	Male gender, younger age, lower HbA1c, higher insulin dose underinsurance, psychiatric disorders
42	U.S.A.	7–16	300	Prospective cohort	1 yr	Coma, seizure, glucagon injection, or IV dextrose	8	Higher HbA1c
181	Sweden	1–18	146	Prospective cohort	3 yr	Coma or seizure	15–19	Lower HbA1c, higher insulin dose
96	France	1–19	2579	Cross-sectional	6 mo	Coma, seizure, or glucagon injection	45	Lower HbA1c, more exercise, number of BG measurements/day
88	Finland	1–24	287	Prospective cohort	2 yr	Coma, seizure, or glucagon injection	3.1	Lower HbA1c level, higher insulin dose
81	Australia	0–18	329 709	Retrospective Prospective cohort	4 yr 4 yr	Coma or seizure	3.6 8	Younger age, lower HbA1c
180	Australia	1–19	268	Retrospective	3 mo	Coma or seizure	25	Younger age, lower HbA1c, number of visits
95	U.S.A., Europe, Japan	1–18	2873	Cross-sectional	5 mo	Coma or seizure	22	Younger age, lower HbA1c
182	Canada, Europe, Japan	0–18	2780	Cross-sectional	5–6 mo	Coma or seizure	7–20	Poor glycemic control

Abbreviation: DCCT, diabetes control and complications trial.

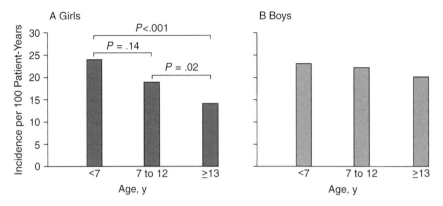

FIGURE 3 Incidence of severe hypoglycemia by age and gender, Colorado, 1996–2001. *Source*: From Ref. 33.

with a notable exception of very low incidence (<4/100 patient-years) in a Finnish study (88).

Incidence in Type 2 Diabetic Patients

Severe hypoglycemia does not occur in patients with T2D treated with diet and exercise and is uncommon in those treated with oral hypoglycemic agents. However, the risk of hyperglycemia increases with transition to insulin dependence. In the United Kingdom Prospective Diabetes Study Group (UKPDS), the risk of severe hypoglycemia was 1/100 patient-years in those intensively treated with chlorpropamide, 1.4/100 patient-years with glibenclamide and 1.8/100 patient-years with insulin (89). Long-acting sulfonylureas confer higher risk compared with shorter-acting ones (90). Additional risk factors include older age, longer duration of diabetes, polypragmasia, and recent hospitalization (91). Reports of an increased risk of hypoglycemia in patients treated with sulfonylurea and ACE inhibitors (92) have not been confirmed by a recent large trial (93).

Risk Factors

Demographic Predictors

Some of the commonly reported predictors of severe hypoglycemia are not modifiable: age (infancy and adolescence) (94,95), male gender (33), or increased duration of diabetes (96). Longer duration of diabetes predicts hypoglycemia regardless of age (33,87).

HLA Genotype, Islet Autoantibodies at Onset of Diabetes,
and Subsequent Risk of Hypoglycemia

The risk of hypoglycemia increases with duration of diabetes, partially due to progressive blunting of α-cell glucagon response to hypoglycemia (97). This process is inversely related to preservation of β cell that often leads to partial remission at 1 to 12 months after diagnosis (97). In the DCCT, presence of residual endogenous insulin secretion predicted 65% lower risk of severe hypoglycemia (98). Abrupt loss of endogenous insulin production is more frequent in patients with the HLA-DR3/4 genotype (99–101) and those positive for multiple islet autoantibodies (100,102).

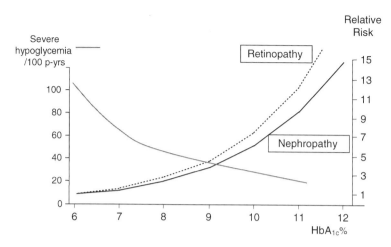

FIGURE 4 Inverse relationship between the risk of microvascular complications and hypoglycemia. DCCT Study. *Source*: From Ref. 183.

Imperfect Insulin Replacement

The relation between severe hypoglycemia and tight glycemic control had been extensively explored (103), especially in children (42,95,104). The DCCT showed clearly that the level of metabolic control needed to prevent development and progression of diabetic microvascular complications increases significantly the risk of hypoglycemia (Fig. 4) (75). As many as 63% of the intensively treated adolescents (age, 13–17 years) participating in the DCCT had coma or seizure during the trial compared with 25% of those treated conventionally (75). Over the past several years, intensive treatment strategies, with the emphasis on improving glycemic control, have been extended to younger children and may have led to hypoglycemia risk even higher than that reported by the DCCT (42). When the DCCT definition of hypoglycemia was applied to a large clinic patient population in Colorado, the incidence of severe hypoglycemia increased from 28/100 patient-years in 1993 to an average of 43/100 patient-years in 1995–1998, reflecting the intensification of diabetes control in the post-DCCT era (105).

Hypoglycemia Unawareness

Inability to recognize symptoms of hypoglycemia is seen in approximately 1 in 10 patients and is more common in those who keep blood glucose generally low (106,107). A single hypoglycemic episode can lead to significant decrease in neurohormonal counterregulatory responses and cause unawareness of hypoglycemia over the subsequent 24 hours (108). The syndrome is usually associated with decreased glucagon or epinephrine output (106,109) and autonomic neuropathy (110). There is evidence that loss of awareness of hypoglycemia can be reversed by avoiding hypoglycemia for two to three weeks (103,111).

Recurrent Severe Hypoglycemia

Unfortunately, severe hypoglycemia is a recurrent problem in some diabetic patients. In our experience, nearly 80% of severe hypoglycemic episodes occur in a relatively small group (14%) of children with recurrent events (33). While unawareness of symptoms is a major factor, we showed that poor medical insurance doubles the risk of recurrence.

Exercise
Acute blood glucose lowering effect of physical activity may result in hypoglycemia, if not matched by decreased insulin delivery and increased ingestion of carbohydrates (112). Higher habitual physical activity is associated with higher insulin sensitivity. While a large body of evidence suggests that exercise is an important trigger of many events of severe hypoglycemia, there is a paucity of epidemiological data to quantitate the magnitude of the problem (113,114).

Alcohol Consumption
Alcohol suppresses gluconeogenesis and glycogenolysis (115) and may induce hypoglycemia unawareness (116). In addition, alcohol ingestion acutely improves insulin sensitivity (117). In combination with exercise, drinking can lead to severe hypoglycemia, often delayed for 10 to 12 hours (118). Despite anecdotal reports of severe hypoglycemic events in the morning after drinking and dancing, this phenomenon has not yet been documented in epidemiological studies.

Family Dynamics, Behavioral, and Psychiatric Factors
The DCCT analyses indicated that conventional risk factors explained only 8.5% of the variance in occurrence of severe hypoglycemia (87). The majority of severe hypoglycemic events may be attributable not as much to intensive insulin treatment, but rather to insufficient diabetes education, low socioeconomic status, inability to pay for standard care, unstable living conditions, behavioral factors, and psychiatric disorders affecting patients and their families. These factors have significant influence on glycemic control and the rate of acute complications, as reviewed above in the context of DKA. Family relationship and personality type have significant effects on adaptation to illness and metabolic control among persons with diabetes. It seems possible that chronic illness points out and fixes perhaps pathological characteristics already present (119). Initial maternal psychopathology, particularly maternal depression, increases the risk of psychiatric disorder in children with T1D (120). Monitoring of the psychological status of the patients and their mothers may help to identify children at risk for psychiatric disorder and facilitate prevention or treatment efforts. Monitoring may be particularly beneficial during the first year of diabetes (120).

Reported prevalence of psychiatric disorders among patients with T1D is high, up to 48% by 10 years of diabetes duration and age 20 years (120,121). The most prevalent are major depressive (28%), conduct, and generalized anxiety disorders (120). In addition, diabetic youths have propensity for more suicidal thoughts (122), protracted depressions, and the higher risk of recurrence of major depression (119). There are indications of lower self-esteem in the T1D patients that could predispose them for future depression or difficulties in adaptation (123). The presence of psychiatric disorders is associated with poor diabetic metabolic control (124,125) and with noncompliance with the medical regimen (122).

It is not clear if increased risk of hypoglycemia is caused by incompliance due to psychiatric illness itself, or whether it is side effect of the medications leading to hypoglycemia unawareness. Hypoglycemia unawareness has been reported in

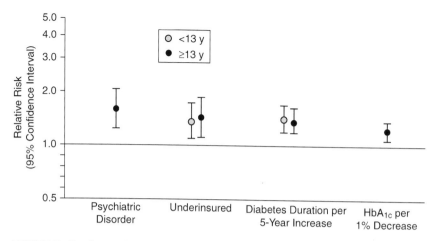

FIGURE 5 Predictors of severe hypoglycemia, Colorado, 1996–2001. *Source*: From Ref. 33.

patients treated with serotonin reuptake inhibitors commonly prescribed for treatment of psychiatric conditions (126). More information regarding the relationship between psychiatric disorders, medications, family dynamics, and the incidence of hypoglycemic events is needed.

In the Colorado children and adolescents with T1D, the presence of psychiatric disorders increased the risk of hypoglycemia by 60% in children aged 13 years and older (33) (Fig. 5).

Health Insurance and Access to Care

In the Colorado study mentioned above (Fig. 5), lack of adequate health insurance was an independent predictor of severe hypoglycemia in children of any age, increasing the risk by approximately 40% (33). A study from Wisconsin found similar associations (127).

Studies from countries with nationalized health care systems have shown that socioeconomic status did not appear to play a major role in the risk of hypoglycemia (124). However, in countries with privatized, largely for profit health care, major economic inequities become barriers in access to care and compliance. In the United States, the cost containment of escalating health care expenditures has left more than a quarter of people with no health insurance and has shifted the others toward managed care organizations. Coverage provided by these plans is similar between the diabetes-affected families and the general population, but out-of-pocket expenses (co-pays, deductibles, and uncovered expenses) have been shown to be 56% higher in the diabetes-affected families. Seventeen percent of the diabetes-affected families had expenses over 10% of their household income (128). Further investigation is needed to clarify the extent of barriers to care, economic decisions regarding health insurance, the use of health care, and health outcomes in relation to the risk of acute complications among patient with diabetes.

Coexisting Autoimmune Conditions

Autoimmune thyroid, celiac, and Addison's disease affect up to 30% of patients with T1D and increase, through different mechanisms, the risk of hypoglycemia. Thyroid autoimmune disease is the most common of the above, affecting 6–18% of the patients (129–131). The clinical presentation of hypothyroidism is associated with increased frequency of severe hypoglycemia (130). Biopsy-confirmed celiac disease (CD) is present in 4–10% of patients with T1D (132). Untreated CD is associated with increased risk of hypoglycemia due to malabsorption. The introduction of a gluten-free diet may reduce the frequency of hypoglycemia (133,134). Primary adrenal insufficiency (Addison's disease) is a rare disorder, although it is more common in T1D mellitus, affecting nearly 1% of the patients by adulthood (135). Recurrent severe hypoglycemia, despite a reduction in insulin dose, and severe hypoglycemia unawareness, has been reported in patients with T1D and undiagnosed Addison's disease (136,137).

Mortality
Hypoglycemia is a significant factor in the excess mortality observed among patients with diabetes (138). Despite recent improvements in therapy, diabetes-related mortality among children has not declined for 14 years (139). Sudden nocturnal death in young persons with T1D has been described, and is known as the "dead in bed" syndrome (140). It appears to be responsible for about 6% of deaths in diabetic patients below age 40 years (141). In these cases, nocturnal hypoglycemia is a likely precipitant consistent with demonstrated impairment of counterregulatory hormone response during sleep (142), high frequency of nocturnal hypoglycemia reported by the DCCT (87) and more recent studies using continuous glucose monitoring (CGM; see section "Prevention").

Consequences of Hypoglycemia
Neuropsychological and Cognitive Functioning
The consequences of hypoglycemia extend from mild neurogenic symptoms to coma and seizures. Previous studies have shown an association between hypoglycemia and a decrease in cognitive functioning in children with T1D (143–145), particularly those diagnosed before age of five to six years (145,146). Hypoglycemic seizures lead to significant declines in verbal abilities (147), memory skills (148), and ability to organize and recall information (149), even after mild hypoglycemia (150). Severe hypoglycemia in children may result in persistent electroencephalographic (EEG) changes (151–154). EEG abnormalities were found in 80% of diabetic children with a history of severe hypoglycemia, compared with only 30% of those without and 24% of healthy control children (154). However, intensive insulin treatment in the DCCT cohort (aged 13–39 years at the baseline), while increasing the incidence of hypoglycemia, has not lead to a significant worsening of neuropsychological or cognitive functioning during the trial (155,156) as well as 18 years after entry into the trial (157). This observation may be further evidence that the effect of severe hypoglycemia on long-term neuropsychological functioning is age dependent.

Quality of Life
Hypoglycemic episodes have a significant influence on the patient's and family's life (103). One third of the events require assistance of people other than parents, and many are associated with patient school or work absence, parent absence from work, increased need for extra transport, and telephone calls (64). Severe hypoglycemia can lead to increased worry, poor sleep, hospital visits, and hospitalizations,

excessive lowering of daily insulin dose, and worsening of subsequent glycemic control (158). Patients with severe hypoglycemia also reported lower global quality of life; on the other hand, some patients may inappropriately deny or disregard warning signs of hypoglycemia (159).

Cost
In 1999, a Swedish study estimated the direct health care cost of severe hypo-glycemic events at Euro 17,400/100 patients per year (104). Using the incidence rate reported for severe hypoglycemia from Colorado (33) and the average annual cost of severe hypoglycemia estimated at $174 per person (42), the direct medical cost of severe hypoglycemia in the U.S. children was at least $26 million per year, in the late 1990s. The personal, family, and societal cost of trauma, of loss of conscious-ness, seizure, long-term disability, and fears are harder to measure. Further studies are needed to update these figures and to estimate, in addition, the indirect costs (e.g., associated with lost productivity and diminished quality of life).

Prevention
Improved Insulin Delivery
While technological advances provide new opportunities to improve glycemic control without undue risk of severe hypoglycemia, it is important to bear in mind that these modalities have limited use without intensified patient education and compliance (96,160,161). Intensive insulin therapy using insulin pumps, multiple daily injections (MDI), and new insulin analogues has been found effective in lowering HbA1c levels, but there has been less evidence for a beneficial effect on the risk of hypoglycemia. Insulin pump treatment may lower HbA1c levels and improve quality of life compared with multiple daily injections of insulin and, of importance, reduce the rate of severe hypoglycemia (162–164).

The introduction of Humalog® has made insulin treatment easier and safer. An ecologic analysis explored the effects of the DCCT report in 1993 and that of the introduction of rapid-acting insulin analogue (lispro) in 1996 on the risk of severe hypoglycemia in type 1 diabetic patients (105). The HbA1c levels declined sig-nificantly during 1993–1996 ($p < 0.001$), following the DCCT report, but the number of severe hypoglycemic events increased ($p < 0.001$) during that time frame. A further decline in HbA1c levels was observed after the introduction of Humalog insulin in 1996 ($p < 0.001$), however, without a concomitant change in the incidence of severe hypoglycemia. The introduction of a long-lasting insulin analogues also suggests a potential for improving glycemic control without an increased risk of hypoglycemia (165–167).

Continuous Glucose Monitoring
Frequent self-blood glucose monitoring has been found to be an important factor in attaining better glucose control for the intensively treated participants in the DCCT and in the UKPDS. However, many patients do not accept frequent blood glucose monitoring, mainly because of pain and inconvenience. The results also give data valid for only a few seconds, without any information on glucose trends before or after the glucose value. In addition, patients infrequently measure blood glucose levels during the night, although over 50% of severe hypoglycemic events occur during sleep (83,87).

CGM holds great promise for prevention of hypoglycemia. Clinical trials of CGM have given reason to believe that tighter glycemic control may not necessarily lead to increased risk of hypoglycemia (168–174). The ultimate goal remains the development of a noninvasive sensor or an implantable sensor with long lifetime and capability to control automatic "close-loop" insulin delivery system (175).

Behavioral Interventions

Interventions integrating intensive medical care, increased access to care, and increased level of psychosocial support, including treatment of psychiatric disorders, should be considered to lower the risk of hypoglycemia. There are preliminary indications suggesting efficacy of this approach (176,177).

SUMMARY

The incidence of the acute complications of diabetes, DKA, and hypoglycemia remain high and are responsible for a major portion of the cost of diabetes care in childhood. Education of the general population, especially those responsible for the care of children, i.e., physicians and teachers, in the signs and symptoms of undiagnosed diabetes can decrease the occurrence of DKA at diagnosis. Improved analogue insulins, insulin infusion systems, and continuous glucose-monitoring devices offer promise for decreasing the complications of both DKA and hypoglycemia; however, these technological advances remain expensive and do not diminish the need for extensive patient education, comprehensive diabetes health care, and support systems required decrease the acute complications of diabetes. Comprehensive diabetes health care, educational, and behavioral support systems also are required to achieve optimal diabetes care as well as to improve the quality of life for children with diabetes and their families. Ongoing investment in patient education and behavioral support will be required in all countries for children to fully achieve the potential benefit of current and future technology.

REFERENCES

1. Wolfsdorf J, Glaser N, Sperling MA. Diabetic ketoacidosis in infants, children, and adolescents: a consensus statement from the American Diabetes Association. Diabetes Care 2006; 29(5):1150–1159.
2. Kitabchi AE, Umpierrez GE, Murphy MB, et al. Hyperglycemic crises in adult patients with diabetes: a consensus statement from the American Diabetes Association. Diabetes Care 2006; 29(12):2739–2748.
3. Wolfsdorf J, Craig ME, Daneman D, et al. Diabetic ketoacidosis. Pediatr Diabetes 2007 February; 8(1):28–43.
4. Dunger DB, Sperling MA, Acerini CL, et al. ESPE/LWPES consensus statement on diabetic ketoacidosis in children and adolescents. Arch Dis Child 2004; 89(2):188–194.
5. Ireland JT, Thomson WS. Euglycemic diabetic ketoacidosis. Br Med J 1973; 3(5871):107.
6. Burge MR, Hardy KJ, Schade DS. Short-term fasting is a mechanism for the development of euglycemic ketoacidosis during periods of insulin deficiency. J Clin Endocrinol Metab 1993; 76(5):1192–1198.
7. Laffel LM, Wentzell K, Loughlin C, et al. Sick day management using blood 3-hydroxybutyrate (3-OHB) compared with urine ketone monitoring reduces hospital visits in young people with T1DM: a randomized clinical trial. Diabet Med 2006; 23(3): 278–284.
8. Rewers A, McFann K, Chase HP. Bedside monitoring of blood beta-hydroxybutyrate levels in the management of diabetic ketoacidosis in children. Diabetes Technol Ther 2006; 8(6):671–676.

9. Rewers A, Klingensmith G, Davis C, et al. Diabetes ketoacidosis at onset of diabetes: the SEARCH for diabetes in Youth Study. Diabetes 54(suppl 1) 2007; A63–A64 (abstr).
10. Mallare JT, Cordice CC, Ryan BA, et al. Identifying risk factors for the development of diabetic ketoacidosis in new onset type 1 diabetes mellitus. Clin Pediatr (Phila) 2003; 42(7):591–597.
11. Quinn M, Fleischman A, Rosner B, et al. Characteristics at diagnosis of type 1 diabetes in children younger than 6 years. J Pediatr 2006; 148(3):366–371.
12. Pinkey JH, Bingley PJ, Sawtell PA, et al. Presentation and progress of childhood diabetes mellitus: a prospective population-based study. The Bart's-Oxford Study Group. Diabetologia 1994; 37(1):70–74.
13. Komulainen J, Lounamaa R, Knip M, et al. Ketoacidosis at the diagnosis of type 1 (insulin dependent) diabetes mellitus is related to poor residual beta cell function. Childhood Diabetes in Finland Study Group. Arch Dis Child 1996; 75(5):410–415.
14. Levy-Marchal C, Patterson CC, Green A. Geographical variation of presentation at diagnosis of type I diabetes in children: the EURODIAB study. European and Diabetes. Diabetologia 2001; 44(suppl 3):B75–B80.
15. Neu A, Willasch A, Ehehalt S, et al. Ketoacidosis at onset of type 1 diabetes mellitus in children—frequency and clinical presentation. Pediatr Diabetes 2003; 4(2):77–81.
16. Roche EF, Menon A, Gill D, et al. Clinical presentation of type 1 diabetes. Pediatr Diabetes 2005; 6(2):75–78.
17. Hekkala A, Knip M, Veijola R. Ketoacidosis at diagnosis of type 1 diabetes in children in Northern Finland: temporal changes over 20 years. Diabetes Care 2007; 30(4): 861–866.
18. Daneman D, Knip M, Kaar ML, et al. Comparison of children with type 1 (insulin-dependent) diabetes in northern Finland and southern Ontario: differences at disease onset. Diabetes Res 1990; 14(3):123–126.
19. Soliman AT, al Salmi I, Asfour M. Mode of presentation and progress of childhood diabetes mellitus in the Sultanate of Oman. J Trop Pediatr 1997; 43(3):128–132.
20. al-Khawari M, Shaltout A, Qabazard M, et al. Incidence and severity of ketoacidosis in childhood-onset diabetes in Kuwait. Kuwait Diabetes Study Group. Diabetes Res Clin Pract 1997; 35(2–3):123–128.
21. Abdul-Rasoul M, Habib H, Al-Khouly M. 'The honeymoon phase' in children with type 1 diabetes mellitus: frequency, duration, and influential factors. Pediatr Diabetes 2006; 7(2):101–107.
22. Hamman RF, Cook M, Keefer S, et al. Medical care patterns at the onset of insulin-dependent diabetes mellitus: association with severity and subsequent complications. Diabetes Care 1985; 8(suppl 1):94–100.
23. Rewers A, Chase P, Bothner J, et al. Medical care patterns at the onset of type I diabetes in Colorado children, 1978–2001. Diabetes 2003; 52(suppl 1):A62.
24. Curtis JR, To T, Muirhead S, et al. Recent trends in hospitalization for diabetic ketoacidosis in ontario children. Diabetes Care 2002; 25(9):1591–1596.
25. HiraSing RA, Reeser HM, de Groot RR, et al. Trends in hospital admissions among children aged 0–19 years with type I diabetes in The Netherlands. Diabetes Care 1996; 19(5):431–434.
26. Levy-Marchal C, Papoz L, de BC, et al. Clinical and laboratory features of type 1 diabetic children at the time of diagnosis. Diabet Med 1992; 9(3):279–284.
27. Komulainen J, Kulmala P, Savola K, et al. Clinical, autoimmune, and genetic characteristics of very young children with type 1 diabetes. Childhood Diabetes in Finland (DiMe) Study Group. Diabetes Care 1999; 22(12):1950–1955.
28. Maniatis AK, Goehrig SH, Gao D, et al. Increased incidence and severity of diabetic ketoacidosis among uninsured children with newly diagnosed type 1 diabetes mellitus. Pediatr Diabetes 2005; 6(2):79–83.
29. Maldonado MR, Chong ER, Oehl MA, et al. Economic Impact of Diabetic Ketoacidosis in a Multiethnic Indigent Population: Analysis of costs based on the precipitating cause. Diabetes Care 2003; 26(4):1265–1269.
30. Alavi IA, Sharma BK, Pillay VK. Steroid-induced diabetic ketoacidosis. Am J Med Sci 1971; 262(1):15–23.

31. Wilson DR, D'Souza L, Sarkar N, et al. New-onset diabetes and ketoacidosis with atypical antipsychotics. Schizophr Res 2003; 59(1):1–6.
32. Likitmaskul S, Santiprabhob J, Sawathiparnich P, et al. Clinical pictures of type 2 diabetes in Thai children and adolescents are highly related to features of metabolic syndrome. J Med Assoc Thai 2005; 88(suppl 8):S169–S175.
33. Rewers A, Chase HP, Mackenzie T, et al. Predictors of acute complications in children with type 1 diabetes. JAMA 2002; 287(19):2511–2518.
34. Golden MP, Herrold AJ, Orr DP. An approach to prevention of recurrent diabetic ketoacidosis in the pediatric population. J Pediatr 1985; 107(2):195–200.
35. Reda E, Von RA, Dunn P. Metabolic control with insulin pump therapy: the Waikato experience. N Z Med J 2007; 120(1248):U2401.
36. Mbugua PK, Otieno CF, Kayima JK, et al. Diabetic ketoacidosis: clinical presentation and precipitating factors at Kenyatta National Hospital, Nairobi. East Afr Med J 2005; 82(suppl 12):S191–S196.
37. Flood RG, Chiang VW. Rate and prediction of infection in children with diabetic ketoacidosis. Am J Emerg Med 2001; 19(4):270–273.
38. Kaufman FR, Halvorson M, Miller D, et al. Insulin pump therapy in type 1 pediatric patients: now and into the year 2000. Diabetes Metab Res Rev 1999; 15(5):338–352.
39. Hanas R, Ludvigsson J. Hypoglycemia and ketoacidosis with insulin pump therapy in children and adolescents. Pediatr Diabetes 2006; 7(suppl 4):32–38.
40. Sulli N, Shashaj B. Long-term benefits of continuous subcutaneous insulin infusion in children with Type 1 diabetes: a 4-year follow-up. Diabet Med 2006; 23(8):900–906.
41. Quinn L. Diabetes emergencies in the patient with type 2 diabetes. Nurs Clin North Am 2001; 36(2):341–360, viii.
42. Levine BS, Anderson BJ, Butler DA, et al. Predictors of glycemic control and short-term adverse outcomes in youth with type 1 diabetes. J Pediatr 2001; 139(2):197–203.
43. Snorgaard O, Eskildsen PC, Vadstrup S, et al. Diabetic ketoacidosis in Denmark: epidemiology, incidence rates, precipitating factors and mortality rates. J Intern Med 1989; 226(4):223–228.
44. Smith CP, Firth D, Bennett S, et al. Ketoacidosis occurring in newly diagnosed and established diabetic children. Acta Paediatr 1998; 87(5):537–541.
45. Polonsky WH, Anderson BJ, Lohrer PA, et al. Insulin omission in women with IDDM. Diabetes Care 1994; 17(10):1178–1185.
46. Meltzer LJ, Johnson SB, Prine JM, et al. Disordered eating, body mass, and glycemic control in adolescents with type 1 diabetes. Diabetes Care 2001; 24(4):678–682.
47. Dumont RH, Jacobson AM, Cole C, et al. Psychosocial predictors of acute complications of diabetes in youth. Diabet Med 1995; 12(7):612–618.
48. Alvi NS, Davies P, Kirk JM, et al. Diabetic ketoacidosis in Asian children. Arch Dis Child 2001; 85(1):60–61.
49. Edge JA, Ford-Adams ME, Dunger DB. Causes of death in children with insulin dependent diabetes 1990–1996. Arch Dis Child 1999; 81(4):318–323.
50. Podar T, Solntsev A, Reunanen A, et al. Mortality in patients with childhood-onset type 1 diabetes in Finland, Estonia, and Lithuania: follow-up of nationwide cohorts. Diabetes Care 2000; 23(3):290–294.
51. Edge JA, Hawkins MM, Winter DL, et al. The risk and outcome of cerebral oedema developing during diabetic ketoacidosis. Arch Dis Child 2001; 85(1):16–22.
52. Lawrence SE, Cummings EA, Gaboury I, et al. Population-based study of incidence and risk factors for cerebral edema in pediatric diabetic ketoacidosis. J Pediatr 2005;146(5):688–692.
53. Glaser N, Barnett P, McCaslin I, et al. Risk factors for cerebral edema in children with diabetic ketoacidosis. The Pediatric Emergency Medicine Collaborative Research Committee of the American Academy of Pediatrics. N Engl J Med 2001; 344(4):264–269.
54. Gutierrez JA, Bagatell R, Samson MP, et al. Femoral central venous catheter-associated deep venous thrombosis in children with diabetic ketoacidosis. Crit Care Med 2003; 31(1):80–83.
55. Roberts MD, Slover RH, Chase HP. Diabetic ketoacidosis with intracerebral complications. Pediatr Diabetes 2001; 2(3):109–114.

56. Atluru VL. Spontaneous intracerebral hematomas in juvenile diabetic ketoacidosis. Pediatr Neurol 1986; 2(3):167–169.
57. Ho J, Mah JK, Hill MD, et al. Pediatric stroke associated with new onset type 1 diabetes mellitus: case reports and review of the literature. Pediatr Diabetes 2006; 7(2):116–121.
58. Kanter RK, Oliphant M, Zimmerman JJ, et al. Arterial thrombosis causing cerebral edema in association with diabetic ketoacidosis. Crit Care Med 1987; 15(2):175–176.
59. Kameh DS, Gonzalez OR, Pearl GS, et al. Fatal rhino-orbital-cerebral zygomycosis. South Med J 1997; 90(11):1133–1135.
60. Gessesse M, Chali D, Wolde-Tensai B, et al. Rhinocerebral mucormycosis in an 11-year-old boy. Ethiop Med J 2001; 39(4):341–348.
61. Dixon AN, Jude EB, Banerjee AK, et al. Simultaneous pulmonary and cerebral oedema, and multiple CNS infarctions as complications of diabetic ketoacidosis: a case report. Diabet Med 2006; 23(5):571–573.
62. Young MC. Simultaneous acute cerebral and pulmonary edema complicating diabetic ketoacidosis. Diabetes Care 1995; 18(9):1288–1290.
63. Javor KA, Kotsanos JG, McDonald RC, et al. Diabetic ketoacidosis charges relative to medical charges of adult patients with type I diabetes. Diabetes Care 1997; 20(3):349–354.
64. Nordfeldt S, Jonsson D. Short-term effects of severe hypoglycaemia in children and adolescents with type 1 diabetes. A cost-of-illness study. Acta Paediatr 2001; 90(2):137–142.
65. Ginde AA, Pelletier AJ, Camargo CA, Jr. National study of U.S. emergency department visits with diabetic ketoacidosis, 1993–2003. Diabetes Care 2006; 29(9):2117–2119.
66. Kim S. Burden of hospitalizations primarily due to uncontrolled diabetes: implications of inadequate primary health care in the United States. Diabetes Care 2007; 30(5):1281–1282.
67. Kitabchi AE, Umpierrez GE, Murphy MB, et al. Management of hyperglycemic crises in patients with diabetes. Diabetes Care 2001; 24(1):131–153.
68. Barker JM, Goehrig SH, Barriga K, et al. Clinical characteristics of children diagnosed with type 1 diabetes through intensive screening and follow-up. Diabetes Care 2004; 27(6):1399–1404.
69. Vanelli M, Chiari G, Ghizzoni L, et al. Effectiveness of a prevention program for diabetic ketoacidosis in children. An 8-year study in schools and private practices. Diabetes Care 1999; 22(1):7–9.
70. Vanelli M, Chiari G, Lacava S, et al. Campaign for diabetic ketoacidosis prevention still effective 8 years later. Diabetes Care 2007; 30(4):e12.
71. Diabetes Prevention Trial—Type 1 Diabetes Study Group. Effects of insulin in relatives of patients with type 1 diabetes mellitus. N Engl J Med 2002; 346(22):1685–1691.
72. Hoffman WH, O'Neill P, Khoury C, et al. Service and education for the insulin-dependent child. Diabetes Care 1978; 1(5):285–288.
73. Drozda DJ, Dawson VA, Long DJ, et al. Assessment of the effect of a comprehensive diabetes management program on hospital admission rates of children with diabetes mellitus. Diabetes Educ 1990; 16(5):389–393.
74. Grey M, Boland EA, Davidson M, et al. Coping skills training for youth with diabetes mellitus has long-lasting effects on metabolic control and quality of life. J Pediatr 2000; 137(1):107–113.
75. The Diabetes Control and Complications Trial Research Group. Effect of intensive diabetes treatment on the development and progression of long-term complications in adolescents with insulin-dependent diabetes mellitus: Diabetes Control and Complications Trial. Diabetes Control and Complications Trial Research Group. J Pediatr 1994; 125(2):177–188.
76. Svoren BM, Butler D, Levine BS, et al. Reducing acute adverse outcomes in youths with type 1 diabetes: a randomized, controlled trial. Pediatrics 2003; 112(4):914–922.
77. Cryer PE. Hypoglycemia in diabetes: pathophysiological mechanisms and diurnal variation. Prog Brain Res 2006; 153:361–365.
78. Kerr D, Macdonald IA, Heller SR, et al. Beta-adrenoceptor blockade and hypoglycaemia. A randomised, double-blind, placebo controlled comparison of metoprolol

CR, atenolol and propranolol LA in normal subjects. Br J Clin Pharmacol 1990; 29(6): 685–693.

79. The Diabetes Control and Complications Trial Research Group. Adverse events and their association with treatment regimens in the diabetes control and complications trial. Diabetes Care 1995; 18(11):1415–1127.

80. Becker DJ, Ryan CM. Hypoglycemia: a complication of diabetes therapy in children. Trends Endocrinol Metab 2000; 11(5):198–202.

81. Davis EA, Keating B, Byrne GC, et al. Impact of improved glycaemic control on rates of hypoglycaemia in insulin dependent diabetes mellitus. Arch Dis Child 1998; 78(2):111–115.

82. Bhatia V, Wolfsdorf JI. Severe hypoglycemia in youth with insulin-dependent diabetes mellitus: frequency and causative factors. Pediatrics 1991; 88(6):1187–1193.

83. Bergada I, Suissa S, Dufresne J, et al. Severe hypoglycemia in IDDM children. Diabetes Care 1989; 12(4):239–244.

84. Daneman D, Frank M, Perlman K, et al. Severe hypoglycemia in children with insulin-dependent diabetes mellitus: frequency and predisposing factors (see comments). J Pediatr 1989; 115:681–685.

85. Aman J, Karlsson I, Wranne L. Symptomatic hypoglycaemia in childhood diabetes: a population-based questionnaire study. Diabet Med 1989; 6(3):257–261.

86. Egger M, Gschwend S, Smith GD, et al. Increasing incidence of hypoglycemic coma in children with IDDM. Diabetes Care 1991; 14(11):1001–1005.

87. DCCT. Epidemiology of severe hypoglycemia in the diabetes control and complications trial. The DCCT Research Group. Am J Med 1991; 90(4):450–459.

88. Tupola S, Rajantie J, Maenpaa J. Severe hypoglycemia in children and adolescents during multiple-dose insulin therapy. Diabet Med 1998; 15(8):695–699.

89. Intensive blood-glucose control with sulphonylureas or insulin compared with conventional treatment and risk of complications in patients with type 2 diabetes (UKPDS 33). UK Prospective Diabetes Study (UKPDS) Group. Lancet 1998; 352(9131):837–853.

90. Shorr RI, Ray WA, Daugherty JR, et al. Individual sulfonylureas and serious hypoglycemia in older people. J Am Geriatr Soc 1996; 44(7):751–755.

91. Shorr RI, Ray WA, Daugherty JR, et al. Incidence and risk factors for serious hypoglycemia in older persons using insulin or sulfonylureas. Arch Intern Med 1997; 157(15):1681–1686.

92. Shorr RI, Ray WA, Daugherty JR, et al. Antihypertensives and the risk of serious hypoglycemia in older persons using insulin or sulfonylureas. JAMA 1997; 278(1):40–43.

93. Effects of ramipril on cardiovascular and microvascular outcomes in people with diabetes mellitus: results of the HOPE study and MICRO-HOPE substudy. Heart Outcomes Prevention Evaluation Study Investigators. Lancet 2000; 355(9200):253–259.

94. Jones TW, Boulware SD, Kraemer DT, Caprio S, Sherwin RS, Tamborlane WV. Independent effects of youth and poor diabetes control on responses to hypoglycemia in children. Diabetes 1991; 40:358–363.

95. Mortensen HB, Hougaard P. Comparison of metabolic control in a cross-sectional study of 2,873 children and adolescents with IDDM from 18 countries. The Hvidore Study Group on Childhood Diabetes. Diabetes Care 1997; 20(5):714–720.

96. Rosilio M, Cotton JB, Wieliczko MC et al. Factors associated with glycemic control. A cross-sectional nationwide study in 2,579 French children with type 1 diabetes. The French Pediatric Diabetes Group. Diabetes Care 1998; 21(7):1146–1153.

97. Fukuda M, Tanaka A, Tahara Y, et al. Correlation between minimal secretory capacity of pancreatic beta-cells and stability of diabetic control. Diabetes 1988; 37(1):81–88.

98. Effect of intensive therapy on residual beta-cell function in patients with type 1 diabetes in the diabetes control and complications trial. A randomized, controlled trial. The Diabetes Control and Complications Trial Research Group. Ann Intern Med 1998; 128(7):517–523.

99. Knip M, Llonen J, Mustonen A, Akerblom HK. Evidence of an accelerated B-cell destruction in HLA-Dw3/Dw4 heterozygous children with type I (insulin-dependent) diabetes. Diabetologia 1986; 29:347–351.

100. Dahlquist G, Blom L, Persson B, et al. The epidemiology of lost residual beta-cell function in short term diabetic children. Acta Paediatr Scand 1988; 77:852–859.

101. Petersen JS, Dyrberg T, Karlsen AE et al. Glutamic acid decarboxylase (GAD65) auto-antibodies in prediction of B-cell function and remission in recent-onset IDDM after cyclosporin treatment. Diabetes 1994; 43(11):1291–1296.

102. Lteif AN, Schwenk WF. Type 1 diabetes mellitus in early childhood: glycemic control and associated risk of hypoglycemic reactions. Mayo Clin Proc 1999; 74(3):211–216.

103. Cryer PE, Fisher JN, Shamoon H. Hypoglycemia. Diabetes Care 1994; 17(7):734–755.

104. Nordfeldt S, Ludvigsson J. Adverse events in intensively treated children and adolescents with type 1 diabetes. Acta Paediatr 1999; 88(11):1184–1193.

105. Chase HP, Lockspeiser T, Peery B, et al. The impact of the diabetes control and complications trial and humalog insulin on glycohemoglobin levels and severe hypoglycemia in type 1 diabetes. Diabetes Care 2001; 24(3):430–434.

106. Simonson DC, Tamborlane WV, DeFronzo RA, Sherwin RS. Intensive insulin therapy reduces counterregulatory hormone responses to hypoglycemia in patients with type I diabetes. Ann Intern Med 1985; 103(2):184–190.

107. Jones TW, Borg WP, Borg MA, et al. Resistance to neuroglycopenia: an adaptive response during intensive insulin treatment of diabetes. J Clin Endocrinol Metab 1997; 82(6):1713–1718.

108. Heller SR, Cryer PE. Reduced neuroendocrine and symptomatic responses to subsequent hypoglycemia after 1 episode of hypoglycemia in nondiabetic humans. Diabetes 1991; 40(2):223–226.

109. Amiel SA, Simonson DC, Sherwin RS, et al. Exaggerated epinephrine responses to hypoglycemia in normal and insulin-dependent diabetic children. J Pediatr 1987; 110(6):832–837.

110. Hepburn DA, Patrick AW, Eadington DW, et al. Unawareness of hypoglycaemia in insulin-treated diabetic patients: prevalence and relationship to autonomic neuropathy. Diabet Med 1990; 7(8):711–717.

111. Cranston I, Lomas J, Maran A, et al. Restoration of hypoglycaemia awareness in patients with long-duration insulin-dependent diabetes. Lancet 1994; 344(8918):283–287.

112. Tsalikian E, Kollman C, Tamborlane WB, et al. Prevention of hypoglycemia during exercise in children with type 1 diabetes by suspending basal insulin. Diabetes Care 2006; 29(10):2200–2204.

113. Tansey MJ, Tsalikian E, Beck RW, et al. The effects of aerobic exercise on glucose and counterregulatory hormone concentrations in children with type 1 diabetes. Diabetes Care 2006; 29(1):20–25.

114. Tsalikian E, Mauras N, Beck RW, et al. Impact of exercise on overnight glycemic control in children with type 1 diabetes mellitus. J Pediatr 2005; 147(4):528–534.

115. van de WA. Diabetes mellitus and alcohol. Diabetes Metab Res Rev 2004; 20(4):263–267.

116. Kerr D, Macdonald IA, Heller SR, et al. Alcohol causes hypoglycaemic unawareness in healthy volunteers and patients with type 1 (insulin-dependent) diabetes. Diabetologia 1990; 33(4):216–221.

117. Avogaro A, Watanabe RM, Dall'Arche A, et al. Acute alcohol consumption improves insulin action without affecting insulin secretion in type 2 diabetic subjects. Diabetes Care 2004; 27(6):1369–1374.

118. Ismail D, Gebert R, Vuillermin PJ, et al. Social consumption of alcohol in adolescents with Type 1 diabetes is associated with increased glucose lability, but not hypoglycaemia. Diabet Med 2006; 23(8):830–833.

119. Bargagna S, Tosi B, Calisti L, et al. [Psychopathological aspects in a group of children and adolescent with insulin-dependent diabetes mellitus]. Minerva Pediatr 1997; 49(3):71–77.

120. Kovacs M, Goldston D, Obrosky DS, et al. Psychiatric disorders in youths with IDDM: rates and risk factors. Diabetes Care 1997; 20(1):36–44.

121. Blanz BJ, Rensch-Riemann BS, Fritz-Sigmund DI, Schmidt MH. IDDM is a risk factor for adolescent psychiatric disorders. Diabetes Care 1993 December; 16(12):1579–1587.

122. Goldston DB, Kovacs M, Ho VY, et al. Suicidal ideation and suicide attempts among youth with insulin-dependent diabetes mellitus. J Am Acad Child Adolesc Psychiatry 1994; 33(2):240–246.

123. Jacobson AM, Hauser ST, Willett JB, et al. Psychological adjustment to IDDM: 10-year follow-up of an onset cohort of child and adolescent patients. Diabetes Care 1997; 20(5):811–818.

124. Nakazato M, Kodama K, Miyamoto S, et al. Psychiatric disorders in juvenile patients with insulin-dependent diabetes mellitus. Diabetes Res Clin Pract 2000; 48(3):177–183.
125. Kovacs M, Mukerji P, Iyengar S, et al. Psychiatric disorder and metabolic control among youths with IDDM. A longitudinal study. Diabetes Care 1996; 19(4):318–323.
126. Sawka AM, Burgart V, Zimmerman D. Loss of hypoglycemia awareness in an adolescent with type 1 diabetes mellitus during treatment with fluoxetine hydrochloride. J Pediatr 2000; 136(3):394–396.
127. Allen C, LeCaire T, Palta M, et al. Risk factors for frequent and severe hypoglycemia in type 1 diabetes. Diabetes Care 2001; 24(11):1878–1881.
128. Songer TJ, LaPorte R, Lave JR, et al. Health insurance and the financial impact of IDDM in families with a child with IDDM. Diabetes Care 1997; 20(4):577–584.
129. Kontiainen S, Schlenzka A, Koskimies S, et al. Autoantibodies and autoimmune diseases in young diabetics. Diabetes Res 1990; 13(4):151–156.
130. Leong KS, Wallymahmed M, Wilding J, et al. Clinical presentation of thyroid dysfunction and Addison's disease in young adults with type 1 diabetes. Postgrad Med J 1999; 75(886):467–470.
131. Roldan MB, Alonso M, Barrio R. Thyroid autoimmunity in children and adolescents with Type 1 diabetes mellitus. Diabetes Nutr Metab 1999; 12(1):27–31.
132. Rewers M, Liu E, Simmons J, et al. Celiac disease associated with type 1 diabetes mellitus. Endocrinol Metab Clin North Am 2004; 33(1):197–214, xi.
133. Mohn A, Cerruto M, Lafusco D, et al. Celiac disease in children and adolescents with type I diabetes: importance of hypoglycemia. J Pediatr Gastroenterol Nutr 2001; 32(1):37–40.
134. Iafusco D, Rea F, Prisco F. Hypoglycemia and reduction of the insulin requirement as a sign of celiac disease in children with IDDM. Diabetes Care 1998; 21(8):1379–1381.
135. Yu L, Brewer KW, Gates S, et al. DRB1*04 and DQ alleles: expression of 21-hydroxylase autoantibodies and risk of progression to Addison's disease. J Clin Endocrinol Metab 1999; 84(1):328–335.
136. McAulay V, Frier BM. Addison's disease in type 1 diabetes presenting with recurrent hypoglycaemia. Postgrad Med J 2000; 76(894):230–232.
137. Phornphutkul C, Boney CM, Gruppuso PA. A novel presentation of Addison disease: hypoglycemia unawareness in an adolescent with insulin-dependent diabetes mellitus. J Pediatr 1998; 132(5):882–884.
138. Nishimura R, Laporte RE, Dorman JS, et al. Mortality trends in type 1 diabetes. The Allegheny County (Pennsylvania) Registry 1965–1999. Diabetes Care 2001; 24(5):823–827.
139. DiLiberti JH, Lorenz RA. Long-term trends in childhood diabetes mortality: 1968–1998. Diabetes Care 2001; 24(8):1348–1352.
140. Weston PJ, Gill GV. Is undetected autonomic dysfunction responsible for sudden death in Type 1 diabetes mellitus? The "dead in bed" syndrome revisited. Diabet Med 1999; 16(8):626–631.
141. Sovik O, Thordarson H. Dead-in-bed syndrome in young diabetic patients. Diabetes Care 1999; 22(suppl 2):B40–B42.
142. Jones TW, Porter P, Sherwin RS, et al. Decreased epinephrine responses to hypoglycemia during sleep. N Engl J Med 1998; 338(23):1657–1662.
143. Golden MP, Ingersoll GM, Brack CJ, et al. Longitudinal relationship of asymptomatic hypoglycemia to cognitive function in IDDM. Diabetes Care 1989; 12:89–93.
144. Rovet JF, Ehrlich RM, Hoppe M. Specific intellectual deficits in children with early onset diabetes mellitus. Child Dev 1988; 59(1):226–234.
145. Rovet JF, Ehrlich RM, Czuchta D. Intellectual characteristics of diabetic children at diagnosis and one year later. J Pediatr Psychol 1990; 15:775–788.
146. Ryan C, Vega A, Drash A. Cognitive deficits in adolescents who developed diabetes early in life. Pediatrics 1985; 75(5):921–927.
147. Rovet JF, Ehrlich RM. The effect of hypoglycemic seizures on cognitive function in children with diabetes: a 7-year prospective study. J Pediatr 1999; 134(4):503–506.
148. Kaufman FR, Epport K, Engilman R, et al. Neurocognitive functioning in children diagnosed with diabetes before age 10 years. J Diabetes Complications 1999; 13(1):31–38.
149. Hagen JW, Barclay CR, Anderson BJ, et al. Intellective functioning and strategy use in children with insulin-dependent diabetes mellitus. Child Dev 1990; 61(6):1714–1727.

150. Ryan CM, Williams TM, Finegold DN, et al. Cognitive dysfunction in adults with Type 1 (insulin-dependent) diabetes mellitus of long duration: effects of recurrent hypoglycaemia and other chronic complications. Diabetologia 1993; 36:329–334.
151. Eeg-Olofsson O, Petersen I. Childhood Diabetic Neuropathy. A clinical and neurophysiological study. Acta Paediatr Scand 55, 163–176. 2001.
152. Schlack H, Palm D, Jochmus I. [Influence of recurrent hypoglycemia on the EEG of the diabetic child]. Monatsschr Kinderheilkd 1969; 117(4):251–253.
153. Gilhaus KH, Daweke H, Lulsdorf HG, et al. [EEG changes in diabetic children]. Dtsch Med Wochenschr 1973; 98(31):1449–1454.
154. Soltesz G, Acsadi G. Association between diabetes, severe hypoglycaemia, and electroencephalographic abnormalities. Arch Dis Child 1989; 64:992–996.
155. DCCT. Effects of intensive diabetes therapy on neuropsychological function in adults in the diabetes control and complications trial. Annals of Internal Medicine 1996; 124(4): 379–388.
156. Austin EJ, Deary IJ. Effects of repeated hypoglycemia on cognitive function: a psychometrically validated reanalysis of the Diabetes Control and Complications Trial data. Diabetes Care 1999; 22(8):1273–1277.
157. Jacobson AM, Musen G, Ryan CM, et al. Long-term effect of diabetes and its treatment on cognitive function. N Engl J Med 2007; 356(18):1842–1852.
158. Tupola S, Rajantie J, Akerblom HK. Experience of severe hypoglycaemia may influence both patient's and physician's subsequent treatment policy of insulin-dependent diabetes mellitus. Eur J Pediatr 1998; 157(8):625–627.
159. Cox DJ, Irvine A, Gonder-Frederick L, et al. Fear of hypoglycemia: quantification, validation, and utilization. Diabetes Care 1987; 10(5):617–621.
160. Karter AJ, Ackerson LM, Darbinian JA, et al. Self-monitoring of blood glucose levels and glycemic control: the Northern California Kaiser Permanente Diabetes registry. Am J Med 2001; 111(1):1–9.
161. Kubiak T, Hermanns N, Schreckling HJ, et al. Evaluation of a self-management-based patient education program for the treatment and prevention of hypoglycemia-related problems in type 1 diabetes. Patient Educ Couns 2006; 60(2):228–234.
162. Boland EA, Grey M, Oesterle A, et al. Continuous subcutaneous insulin infusion. A new way to lower risk of severe hypoglycemia, improve metabolic control, and enhance coping in adolescents with type 1 diabetes. Diabetes Care 1999; 22(11):1779–1784.
163. Maniatis AK, Klingensmith GJ, Slover RH, et al. Continuous subcutaneous insulin infusion therapy for children and adolescents: an option for routine diabetes care. Pediatrics 2001; 107(2):351–356.
164. Bulsara MK, Holman CD, Davis EA, et al. The impact of a decade of changing treatment on rates of severe hypoglycemia in a population-based cohort of children with type 1 diabetes. Diabetes Care 2004; 27(10):2293–2298.
165. Ratner RE, Hirsch IB, Neifing JL, et al. Less hypoglycemia with insulin glargine in intensive insulin therapy for type 1 diabetes. U.S. Study Group of Insulin Glargine in Type 1 Diabetes. Diabetes Care 2000; 23(5):639–643.
166. Raskin P, Klaff L, Bergenstal R, et al. A 16-week comparison of the novel insulin analog insulin glargine (HOE 901) and NPH human insulin used with insulin lispro in patients with type 1 diabetes. Diabetes Care 2000; 23(11):1666–1671.
167. Mohn A, Strang S, Wernicke-Panten K, et al. Nocturnal glucose control and free insulin levels in children with type 1 diabetes by use of the long-acting insulin HOE 901 as part of a three-injection regimen. Diabetes Care 2000; 23(4):557–559.
168. Boland E, Monsod T, Delucia M, et al. Limitations of conventional methods of self-monitoring of blood glucose: Lessons learned from 3 days of continuous glucose sensing in pediatric patients with type 1 diabetes. Diabetes Care 2001; 24(11):1858–1862.
169. Chase HP, Kim LM, Owen SL, et al. Continuous subcutaneous glucose monitoring in children with type 1 diabetes. Pediatrics 2001; 107(2):222–226.
170. UK Hypoglycaemia Study Group. Risk of hypoglycaemia in types 1 and 2 diabetes: effects of treatment modalities and their duration. Diabetologia 2007; 50(6):1140–1147.

171. Clarke WL, Anderson S, Farhy L, et al. Evaluating the clinical accuracy of two continuous glucose sensors using continuous glucose-error grid analysis. Diabetes Care 2005; 28(10):2412–2417.

172. Fayolle C, Brun JF, Bringer J, et al. Accuracy of continuous subcutaneous glucose monitoring with the GlucoDay in type 1 diabetic patients treated by subcutaneous insulin infusion during exercise of low versus high intensity. Diabetes Metab 2006; 32(4):313–320.

173. Maia FF, Araujo LR. Efficacy of continuous glucose monitoring system to detect unrecognized hypoglycemia in children and adolescents with type 1 diabetes. Arq Bras Endocrinol Metabol 2005; 49(4):569–574.

174. Streja D. Can continuous glucose monitoring provide objective documentation of hypoglycemia unawareness? Endocr Pract 2005; 11(2):83–90.

175. Renard E, Costalat G, Chevassus H, et al. Artificial beta-cell: clinical experience toward an implantable closed-loop insulin delivery system. Diabetes Metab 2006; 32(5 pt 2): 497–502.

176. Halvorson M, Carpenter S, Kaiserman K, et al. A pilot trial in pediatrics with the sensor-augmented pump: combining real-time continuous glucose monitoring with the insulin pump. J Pediatr 2007; 150(1):103–105.

177. Svoren BM, Volkening LK, Butler DA, et al. Temporal trends in the treatment of pediatric type 1 diabetes and impact on acute outcomes. J Pediatr 2007; 150(3):279–285.

178. The Diabetes Control and Complications Trial Research Group. Effect of intensive diabetes treatment on the development and progression of long-term complications in adolescents with insulin-dependent diabetes mellitus: Diabetes Control and Complications Trial. Diabetes Control and Complications Trial Research Group. J Pediatr 1994; 125(2):177–188.

179. Smith CP, Firth D, Bennett S, et al. Ketoacidosis occurring in newly diagnosed and established diabetic children. Acta Paediatr 1998; 87(5):537–541.

180. Thomsett M, Shield G, Batch J, et al. How well are we doing? Metabolic control in patients with diabetes. J Paediatr Child Health 1999; 35(5):479–482.

181. Nordfeldt S, Ludvigsson J. Severe hypoglycemia in children with IDDM. A prospective population study, 1992–1994. Diabetes Care 1997; 20(4):497–503.

182. Danne T, Mortensen HB, Hougaard P, et al. Persistent differences among centers over 3 years in glycemic control and hypoglycemia in a study of 3,805 children and adolescents with type 1 diabetes from the Hvidore Study Group. Diabetes Care 2001; 24(8): 1342–1347.

183. Skyler J, Diabetic complications. The importance of glucose control. Endocrinol Metab Clin North Am 1996; 25(2):243–254.

17 Dietary Factors in Youth with Diabetes

Elizabeth J. Mayer-Davis
Department of Epidemiology and Biostatistics and Center for Research in Nutrition and Health Disparities, Arnold School of Public Health, University of South Carolina, Columbia, South Carolina, U.S.A.

Franziska K. Bishop
Barbara Davis Center for Childhood Diabetes, University of Colorado at Denver and Health Sciences Center, Aurora, Colorado, U.S.A.

INTRODUCTION

Nutrition is commonly regarded as the cornerstone of treatment of childhood diabetes mellitus (DM) (1,2). However, due to a paucity of data on dietary intake and metabolic status among youth with either type 1 diabetes mellitus (T1DM) or type 2 diabetes mellitus (T2DM), current American Diabetes Association (ADA) nutrition recommendations for youth with diabetes are based primarily on expert consensus based almost entirely on studies of adults with diabetes and on studies of healthy children, incorporating recommendations from government or other professional organizations (1). Current recommendations have been distilled and are presented in Table 1 reprinted from Mayer-Davis, 2006 (3).

Whatever the recommendations, medical nutrition therapy (MNT) refers to specific nutrition recommendations and the process by which these recommendations are provided to patients and their families, typically delivered by a registered dietitian as an integral part of diabetes self-management education. Details of optimal delivery of MNT and diabetes self-management education in general have been discussed recently (1,13).

Key goals of MNT for youth with diabetes are: (1) to promote normal growth and development with appropriate weight gain, (2) to optimize glycemic control, (3) to optimize cardiovascular risk profile including lipid profile and blood pressure. Goals are to be accomplished through healthy food choices and physical activity, with consideration of individual metabolic status and treatment regimen as well as community and family culture, individual preferences and willingness to change. Wysocki has recently reviewed extensively behavioral and psychosocial aspects of self-management approaches for youth with diabetes in general (14). Although not necessarily specific to MNT, behavioral interventions that consider family support and communications, stress and anxiety management, coping and social skills, and problem solving may be useful.

ESTIMATES OF DIETARY INTAKE IN YOUTH

From national survey data, a majority of youth consumed higher than recommended levels of total and saturated fat, and fewer than 50% of youth met recommendations for intake of calcium, fiber, fruits, and vegetables (15–19). It would seem reasonable to think that youth at high risk for a nutrition-related chronic disease might have dietary intakes that more closely reflected current nutrition recommendations. However, Kelley et al. (20) compared usual dietary intake in

TABLE 1 Recommended Dietary Intake for Children and Adolescents with Diabetes

Nutrients	Source	Age 9–13 yr Males	Age 9–13 yr Females	Age 14–18 yr Males	Age 14–18 yr Females	Age 19+ yr Males	Age 19+ yr Females
% Total fat	AHA[a] and HP[b] 2010	30% total energy (AHA)					
		Target: 75% ≤ 30% total energy (HP 2010)					
% Saturated fat	AHA, ADA[c] and HP 2010	<10% total energy (AHA and ADA)					
		Target: 75% < 10% total energy (HP 2010)					
Calcium (mg)	IOM DRI–AI[d]	75% consuming ≥ 1300 mg/day					
Vitamin C (mg)	IOM DRI–EAR[e]	39	39	63	56	75	60
Vitamin E (α-tocopherol, mg)	IOM DRI–EAR[e]	9	9	12	12	12	12
Iron (mg)	IOM DRI–EAR[e]	5.9	5.7	7.7	7.9	6	8.1
Fiber (g)	IOM DRI–AI[d]	23.9	20	29.3	29.3	29.3	19.2
Food groups							
Fruits	HP 2010			Target: 75% ≥ 2 servings/day			
Vegetables	HP 2010			Target: 50% ≥ 3 servings/day			
Grains (total)	HP 2010			Target: 50% ≥ 6 servings/day			
Whole grains	HP 2010			Target: 50% ≥ 3 servings/day			

[a]AHA, American Heart Association (4).
[b]HP 2010, Healthy People 2010 (5).
[c]ADA, American Diabetes Association (6).
[d]IOM DRI–AI, Institute of Medicine, Dietary Reference Intakes based on 0.77* Adequate Intake (7) for calcium (8) or fiber (9).
[e]IOM DRI, based on estimated average requirement for Vitamin C (10) or Vitamin E (11) or iron (12).

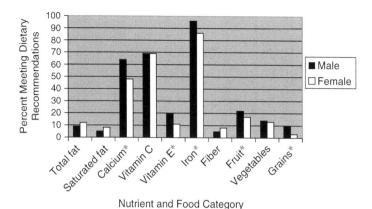

Nutrient and Food Category

* p <0.01 for comparison of Male versus Female, adjusted for clinical site, race/ethnicity, and parental education

FIGURE 1 Percent of males and females with diabetes who meet Dietary Recommendations: SEARCH for Diabetes in Youth Participants in the Dietary Assessment Protocol, Prevalent 2001 and Incident 2002.

children with a family history of early cardiovascular disease (CVD) to children without such a family history and found no difference in reported intake of dietary fats, cholesterol, or fiber.

Remarkably few data have been published on dietary intake among youth with DM. SEARCH for Diabetes in Youth investigators have shown that dietary intake of adolescents with either T1DM ($n = 1531$) or T2DM ($n = 186$) is high in total and saturated fat, low in vitamin E, and low in fiber, fruits, and vegetables compared with current nutrition recommendations (3). Specifically, percent energy from dietary fat did not differ according to DM type and ranged from 36.9 to 38.2 for youth with T1DM or T2DM, aged 10 to 14 years, or 15 years, or older, compared with the recommended 30% or less. Similarly, compared with the recommended intake of 10% or less from saturated fat, youth with DM reported intakes of about 13%. The finding of high intake of dietary fat is consistent with results of Helgeson et al. (21) among 132 adolescents with T1DM. Although dietary fat intake did not differ according to DM type, youth with T2DM in the SEARCH study consumed less calcium, magnesium, and vitamin E than youth with T1DM ($p < 0.01$ for each) (3). Intake of soda among older (aged 15+ years) youth with T2DM was twice that of older youth with T1DM ($p < 0.01$).

A useful way to describe dietary intake is to consider the percent of individuals who meet nutrition guidelines. As shown in Figure 1, only 6.5% of the SEARCH cohort met ADA recommendation for percent of energy from saturated fat. Less than 50% met recommendations for total fat, vitamin E, fiber, fruits, vegetables, and grains, although a majority met recommendations for vitamin C, calcium, and iron. Without a doubt, there is a great need to develop, evaluate, and disseminate effective approaches to improve dietary intake in youth with diabetes.

DIETARY APPROACHES TO OPTIMAL GLYCEMIC CONTROL

The key dietary factor influencing glycemic control is the total amount of carbohydrate. Increased fiber, fructose, lactose, and fat are dietary constituents that tend to lower glycemic response. Other characteristics of food such as type of starch (i.e., proportion of amylase vs. amylopectin), cooking style and time, and ripeness of fruit impact the glycemic effect of the food. Because carbohydrate-containing foods provide important nutrients and dietary fiber, very low carbohydrate diets (less than 130 g/day) are not recommended, and consistent with current US Department of Agriculture (USDA), intake of at least 14 gm/1000 kcal dietary fiber and selection of whole grain products (at least half of all grain servings) is recommended by the ADA.

The most recent guidelines published by the ADA note the importance of adjustment of premeal insulin based on the (anticipated) carbohydrate content of the meal. Currently, there are three main dietary approaches to accounting for the carbohydrate content of meals: food exchanges, carbohydrate counting, and selection of low glycemic index (GI) foods. It is now well recognized that use of carbohydrate counting provides considerably more flexibility in food choices than the exchange system and is often preferred. Particularly for youth with diabetes, such flexibility is critical given variable schedules and appetites of youth. Carbohydrate counting (or use of exchanges) and inclusion of low-GI foods are not mutually exclusive. In fact, as a result of pre- and postprandial glucose testing over time, some individuals develop what is referred to as "experience-based estimation" which essentially considers both amount and type of carbohydrate as well as other factors (e.g., premeal fasting or non-fasting, other constituents of the meal, physical activity) in order that food, physical activity, and insulin are balanced to attain appropriate glycemic control.

The remarkable lack of empiric evidence as to the effectiveness of these and related approaches, including approaches to nutrition education for youth with diabetes, has been highlighted by Waldron et al. (22). These authors also note a potential concern with undue focus on carbohydrate in nutrition education that intake of dietary fat (particularly saturated fat) may increase to the detriment of cardiovascular risk management. However, one clinical trial conducted among 104 youth with T1DM compared traditional food exchange system with a more flexible approach focused on selection of low-GI foods. Macronutrient content did not differ between these approaches (23), and glycemic control was improved among those on the low-GI intervention compared with the traditional exchange group (23). A trial of "dose-adjustment for normal eating (DAFNE)" (24) conducted among adults using intensified insulin therapy demonstrated improved glycemic control and improved quality of life, however educational approaches were specific to adult education thus findings are not directly applicable to youth.

Carbohydrate Counting

Carbohydrate counting was used successfully (although not exclusively) in the Diabetes Control and Complications Trial (25) and has been promoted for widespread use in clinical practice since that time. The basics of carbohydrate counting have been described (26) as a progression of three levels of complexity. The first level considers total carbohydrate content of meals and focuses on consistency of carbohydrate intake from day-to-day, relative to the patient's diabetes medication regimen. Instruction on carbohydrate content of commonly consumed foods, and portion size estimation, is emphasized. The second level introduces the combined impacts of carbohydrate intake and other meal constituents, insulin or other diabetes medication, physical activity, and glucose monitoring on attaining optimal glycemic control. Finally, patients using multiple daily insulin injections or an insulin pump are instructed how they can match short-acting insulin to carbohydrate intake using carbohydrate to insulin ratios.

Glycemic Index
Current ADA nutrition recommendations suggest that, "The use of GI and load may provide a modest additional benefit over that observed when total carbohydrate is considered alone (1)." The Canadian nutrition guidelines more explicitly encourage selection of low-GI foods (2). However, there is considerable debate as to merit of the GI as an approach to reduce postprandial glucose excursions and thus improve overall glycemic control. The premise of GI is that glucose excursion due to ingestion of a carbohydrate containing food, relative to that of a standard food, is fairly constant across individuals and thus can be quantified as GI for that food (27,28). The rationale for use of GI as a part of MNT is that slowed digestion and absorption of carbohydrate from food, accomplished via choice of low-GI foods, will yield long term metabolic benefits initiated by blunted glucose excursions following consumption of carbohydrate-containing foods (29). A meta-analysis demonstrated modest benefit of low- versus high-GI diets to reduce hemoglobin A1c (HbA1c) in persons with diabetes (30). There are no published studies at this time that specifically evaluated use of GI to improve glycemic control in youth with diabetes not taking insulin, however in nondiabetic adults, GI as a function of usual dietary intake does not appear to be associated with glycemia (31).

GI values currently utilized have been determined based on glucose excursion following ingestion of test foods or meals administered in the fasting state (32). The glycemic loads of foods, meals, and diets are calculated by multiplying the GI of the constituent foods by the amounts of carbohydrate in each food and then totaling the values for all foods. Foods with low glycemic indices include oats, lentils, legumes, pasta, pumpernickel (coarse rye) bread, apples, oranges, and milk. However, several potential methodological problems with the GI have been noted (31). For example, macronutrients in mixed meals often elicit glucose and insulin excursions well beyond the time used to establish the GI (33,34). Moreover, it has been shown that glycemic response to the same meal consumed serially through the day (4 hours apart) can vary considerably (33,35,36). Debate continues regarding the impact of dietary protein and fat in the overall diet on glycemia (34,37–39). Finally, recent studies demonstrate that on an individual (40) and group basis (41), glycemic response to food may be quite variable.

The summary of Gannon and Nuttall in 1987 (33) remains true today that considerable methodological work will be needed to generate a dietary measure or set of measures that capture the known nutrient and nonnutrient determinants of carbohydrate digestion and absorption rates, and their metabolic effects. Thus, carbohydrate counting, either explicitly or experience-based estimation, along with selection of high fiber, whole grain products, and recognition of individual-level response to commonly consumed foods (potentially reflecting selection of low versus high GI foods), is the most appropriate overall focus for MNT toward the critical goal of optimal glucose control.

DIETARY APPROACHES TO OPTIMAL CVD RISK PROFILE

The metabolic syndrome (MetS), previously known as the insulin resistance syndrome, is characterized by a clustering of CVD risk factors, including glucose intolerance, abdominal obesity, hypertriglyceridemia, low high-density lipoprotein cholesterol (HDL-C), and high blood pressure (42,43), as well as elevated levels of inflammatory cytokines (44). Although the notion of the MetS being a true syndrome has recently been challenged (45,46), components of the syndrome, as well as low-density lipoprotein cholesterol (LDL-C), have been associated with an increased risk of cardiovascular disease (47–49). These risk factors are important predictors of CVD specifically among individuals with DM as well (50,51).

The presence of insulin resistance in individuals with T2DM is well documented, and insulin resistance has also been observed in individuals with T1DM (52,53). Dabelea et al. (54) reported associations among markers of insulin resistance and coronary artery calcification in young adults with T1DM. The SEARCH for Diabetes in Youth study reported that CVD risk profile is worse for youth with either T1DM or T2DM compared with nondiabetic youth (55). Thus, for youth with DM it is critically important to identify modifiable factors that can contribute to, and conversely be used to ameliorate, an already adverse CVD risk profile. Potential nutritional approaches that may be relevant are considered below, and include weight management, macronutrients, micronutrients, and dietary patterns.

Weight Management

It is well known that the prevalence of overweight in childhood has increased dramatically in recent years (56), particularly among race/ethnic groups at high risk for T2DM such as African-Americans (57). Of importance to cardiovascular health, measures of central adiposity have also increased dramatically in nondiabetic U.S. children and adolescents (58). Further, overweight in youth has been associated with adverse levels of blood pressure, HDL-C, and triglycerides (56), and overweight in adolescents tracks into adulthood (56,59). The prevalence of overweight among youth with T2DM is extremely high and (55), in fact, excess adiposity is considered a major risk factor for development of T2DM in youth (60,61). Less well recognized is the prevalence of excess adiposity among youth with T1DM. Using the Centers for Disease Control and Prevention definitions for "at risk for overweight" and "overweight," the SEARCH for Diabetes in Youth study reported that the prevalence of overweight among youth with T1DM is similar to that of the nondiabetic population. However, the prevalence of being "at risk for overweight" was significantly higher among youth with T1DM than among nondiabetic youth (62).Thus, it is important to incorporate consideration of weight management strategies not only for patients with T2DM, but also for selected patients with T1DM.

It is beyond the scope of this chapter to comprehensively review the extensive literature dealing with obesity treatment in children and adolescents. Individual and family based approaches have been reviewed recently (63–65) and demonstrate modest success at best. Considerable work has been done to advance understanding of various aspects of parenting styles and degree of parental direction of weight management strategies that may be supportive, or not supportive, of success in adoption of appropriate diet and physical activity behaviors (66–70). Particularly, given limited success with individual-level interventions to address a major public health problem, schools have become an important venue to provide education on healthy lifestyles, appropriate food and beverage choices, and opportunities for physical activity (71).

In terms of specific findings from recent research, longitudinal studies in nondiabetic children (72,73) have shown that lower intake of calcium and dairy products predict increased risk for obesity. This finding takes on particular importance given the recent observation that only 9% of children aged 7 to 14 years met the national recommendations for dairy consumption (74). A partial explanation for the association of low dairy intake with obesity may be that soft drinks have largely replaced milk as a beverage (16) and prospectively, increased soft drink consumption has been associated with increased weight gain and obesity in youth (75). Low intake of whole grains has been associated with higher BMI and worse insulin sensitivity (76). Although fruit and vegetable consumption has been promoted in the context of obesity prevention in youth (77), intake of fruits and vegetables in adolescents was not associated with one year change in BMI in a large observational cohort of U.S. youth (78). A school-based intervention that resulted in reduced percent calories from total and saturated fat (79) did not lead to statistically significant change in blood pressure, body size, or cholesterol concentrations (80). More recently, Planet Health was a two-year, school-based intervention to decrease television viewing, decrease intake of high-fat foods, increase intake of fruits and vegetables, and increase physical activity in middle-school youth (81). Favorable effects on obesity were observed among girls, but not boys.

Whether individual, family, or school based, some specific behaviors commonly targeted for change are reduced consumption of sweetened beverages (soda in particular); reduced consumption of high-fat foods commonly purchased from fast food restaurants; reduced portion sizes; increased consumption of low-fat milk, fruits, vegetables and whole grain products; reduced time spent in physical inactivity (e.g., TV viewing, computer); and increased time spent on physical activity including team and individual pursuits.

There is a notable paucity of data on efficacy of weight management interventions for youth with diabetes. For youth with T2DM, the Treatment Options for type 2 Diabetes in Adolescents and Youth (TODAY) is ongoing and includes an intensive lifestyle intervention arm that is likely to yield critical information (82). Among adolescent girls with T1DM, increased intake of dietary fat has been associated with increased gain in percentage of body fat over one year (83). Also of interest, increased number of daily insulin injections (6 vs. 4) was positively associated with gain in body fat, thus underscoring the need to consider weight management for youth with diabetes not in isolation, but rather as part of overall strategies for diabetes self-management.

Macronutrients

From studies of nondiabetic adults, diets high in fat appear to promote obesity (84), but whether this is due to metabolic or behavioral effects (i.e., palatability, satiety) is controversial (85–87). Several studies have identified dietary fat as a contributor to insulin resistance independent of obesity (88–96), but other studies do not support this (97–99). All types of dietary fat, except n-3 fatty acids, may have an adverse effect on insulin sensitivity, with the most consistent findings for saturated fat. N-3 fatty acids may have beneficial effects on inflammatory markers (100–102).

Increased intake of trans fatty acids have been associated consistently with higher LDL-C (103), and with increased concentration of inflammatory markers

(104); however, studies of effects of trans fatty acids on insulin resistance have been equivocal (98,105–106). Diets high in monounsaturated fats (107–111) or low in fat and high in total carbohydrates (53,112–118) can reduce LDL-C compared with diets high in saturated fat. However, low saturated fat, high-carbohydrate diets may increase plasma triglycerides (107), and may decrease plasma HDL-C compared with isocaloric, high monounsaturated fat diets (119,120). A recent meta-analysis (121) of the metabolic impact of low-carbohydrate versus low-fat approaches to weight management suggested that low-carbohydrate diets may result in better triglyceride and HDL-C concentrations, but worse LDL-C concentration, with no difference in weight after one year. From two large studies that included adults with DM, Mayer-Davis et al. (122) reported that higher total dietary fat intake was associated consistently with higher LDL-C.

The action of dietary carbohydrate on lipid profile is complex and is influenced by energy balance, type of carbohydrate (e.g., starch vs. fructose or sucrose), and fiber (123). Recently, Bray et al. reported a remarkable increase of >1000% in consumption of high fructose corn syrup, the sole caloric sweetener used in soft drinks in the United States (124). Fructose may be particularly detrimental to energy balance and related CVD risk factors because fructose does not substantially stimulate insulin production (an important signal of the "fed" state) and stimulates de novo lipogenesis. Increased fiber intake has been associated with lower serum C-reactive protein (CRP) in both cross-sectional and longitudinal analyses (125). McKeown et al. (126) showed that increased whole-grain intake was negatively associated, and a high GI was positively associated with the prevalence of the MetS in the Framingham Offspring Cohort. In contrast, Liese et al. (127) showed no association of GI with insulin sensitivity measured directly by an intravenous glucose tolerance test. Among individuals with DM, Mayer-Davis et al. (122) reported that higher carbohydrate intake was associated with increased triglyceride concentrations only among those with previously undiagnosed DM and only among those who gained weight during the previous year.

There are surprisingly few studies of the effect of nutritional factors on CVD risk profile in youth with DM. Among 58 youth with T1DM, percent energy from complex carbohydrates was associated inversely with HDL-C and positively with triglyceride concentrations; however, no associations were seen for dietary fat intake and hyperlipidemia (128). Umpaichitra et al. showed that an oral fat load designed to mimic a high-fat, fast-food meal led to enhanced postprandial lipemia in 12 minority youth with type 2 DM, compared with matched nondiabetic normal weight, or nondiabetic obese control youth (129). Substantially more research is needed in order to elucidate the role of macronutrients in promoting appropriate weight and optimizing CVD risk profile youth with DM.

Micronutrients

There has been considerable interest recently in the potential role of calcium, magnesium, and dairy products on development of obesity, insulin resistance, and the MetS in adults. Dietary magnesium has been inversely related to systolic and diastolic blood pressure (130), but not with incident hypertension (131); however, a protective effect of magnesium on development of coronary heart disease has been reported (132). It has been suggested that intracellular magnesium concentrations (reduced in both DM and hypertension) may explain some of the association of DM with hypertension via simultaneous effects on insulin action and vascular tone

(133). Basic research has suggested a role of calcium in energy partitioning to reduce fat storage (134,135) and epidemiologic studies have now shown an inverse association of calcium intake with obesity and with dyslipidemia (136,137). Low intake of dairy products (rich in both calcium and magnesium) has been linked to obesity, to components of the MetS, and to the MetS itself (135,137−139). However, Al-Delaimy et al. found no association between calcium intake and risk for ischemic heart disease among men (140).

Plasma vitamin C, fruit intake, and dietary vitamin C intake were significantly inversely associated with CRP in healthy adults (141). Among adults with T2DM, supplementation with vitamin E reduced CRP (142). However, high dose supplementation with vitamin E or beta carotene does not appear to provide protection against coronary heart disease (143). Most previous studies were constrained by limited methods to evaluate the dose response effects. Effects below a threshold of high-dose supplementation may have been missed. Careful consideration of potential dose response effects within intake available from food, as well as supplementation, is needed to fully understand whether or not micronutrients can improve CVD risk profiles in patients with DM.

Dietary Patterns

Studies of whole diets have yielded generally consistent results, although again research conducted among youth with diabetes are lacking. The Dietary Approaches to Stop Hypertension (DASH) trial provided critical evidence of the efficacy of a diet rich in fruits, vegetables, and low-fat dairy products with reduced total and saturated fat to substantially reduce blood pressure (144) and to reduce total, LDL-C, and HDL-C without an adverse impact on triglycerides (145). Interestingly, individuals with high CRP experienced less improvement in lipid profile than those with low CRP (146). Intake of fiber (147) and of fruits and vegetables has been associated inversely with CRP (148). Using data from the EPIC-Potsdam study, a dietary pattern was constructed based on the DASH diet, and was associated with reduced incidence of hypertension (149). Consumption of a "Mediterranean diet" (defined as high in whole grains, vegetables, fruits, olive oil, dairy, fish, and moderate alcohol intake) was associated with lower prevalence of the MetS in a Greek population (150). Food patterns derived from cluster analyses of the Malmo Diet and Cancer Cohort showed diets characterized by high fiber bread were associated with lower central obesity and hyperglycemia in men, whereas in women, dietary patterns characterized by white bread (positively) and by milk fat (negatively) were associated with hyperinsulinemia and dyslipidemia (151). Clinical trial data support a reduction in several markers of inflammation following ingestion of a Mediterranean diet compared with a prudent diet (<30% calories from fat); however, the observed beneficial effects may have been largely due to significantly greater weight loss in individuals consuming the Mediterranean diet (152).

SUMMARY

Current nutrition recommendations for youth with diabetes are designed to optimize both short- and long-term health, and include strategies to integrate dietary intake as part of overall diabetes self-management for optimal glycemic control and reduced risk for chronic complications of diabetes, particularly CVD risk reduction. Recommendations to date derive predominantly from studies of healthy children or adults with diabetes, thus research is needed to elucidate specific nutritional factors that may impact specifically on health of youth with diabetes. Dietary behavior is inherently complex, influenced by a myriad of individual, family, and sociocultural factors. On the basis of available data, youth with diabetes generally do not meet nutrition recommendations. Research is, therefore, sorely needed to identify strategies to enable youth with diabetes to attain improved health through nutrition.

REFERENCES

1. Bantle JP, Wylie-Rosett J, Albright AL, et al. Nutrition recommendations and interventions for diabetes—2006: a position statement of the American Diabetes Association. Diabetes Care 2006; 29(9):2140–2157.
2. Canadian Diabetes Association. 2003 Clinical Practice Guidelines for the prevention and management of diabetes in Canada. Can J Diab 2003; 27(suppl 2):S1–S152.
3. Mayer-Davis EJ, Nichols M, Liese AD, et al. Dietary intake among youth with diabetes: the SEARCH for Diabetes in Youth Study. J Am Diet Assoc 2006; 106(5):689–697.
4. Krauss RM, Eckel RH, Howard B, et al. AHA Dietary Guidelines: revision 2000: A statement for healthcare professionals from the Nutrition Committee of the American Heart Association. Circulation 2000; 102(18):2284–2299.
5. US Department of Health and Human Services. Healthy people 2010: understanding and improving health. 2000. Washington, D.C., US Department of Health and Human Services.
6. Franz MJ, Bantle JP, Beebe CA, et al. Nutrition principles and recommendations in diabetes. Diabetes Care 2004; 27(suppl 1):S36–S46.
7. Institute of Medicine. Using the estimated average requirement for nutrient assessment of groups. In: Institute of Medicine, ed. Dietary Reference Intakes: Application in Dietary Assessment. Washington, D.C.: National Academy Press, 2000:73–105.
8. Institute of Medicine. Calcium. In: Institute of Medicine, ed. Dietary Reference Intakes for Calcium, Phosphorus, Magnesium, Vitamin D, and Fluoride. Washington, D.C.: National Academy Press, 1997:71–145.
9. Institute of Medicine. Dietary, functional, and total fiber. In: Institute of Medicine, ed. Dietary Reference Intakes for Energy, Carbohydrate, Fiber, Fat, Fatty Acids, Cholesterol, Protein, and Amino Acids (Macronutrients). Washington, D.C.: National Academies of Press, 2002:265–334.
10. Institute of Medicine. Vitamin C. In: Institute of Medicine, ed. Dietary Reference Intakes for Vitamin C, Vitamin E, Selenium, and Carotenoids. Washington, D.C.: National Academy Press, 2000:95–185.
11. Institute of Medicine. Vitamin E. In: Institute of Medicine, ed. Dietary Reference Intakes for Vitamin C, Vitamin E, Selenium, and Carotenoids. Washington, D.C.: National Academy Press, 2000:186–283.
12. Institute of Medicine, Food and Nutrition Board. Iron. In: Institute of Medicine, ed. Dietary Reference Intakes for Vitamin A, Vitamin K, Arsenic, Boron, Chromium, Copper, Iodine, Iron, Manganese, Molybdenum, Nickel, Silicon, Vanadium, and Zinc. Washington, D.C.: National Academy Press, 2000:290–393.
13. Mensing C, Boucher J, Cypress M, et al. National standards for diabetes self-management education. Diabetes Care 2007; 30(suppl 1):S96–S103.
14. Wysocki T. Behavioral assessment and intervention in pediatric diabetes. Behav Modif 2006; 30(1):72–92.
15. Munoz KA, Krebs-Smith SM, Ballard-Barbash R, et al. Food intakes of US children and adolescents compared with recommendations. Pediatrics 1997; 100(3 pt 1):323–329.
16. Troiano RP, Briefel RR, Carroll MD, et al. Energy and fat intakes of children and adolescents in the United States: data from the national health and nutrition examination surveys. Am J Clin Nutr 2000; 72(5 suppl):1343S–1353S.
17. Neumark-Sztainer D, Story M, Hannan PJ, et al. Overweight status and eating patterns among adolescents: where do youths stand in comparison with the healthy people 2010 objectives? Am J Public Health 2002; 92(5):844–851.

18. McDowell MA, Briefel RR, Alaimo K, et al. Energy and macronutrient intakes of persons ages 2 months and over in the United States: Third National Health and Nutrition Examination Survey, Phase 1, 1988–91. Adv Data 1994; 255:1–24.

19. Briefel RR, Johnson CL. Secular trends in dietary intake in the United States. Annu Rev Nutr 2004; 24:401–431.

20. Kelley DE, Kuller LH, McKolanis TM, et al. Effects of moderate weight loss and orlistat on insulin resistance, regional adiposity, and fatty acids in type 2 diabetes. Diabetes Care 2004; 27(1):33–40.

21. Helgeson VS, Viccaro L, Becker D, et al. Diet of adolescents with and without diabetes: trading candy for potato chips? Diabetes Care 2006; 29(5):982–987.

22. Waldron S, Hanas R, Palmvig B. How do we educate young people to balance carbohydrate intake with adjustments of insulin? Horm Res 2002; 57(suppl 1):62–65.

23. Gilbertson HR, Thorburn AW, Brand-Miller JC, et al. Effect of low-glycemic-index dietary advice on dietary quality and food choice in children with type 1 diabetes. Am J Clin Nutr 2003; 77(1):83–90.

24. DAFNE Study Group. Training in flexible, intensive insulin management to enable dietary freedom in people with type 1 diabetes: dose adjustment for normal eating (DAFNE) randomised controlled trial. BMJ 2002; 325(7367):746.

25. Anderson EJ, Richardson M, Castle G, et al. Nutrition interventions for intensive therapy in the Diabetes Control and Complications Trial. The DCCT Research Group. J Am Diet Assoc 1993; 93(7):768–772.

26. Gillespie SJ, Kulkarni KD, Daly AE. Using carbohydrate counting in diabetes clinical practice. J Am Diet Assoc 1998; 98(8):897–905.

27. Jenkins DJ, Wolever TM, Taylor RH, et al. Glycemic index of foods: a physiological basis for carbohydrate exchange. Am J Clin Nutr 1981; 34(3):362–366.

28. Wolever TM, Jenkins DJ, Jenkins AL, et al. The glycemic index: methodology and clinical implications. Am J Clin Nutr 1991; 54(5):846–854.

29. Wolever TM. The glycemic index. World Rev Nutr Diet 1990; 62:120–185.

30. Brand-Miller JC, Thomas M, Swan V, et al. Physiological validation of the concept of glycemic load in lean young adults. J Nutr 2003; 133(9):2728–2732.

31. Mayer-Davis EJ, Dhawan A, Liese AD, et al. Towards understanding of glycaemic index and glycaemic load in habitual diet: associations with measures of glycaemia in the Insulin Resistance Atherosclerosis Study. Br J Nutr 2006; 95(2):397–405.

32. Foster-Powell K, Holt SH, Brand-Miller JC. International table of glycemic index and glycemic load values: 2002. Am J Clin Nutr 2002; 76(1):5–56.

33. Gannon MC, Nuttall FQ. Factors affecting interpretation of postprandial glucose and insulin areas. Diabetes Care 1987; 10(6):759–763.

34. Nuttall FQ, Gannon MC. Plasma glucose and insulin response to macronutrients in nondiabetic and NIDDM subjects. Diabetes Care 1991; 14(9):824–838.

35. Ercan N, Gannon MC, Nuttall FQ. Effect of added fat on the plasma glucose and insulin response to ingested potato given in various combinations as two meals in normal individuals. Diabetes Care 1994; 17(12):1453–1459.

36. Nuttall FQ, Gannon MC, Wald JL, et al. Plasma glucose and insulin profiles in normal subjects ingesting diets of varying carbohydrate, fat, and protein content. J Am Coll Nutr 1985; 4(4):437–450.

37. Gannon MC, Nuttall FQ, Saeed A, et al. An increase in dietary protein improves the blood glucose response in persons with type 2 diabetes. Am J Clin Nutr 2003; 78(4):734–741.

38. Gannon MC, Nuttall FQ. Effect of a high-protein, low-carbohydrate diet on blood glucose control in people with type 2 diabetes. Diabetes 2004; 53(9):2375–2382.

39. Eckel RH. A new look at dietary protein in diabetes. Am J Clin Nutr 2003; 78(4):671–672.

40. Vega-Lopez S, Ausman LM, Griffith JL, et al. Inter-individual variability and intra-individual reproducibility of glycemic index values for commercial white bread. Diabetes Care 2007; 30(6):1412–1417.

41. Brillon DJ, Sison CP, Salbe AD, et al. Reproducibility of a glycemic response to mixed meals in type 2 diabetes mellitus. Horm Metab Res 2006; 38(8):536–542.

42. Reaven GM. Banting lecture 1988. Role of insulin resistance in human disease. Diabetes 1988; 37(12):1595–1607.

43. Grundy SM, Brewer HB Jr., Cleeman JI, et al. Definition of metabolic syndrome: report of the National Heart, Lung, and Blood Institute/American Heart Association conference on scientific issues related to definition. Arterioscler Thromb Vasc Biol 2004; 24(2): e13–e18.

44. Meigs JB. Invited commentary: insulin resistance syndrome? Syndrome X? Multiple metabolic syndrome? A syndrome at all? Factor analysis reveals patterns in the fabric of correlated metabolic risk factors. Am J Epidemiol 2000; 152(10):908–911.

45. Reaven GM. The metabolic syndrome: requiescat in pace. Clin Chem 2005; 51(6): 931–938.

46. Kahn R, Buse J, Ferrannini E, et al. The metabolic syndrome: time for a critical appraisal: joint statement from the American Diabetes Association and the European Association for the Study of Diabetes. Diabetes Care 2005; 28(9):2289–2304.

47. Bonora E, Kiechl S, Willeit J, et al. Carotid atherosclerosis and coronary heart disease in the metabolic syndrome: prospective data from the Bruneck study. Diabetes Care 2003; 26(4):1251–1257.

48. Lakka HM, Laaksonen DE, Lakka TA, et al. The metabolic syndrome and total and cardiovascular disease mortality in middle-aged men. JAMA 2002; 288(21):2709–2716.

49. Isomaa B, Almgren P, Tuomi T, et al. Cardiovascular morbidity and mortality associated with the metabolic syndrome. Diabetes Care 2001; 24(4):683–689.

50. Lehto S, Ronnemaa T, Haffner SM, et al. Dyslipidemia and hyperglycemia predict coronary heart disease events in middle-aged patients with NIDDM. Diabetes 1997; 46:1354–1359.

51. Jiang R, Schulze MB, Rifai N, et al. Non-HDL cholesterol and apolipoprotein B predict cardiovascular disease events among men with type 2 diabetes. Diabetes Care 2004; 27(8):1991–1997.

52. Williams KV, Erbey JR, Becker D, et al. Can clinical factors estimate insulin resistance in type 1 diabetes? Diabetes 2000; 49(4):626–632.

53. Yu-Poth S, Zhao G, Etherton T, et al. Effects of the National Cholesterol Education Program's Step I and Step II dietary intervention programs on cardiovascular disease risk factors: a meta-analysis. Am J Clin Nutr 1999; 69(4):632–646.

54. Dabelea D, Kinney G, Snell-Bergeon JK, et al. Effect of type 1 diabetes on the gender difference in coronary artery calcification: a role for insulin resistance? The Coronary Artery Calcification in Type 1 Diabetes (CACTI) Study. Diabetes 2003; 52(11):2833–2839.

55. Rodriguez BL, Fujimoto W, Mayer-Davis E, et al. Prevalence of cardiovascular disease risk factors in U.S. children and adolescents with diabetes: the SEARCH for Diabetes in Youth Study. Diabetes Care 2006; 29(8):1891–1896.

56. Thompson DR, Obarzanek E, Franko DL, et al. Childhood overweight and cardiovascular disease risk factors: the National Heart, Lung, and Blood Institute Growth and Health Study. J Pediatr 2007; 150(1):18–25.

57. Freedman DS, Khan LK, Serdula MK, et al. Racial and ethnic differences in secular trends for childhood BMI, weight, and height. Obesity (Silver Spring) 2006; 14(2):301–308.

58. Li C, Ford ES, Mokdad AH, et al. Recent trends in waist circumference and waist-height ratio among US children and adolescents. Pediatrics 2006; 118(5):e1390–e1398.

59. Shmukh-Taskar P, Nicklas TA, Morales M, et al. Tracking of overweight status from childhood to young adulthood: the Bogalusa Heart Study. Eur J Clin Nutr 2006; 60(1): 48–57.

60. Libman IM, Arslanian SA. Prevention and treatment of type 2 diabetes in youth. Horm Res 2007; 67(1):22–34.

61. Vikram NK, Tandon N, Misra A, et al. Correlates of Type 2 diabetes mellitus in children, adolescents and young adults in north India: a multisite collaborative case-control study. Diabet Med 2006; 23(3):293–298.

62. Liu LL, Lawrence JM, Liese A, et al. Prevalence of overweight among US diabetic youth. Diabetes 2005; 54(suppl 1):A450.

63. Kirk S, Scott BJ, Daniels SR. Pediatric obesity epidemic: treatment options. J Am Diet Assoc 2005; 105(5 suppl 1):S44–S51.

64. Summerbell CD, Waters E, Edmunds LD, et al. Interventions for preventing obesity in children. Cochrane Database Syst Rev 2005; 3:CD001871.

65. Gibson LJ, Peto J, Warren JM, et al. Lack of evidence on diets for obesity for children: a systematic review. Int J Epidemiol 2006; 35(6):1544–1552.
66. Stein RI, Epstein LH, Raynor HA, et al. The influence of parenting change on pediatric weight control. Obes Res 2005; 13(10):1749–1755.
67. Wrotniak BH, Epstein LH, Paluch RA, et al. The relationship between parent and child self-reported adherence and weight loss. Obes Res 2005; 13(6):1089–1096.
68. Golan M, Kaufman V, Shahar DR. Childhood obesity treatment: targeting parents exclusively v. parents and children. Br J Nutr 2006; 95(5):1008–1015.
69. Golley RK, Magarey AM, Baur LA, et al. Twelve-month effectiveness of a parent-led, family-focused weight-management program for prepubertal children: a randomized, controlled trial. Pediatrics 2007; 119(3):517–525.
70. Young KM, Northern JJ, Lister KM, et al. A meta-analysis of family-behavioral weight-loss treatments for children. Clin Psychol Rev 2007; 27(2):240–249.
71. Peterson KE, Fox MK. Addressing the epidemic of childhood obesity through school-based interventions: what has been done and where do we go from here? J Law Med Ethics 2007; 35(1):113–130.
72. Skinner JD, Bounds W, Carruth BR, et al. Longitudinal calcium intake is negatively related to children's body fat indexes. J Am Diet Assoc 2003; 103(12):1626–1631.
73. Carruth BR, Skinner JD. The role of dietary calcium and other nutrients in moderating body fat in preschool children. Int J Obes Relat Metab Disord 2001; 25(4):559–566.
74. Brady LM, Lindquist CH, Herd SL, et al. Comparison of children's dietary intake patterns with US dietary guidelines. Br J Nutr 2000; 84(3):361–367.
75. Ludwig DS, Ebbeling CB. Type 2 diabetes mellitus in children: primary care and public health considerations. JAMA 2001; 286(12):1427–1430.
76. Steffen LM, Jacobs DR Jr., Murtaugh MA, et al. Whole grain intake is associated with lower body mass and greater insulin sensitivity among adolescents. Am J Epidemiol 2003; 158(3):243–250.
77. Krebs NF, Jacobson MS. Prevention of pediatric overweight and obesity. Pediatrics 2003; 112(2):424–430.
78. Field AE, Gillman MW, Rosner B, et al. Association between fruit and vegetable intake and change in body mass index among a large sample of children and adolescents in the United States. Int J Obes Relat Metab Disord 2003; 27(7):821–826.
79. Lytle LA, Stone EJ, Nichaman MZ, et al. Changes in nutrient intakes of elementary school children following a school-based intervention: results from the CATCH Study. Prev Med 1996; 25(4):465–477.
80. Luepker RV, Perry CL, McKinlay SM, et al. Outcomes of a field trial to improve children's dietary patterns and physical activity. JAMA 1996; 275(10):768–776.
81. Gortmaker SL, Peterson K, Wiecha J, et al. Reducing obesity via a school-based inter-disciplinary intervention among youth: Planet Health. Arch Pediatr Adolesc Med 1999; 153(4):409–418.
82. Zeitler P, Epstein L, Grey M, et al. Treatment options for type 2 diabetes in adolescents and youth: a study of the comparative efficacy of metformin alone or in combination with rosiglitazone or lifestyle intervention in adolescents with type 2 diabetes. Pediatr Diab 2007; 8(2):74–87.
83. Willett WC, Howe GR, Kushi LH. Adjustment for total energy intake in epidemiologic studies. Am J Clin Nutr 1997; 65(suppl 4):1220S–1228S.
84. Astrup A, Grunwald G, Melanson E, et al. The role of low-fat diets in body weight control: a meta-analysis of *ad libitum* dietary intervention studies. Int J Obes 2000; 24:1545–1552.
85. Bray GA, Popkin BM. Dietary fat affects obesity rate. Am J Clin Nutr 1999; 70(4):572–573.
86. Bray GA, Popkin BM. Dietary fat intake does affect obesity! Am J Clin Nutr 1998; 68(6):1157–1173.
87. Willett WC. Dietary fat and obesity: an unconvincing relation. Am J Clin Nutr 1998; 68(6):1149–1150.
88. Manson J, Spelsberg A. Primary prevention of non-insulin dependent diabetes mellitus. Am J Prev Med 1994; 10:172–184.

89. Marshall J, Bessesen DH, Hamman R. High saturated fat and low starch and fiber are associated with hyperinsulinaemia in a non-diabetic population: The San Luis Valley Diabetes Study. Diabetologia 1997; 40(4):430–438.

90. Feskens EJM, Loeber JG, Kromhout D. Diet and physical activity as determinants of hyperinsulinemia: the Zutphen Elderly Study. Am J Epidemiol 1994; 140:350–360.

91. Folsom AR, Ma J, McGovern PG, et al. Relation between plasma phospholipid saturated fatty acids and hyperinsulinemia. Metabolism 1996; 45(2):223–228.

92. Lovejoy J, DiGirolamo M. Habitual dietary intake and insulin sensitivity in lean and obese adults. Am J Clin Nutr 1992; 55:1174–1179.

93. Lovejoy J, Windhauser M, Rood J, et al. Effect of a controlled high-fat versus low-fat diet on insulin sensitivity and leptin levels in African-American and Caucasian women. Metabolism 1998; 47(12):1520–1524.

94. Mayer EJ, Newman B, Quesenberry CP, et al. Usual dietary fat intake and insulin concentrations in healthy women twins. Diabetes Care 1993; 16:1459–1469.

95. Mayer-Davis EJ, Monaco JH, Hoen HM, et al. Dietary fat and insulin sensitivity in a triethnic population: the role of obesity. The Insulin Resistance Atherosclerosis Study (IRAS). Am J Clin Nutr 1997; 65:79–87.

96. Maron DJ, Fair JM, Haskell WL. Saturated fat intake and insulin resistance in men with coronary artery disease. Circulation 1991; 84:2020–2027.

97. Hughes VA, Fiatarone MA, Fielding RA, et al. Long-term effects of a high-carbohydrate diet and exercise on insulin action in older subjects with impaired glucose tolerance. Am J Clin Nutr 1995; 62(2):426–433.

98. Louheranta AM, Turpeinen AK, Vidgren HM, et al. A high-trans fatty acid diet and insulin sensitivity in young healthy women. Metabolism 1999; 48(7):870–875.

99. Sarkkinen E, Schwab U, Niskanen L, et al. The effects of monounsaturated-fat enriched diet and polyunsaturated-fat enriched diet on lipid and glucose metabolism in subjects with impaired glucose tolerance. Eur J Clin Nutr 1996; 50(9):592–598.

100. Zhao G, Etherton TD, Martin KR, et al. Dietary alpha-linolenic acid reduces inflammatory and lipid cardiovascular risk factors in hypercholesterolemic men and women. J Nutr 2004; 134(11):2991–2997.

101. Lopez-Garcia E, Schulze MB, Manson JE, et al. Consumption of (n-3) fatty acids is related to plasma biomarkers of inflammation and endothelial activation in women. J Nutr 2004; 134(7):1806–1811.

102. Wu D, Han SN, Meydani M, et al. Effect of concomitant consumption of fish oil and vitamin E on production of inflammatory cytokines in healthy elderly humans. Ann N Y Acad Sci 2004; 1031:422–424.

103. Sacks FM, Katan M. Randomized clinical trials on the effects of dietary fat and carbohydrate on plasma lipoproteins and cardiovascular disease. Am J Med 2002; 113 (suppl 9B):13S–24S.

104. Mozaffarian D, Pischon T, Hankinson SE, et al. Dietary intake of trans fatty acids and systemic inflammation in women. Am J Clin Nutr 2004; 79(4):606–612.

105. Bray GA, Lovejoy JC, Smith SR, et al. The influence of different fats and fatty acids on obesity, insulin resistance and inflammation. J Nutr 2002; 132(9):2488–2491.

106. Lovejoy JC, Smith SR, Champagne CM, et al. Effects of diets enriched in saturated (palmitic), monounsaturated (oleic), or trans (elaidic) fatty acids on insulin sensitivity and substrate oxidation in healthy adults. Diabetes Care 2002; 25(8):1283–1288.

107. Garg A, Bantle JP, Henry RR, et al. Effects of varying carbohydrate content of diet in patients with non-insulin-dependent diabetes mellitus. JAMA 1994; 271(18):1421–1428.

108. Walker KZ, O'Dea K, Johnson L, et al. Body fat distribution and non-insulin-dependent diabetes: comparison of a fiber-rich, high-carbohydrate, low-fat (23%) diet and a 35% fat diet high in monounsaturated fat. Am J Clin Nutr 1996; 63(2):254–260.

109. Parillo M, Rivellese AA, Ciardullo AV, et al. A high-monounsaturated fat/low carbohydrate diet improves peripheral insulin sensitivity in non-insulin-dependent diabetic patients. Metabolism 1992; 41:1373–1378.

110. Rasmussen OW, Thomsen C, Hansen KW, et al. Effects on blood pressure, glucose, and lipid levels of a high-monounsaturated fat diet compared with a high-carbohydrate diet in NIDDM subjects. Diabetes Care 1993; 16(12):1565–1571.

111. Campbell LV, Marmot PE, Dyer JA, et al. The high-monounsaturated fat diet as a practical alternative for NIDDM. Diabetes Care 1994; 17(3):177–182.

112. Stone DB, Connor WE. The prolonged effects of a low cholesterol, high carbohydrate diet upon the serum lipids in diabetic patients. Diabetes 1963; 12:127–132.

113. Hjollund E, Pedersen O, Richelsen B, et al. Increased insulin binding to adipocytes and monocytes and increased insulin sensitivity of glucose transport and metabolism in adipocytes from non-insulin-dependent diabetics after a low-fat/high-starch/high-fiber diet. Metabolism 1983; 32(11):1067–1075.

114. Simpson RW, Mann JI, Eaton J, et al. Improved glucose control in maturity-onset diabetes treated with high-carbohydrate-modified fat diet. Br Med J 1979; 1(6180): 1753–1756.

115. Abbott WGH, Boyce VL, Grundy SM, et al. Effects of replacing saturated fat with complex carbohydrate in diets of subjects with NIDDM. Diabetes Care 1989; 12:102–107.

116. Brunzell JD, Lerner RL, Hazzard WR, et al. Improved glucose tolerance with high carbohydrate feeding in mild diabetes. N Engl J Med 1971; 284(10):521–524.

117. Brunzell JD, Lerner RL, Porte D Jr., et al. Effect of a fat free, high carbohydrate diet on diabetic subjects with fasting hyperglycemia. Diabetes 1974; 23(2):138–142.

118. Hales CN, Randle PJ. Effects of low-carbohydrate diet and diabetes mellitus on plasma concentrations of glucose, non-esterified fatty acid, and insulin during oral glucose-tolerance tests. Lancet 1963; 1:790–794.

119. Garg A. High-monounsaturated-fat diets for patients with diabetes mellitus: a meta-analysis. Am J Clin Nutr 1998; 67(suppl):577S–582S.

120. Lichtenstein A, Ausman L, Carrasco W, et al. Short-term consumption of a low fat diet beneficially affects plasma lipid concentrations only when accompanied by weight loss. Arterioscl Throm 1994; 14:1751–1760.

121. Nordmann AJ, Nordmann A, Briel M, et al. Effects of low-carbohydrate vs low-fat diets on weight loss and cardiovascular risk factors: a meta-analysis of randomized controlled trials. Arch Dis Child 2006; 166(3):285–293.

122. Mayer-Davis EJ, Levin S, Marshall JA. Heterogeneity in associations between macronutrient intake and lipoprotein profile in individuals with type 2 diabetes. Diabetes Care 1999; 22(10):1632–1639.

123. Fried SK, Rao SP. Sugars, hypertriglyceridemia, and cardiovascular disease. Am J Clin Nutr 2003; 78(4):873S–880S.

124. Bray GA, Nielsen SJ, Popkin BM. Consumption of high-fructose corn syrup in beverages may play a role in the epidemic of obesity. Am J Clin Nutr 2004; 79(4):537–543.

125. Ma Y, Griffiths JA, Chasan-Taber L, et al. Association between dietary fiber and serum C-reactive protein. Am J Clin Nutr 2006; 83(4):760–766.

126. McKeown NM, Meigs JB, Liu S, et al. Carbohydrate nutrition, insulin resistance, and the prevalence of the metabolic syndrome in the Framingham Offspring Cohort. Diabetes Care 2004; 27(2):538–546.

127. Liese AD, Schulz M, Fang F, et al. Dietary glycemic index and glycemic load, carbohydrate and fiber intake, and measure of insulin sensitivity, secretion, and adiposity in the Insulin Resistance Atherosclerosis Study. Diabetes Care 2005; 28:2832–2838.

128. Wiltshire EJ, Hirte C, Couper JJ. Dietary fats do not contribute to hyperlipidemia in children and adolescents with type 1 diabetes. Diabetes Care 2003; 26(5):1356–1361.

129. Umpaichitra V, Banerji MA, Castells S. Postprandial hyperlipidemia after a fat loading test in minority adolescents with type 2 diabetes mellitus and obesity. J Pediatr Endocrinol Metab 2004; 17(6):853–864.

130. Ma J, Folsom AR, Melnick SL, et al. Associations of serum and dietary magnesium with cardiovascular disease, hypertension, diabetes, insulin, and carotid arterial wall thickness: the ARIC study. Atherosclerosis Risk in Communities Study. J Clin Epidemiol 1995; 48(7):927–940.

131. Peacock JM, Folsom AR, Arnett DK, et al. Relationship of serum and dietary magnesium to incident hypertension: the Atherosclerosis Risk in Communities (ARIC) Study. Ann Epidemiol 1999; 9(3):159–165.

132. Abbott RD, Ando F, Masaki KH, et al. Dietary magnesium intake and the future risk of coronary heart disease (the Honolulu Heart Program). Am J Cardiol 2003; 92(6): 665–669.

133. Paolisso G, Galderisi M, Tagliamonte MR, et al. Myocardial wall thickness and left ventricular geometry in hypertensives. Relationship with insulin. Am J Hypertens 1997; 10(11):1250–1256.

134. Shi H, Norman AW, Okamura WH, et al. 1Alpha,25-dihydroxyvitamin D3 modulates human adipocyte metabolism via nongenomic action. FASEB J 2001; 15(14):2751–2753.

135. Zemel MB, Shi H, Greer B, et al. Regulation of adiposity by dietary calcium. FASEB J 2000; 14(9):1132–1138.

136. Jacqmain M, Doucet E, Despres JP, et al. Calcium intake and body composition in adults. Obes Res 2001; 9:175S.

137. Pereira MA, Jacobs DR Jr., Van Horn L, et al. Dairy consumption, obesity, and the insulin resistance syndrome in young adults: the CARDIA Study. JAMA 2002; 287 (16):2081–2089.

138. Teegarden D. Calcium intake and reduction in weight or fat mass. J Nutr 2003; 133 (1):249S–251S.

139. Fleming KH, Heimbach JT. Consumption of calcium in the U.S.: food sources and intake levels. J Nutr 1994; 124(8 suppl):1426S–1430S.

140. Al-Delaimy WK, Rimm E, Willett WC, et al. A prospective study of calcium intake from diet and supplements and risk of ischemic heart disease among men. Am J Clin Nutr 2003; 77(4):814–818.

141. Wannamethee S, Lowe GD, Rumley A, et al. Associations of vitamin C status, fruit and vegetable intakes, and markers of inflammation and hemostasis. Am J Clin Nutr 2006; 83(3):525–526.

142. Upritchard JE, Sutherland WH, Mann JI. Effect of supplementation with tomato juice, vitamin E, and vitamin C on LDL oxidation and products of inflammatory activity in type 2 diabetes. Diabetes Care 2000; 23(6):733–738.

143. Tornwall ME, Virtamo J, Korhonen PA, et al. Effect of alpha-tocopherol and beta-carotene supplementation on coronary heart disease during the 6-year post-trial follow-up in the ATBC study. Eur Heart J 2004; 25(13):1171–1178.

144. Appel LJ, Moore TJ, Obarzanek E, et al. A clinical trial of the effects of dietary patterns on blood pressure. DASH Collaborative Research Group. N Engl J Med 1997; 336 (16):1117–1124.

145. Obarzanek E, Sacks FM, Vollmer WM, et al. Effects on blood lipids of a blood pressure-lowering diet: the Dietary Approaches to Stop Hypertension (DASH) Trial. Am J Clin Nutr 2001; 74(1):80–89.

146. Erlinger TP, Miller ER III, Charleston J, et al. Inflammation modifies the effects of a reduced-fat low-cholesterol diet on lipids: results from the DASH-sodium trial. Circulation 2003; 108(2):150–154.

147. Ajani UA, Ford ES, Mokdad AH. Dietary fiber and C-reactive protein: findings from national health and nutrition examination survey data. J Nutr 2004; 134(5):1181–1185.

148. Gao X, Bermudez OI, Tucker KL. Plasma C-reactive protein and homocysteine concentrations are related to frequent fruit and vegetable intake in Hispanic and non-Hispanic white elders. J Nutr 2004; 134(4):913–918.

149. Schulze MB, Hoffmann K, Kroke A, et al. Risk of hypertension among women in the EPIC-Potsdam Study: comparison of relative risk estimates for exploratory and hypothesis-oriented dietary patterns. Am J Epidemiol 2003; 158(4):365–373.

150. Panagiotakos DB, Pitsavos C, Chrysohoou C, et al. Impact of lifestyle habits on the prevalence of the metabolic syndrome among Greek adults from the ATTICA study. Am Heart J 2004; 147(1):106–112.

151. Wirfalt E, Hedblad B, Gullberg B, et al. Food patterns and components of the metabolic syndrome in men and women: a cross-sectional study within the Malmo Diet and Cancer cohort. Am J Epidemiol 2001; 154(12):1150–1159.

152. Esposito K, Marfella R, Ciotola M, et al. Effect of a mediterranean-style diet on endothelial dysfunction and markers of vascular inflammation in the metabolic syndrome: a randomized trial. JAMA 2004; 292(12):1440–1446.

18 Health Care Cost and Utilization

Reena Oza-Frank
Nutrition and Health Sciences Program, Hubert Department of Global Health,
The Rollins School of Public Health, Atlanta, Georgia, U.S.A.

Ping Zhang and Giuseppina Imperatore
Division of Diabetes Translation, Centers for Disease Control and Prevention,
Atlanta, Georgia, U.S.A.

K.M. Venkat Narayan
Hubert Department of Global Health, The Rollins School of Public Health,
Atlanta, Georgia, U.S.A.

INTRODUCTION

Diabetes imposes large economic burdens worldwide on nations, individuals, and their families (1). The disease lowers people's quality of life in many ways, including their physical and social functioning and their perceived physical and mental well-being (1). If these issues affect a patient's ability/motivation for disease self-management, costs can be even greater.

The medical costs of diabetes have risen substantially during the past 25 years (2) due to advancements in technology and treatment. These medical advancements not only help in identifying new cases of diabetes but also enable people with the disease to live longer lives, thereby requiring additional years of treatment, all of which further increase diabetes-related costs.

Although extensive information is available on health care cost and utilization in diabetes, little differentiation is made by diabetes type. In addition, limited data are available on diabetes among children and youth, because national surveys on health care cost and utilization typically and more accurately represent adults. Type 1 diabetes accounts for the majority of cases of total diabetes in children and adolescents. Because 90–95% of all adult diabetes cases are type 2, much of the costs data apply to this population. Consequently, adults and children with type 1 diabetes, children with non–type 1 diabetes, and women with gestational diabetes comprise the majority of the remaining proportion of people with the disease. This chapter uses existing data to describe health care cost and utilization among youth with diabetes (Table 1).

TYPES OF COSTS

Overall Costs
During 2002, the estimated total (i.e., direct and indirect) cost attributable to diabetes in the United States was US $132 billion. Of this amount, $92 billion was direct medical costs and $40 billion was indirect costs (3). The average annual health care cost for a person with diabetes in 2002 was US $13,243 (unadjusted for age and sex), compared with an average annual cost of US $2560 for a person without the disease (3). Between 1997 and 2002, the average annual health care cost for a person with diabetes rose by 30% (3). These figures provide an overall picture

TABLE 1 Examples of Current U.S. Surveys Collecting Health Care Cost and Utilization
Information on Children with Diabetes

References	Survey	Data source	Age range available	Variables collected
35	National Health Interview Survey	Self-report	<18 yr	Health insurance, number and sources of outpatient contacts, hospitalizations, and potential productivity lost due to morbidity and mortality
36	Medical Expenditure Panel Survey	Self-report, medical providers, private- and public-sector employers	<18 yr	Specific health services used, frequency of use, cost of services and how they are paid for, and data on cost, scope, and breadth of private health insurance held by and available to the U.S. population
37	National Hospital Discharge Survey	Inpatient hospital records	All for only hospitals with an average length of stay of <30 days, general hospitals, or children's general hospitals	Inpatients discharged from nonfederal, short-stay hospitals in the United States
38	NAMCS	Physician's office fill out patient record forms	All	Visits (not inpatients) to office-based physicians, reasons for visit, ICD-CM for diagnoses, causes of injury and procedures, and medication use
	NHAMCS	Hospital staff fill out patient record forms	All	Visits (not inpatients) to hospital emergency and outpatient departments, reasons for visit, ICD-CM for diagnoses, causes of injury and procedures, and medication use
39	SEARCH for Diabetes in Youth	Self-report	<20 yr	Health care utilization, processes of care, and quality of life

Abbreviations: ICD-CM, international classification of diseases, clinical modification; NAMCS, National Ambulatory Medical Care Survey; NHAMCS, National Hospital Ambulatory Medical Care Survey.

of the economic burden of diabetes in the United States. The next sections separate costs by category (i.e., direct and indirect).

Direct Medical Costs
Direct medical costs include resources used to treat disease and provide medical care (2). These types of costs can be estimated from survey data or studies of

medical or billing records (2). For example, among private insurance claims in a large multisource database, total medical costs of inpatient/outpatient care and prescribed drugs and medical supplies were lowest among people aged 0 to 18 years and highest among those aged 35 to 64 years; however, the three medical cost categories together were above US $5000 for youth with diabetes (4). The following subsections provide specific information on different categories within direct medical costs.

Outpatient Visits

Children and adolescents with chronic diseases, particularly diabetes, are more likely than those without such diseases to visit physicians' offices (5). For example, the growth and hormonal changes associated with moving from childhood to adolescence, and eventually to adulthood, require adjustment of medication regimens in children with diabetes; resulting in increased medical office visits. For privately insured people with diabetes, among all age groups and diabetes types, outpatient visits cost more than inpatient care, prescribed drugs, and medical supplies (4).

Medication

The average annual cost of insulin treatment during 2002 was reported to be US $1778 per patient. This figure includes glucose monitoring supplies, insulin delivery supplies, and insulin (3). One study found that, regardless of sex, the cost of insulin and diabetes supplies was the highest for persons aged 0 to 18 years (4).

Hospitalizations

The largest component of direct medical costs is generally diabetes-related hospital care (6). Hospitalization is 6.5 times more common among people with than without the disease (7). Hospitalizations account for 63–80% of all direct costs for all people with type 1 diabetes (8). In the United States, childhood diabetes is one of the 10 leading causes of preventable hospitalization among people younger than 18 years of age (9). During 2000, in hospital discharges among children and adolescents aged 0 to 17 years, approximately 75% of the discharges that included diabetes as any listed diagnosis, cited diabetes as the first-listed diagnosis, of which about 60% of these were for diabetic ketoacidosis (DKA) (10).

Studies suggest that prevention activities, quality outpatient care, and patient self-management may prevent or reduce the prevalence of acute complications such as multiple hospitalizations due to DKA and chronic complications such as cardiovascular disease and lower extremity amputations (12). In a projection of costs associated with controlling glycosylated hemoglobin values in patients with uncontrolled type 1 diabetes, one study found that US $3.6 billion could be saved over 10 years by reaching the recommended glycosylated hemoglobin target of 6.5% (13). The inclusion of indirect costs in this figure increased savings to US $5.2 billion.

Patient self-management including taking medications appropriately, controlling blood glucose levels, managing diet, and engaging in regular exercise are all important components of diabetes care (12). Although each of these items is associated with monetary costs as well as costs in time, both of which increase the overall health costs of diabetes, without these inputs into self-management and care, the overall costs of diabetes could potentially be even greater.

Direct Nonmedical Costs

Youth with diabetes need assistance from parents, guardians, or other adults in managing their disease. Disease-management assistance is one of the more important costs associated with diabetes in children and adolescents, although it is also one of the most difficult to measure.

Indirect Costs

Indirect costs are associated with loss of productivity due to disease. Productivity loss can result from morbidity, disability, and/or premature mortality. Traditional productivity, however, is not a very good measure for children and adolescents, because most likely they are not yet in the labor force. Nonetheless, one can assume that projected lifetime indirect costs for children with diabetes would be high because of the early onset of acute and chronic complications. Although many studies have found no difference in the academic performance between children with and without diabetes (14), other studies have shown that poor control of the disease might have a negative impact on a child's school performance (15), possibly leading to decreased productivity later in life. A recent systematic review showed that children with type 1 diabetes were more likely than other children to miss school (14). In addition, parents or guardians who provide care for children with diabetes may miss work when their children are sick, which also could be considered an indirect cost.

Quality of life is another measure of indirect costs. Children with diabetes most likely experience more pain and suffering, both physiological and psychological, than other children, thereby reducing their quality of life. Pain and suffering, however, are difficult to measure, and little information has been published on their associated indirect costs.

FACTORS INFLUENCING HEALTH CARE UTILIZATION

Age

The risk of diabetes-associated complications increases with the disease's duration, which subsequently increases the probability of health care utilization. Health care cost and utilization may also increase separately from diabetes costs because of other aging-related health problems. Regardless of age, however, women spend more in total medical costs than men do because of a high number of outpatient visits (4).

Ethnic Group

A few studies address differences in health care utilization by race/ethnicity. Overall, minority children utilize health care differently than do white children (studies referred to did not specify whether they meant all white children or only non-Hispanic white children). This finding could be attributed to a variety of factors including, but not limited to, socioeconomic status and language/cultural barriers. For example, in a Wisconsin cohort of newly diagnosed cases of diabetes among people younger than 30 years old, blacks had a higher hospitalization rate than whites did (11). Other investigations have found that blacks (both adults and children) have worse metabolic control than whites do and that black children are hospitalized for DKA more frequently than white children are (16,17). Research also shows that black and Hispanic children use less health care than do children from other racial/ethnic groups (18,19). However, another study found that use and expenditure patterns for most services were not significantly different between low-income and middle- to high-income black children and were lower than those for white children (20).

Insurance

Among factors that could influence health care utilization, insurance coverage is the most studied. Overall, the U.S. Census reports that 34.1% of children younger than 18 years of age were, at some point during 2003, not covered by private health insurance. One-third of the children who were not continuously covered by private insurance went without any health insurance, and the remaining children had some coverage through public health insurance programs such as Medicaid or State Children's Health Insurance Program (SCHIP) (21). Children from low-income families were more likely than children from middle- to high-income families to be uninsured (13.0% vs. 5.8%) or covered by public insurance (50.8% vs. 7.3%) and less likely to be privately insured (36.2% vs. 87.0%) (20). In addition, approximately 15% of families with children with type 1 diabetes had difficulty obtaining coverage or had to wait for insurance approval because of preexisting illness clauses (22).

Although a large portion of medical expenses are usually covered by private and public health insurance programs for individuals with such coverage, persons with diabetes may still incur substantial out-of-pocket expenses for physician services, medications, laboratory tests, and other services that require co-payments. In the United States, out-of-pocket costs for patients younger than age 65 are roughly two times higher for a person with diabetes than without diabetes (23). In one study, nearly one-third of the families with a child with diabetes spent more than $1000 of their own money on health care (22). A case-control study of families with and without children with diabetes showed that out-of-pocket expenses were 56% higher in the diabetes-affected families than in the control families, despite similarities in percentage of families with or without insurance in both groups (22). Seventeen percent of diabetes-affected families, particularly those of low income, had expenses that were more than 10% of their household income (22). People in the United States with type 1 diabetes who do not have health insurance visit physicians (24) and test their blood glucose (22) less frequently than those who have insurance. In a follow-up study to the Diabetes Control and Complication Trial, persons without insurance coverage had worse levels of glycemic control than those with insurance (25), further indicating that the relationships between access to care, health care utilization, and poor health outcomes in diabetes are legitimate. Finally, the number of multiple hospitalizations is 80% higher for pediatric patients enrolled in Medicaid than for their privately insured counterparts (12).

Socioeconomic Status

Observational studies have shown that children with diabetes use more health care if they come from households with higher, as opposed to lower, incomes and parents with more, as opposed to less, years of education (18,19), possibly because this group can better afford out-of-pocket expenses or are better equipped to navigate the health care system. The burden of out-of-pocket expenses is more profound among the lowest income type 1 diabetes families (2). Some studies suggest that persons of low socioeconomic status who have type 1 diabetes have higher hospitalization rates than persons of higher socioeconomic status (11). Some studies conducted in the 1990s suggest that low socioeconomic status and poor metabolic control increase risk of hospitalizations (26); however, these studies do not reflect current practices in diabetes care. Finally, children with diabetes from low-income families, compared with those from middle- to high-income families, were less likely to have had a medical or dental office visit (63.7% vs. 76.5% for office-based visits), less likely to have medicines prescribed (45.1% vs. 56.4%), and more likely to have made trips to an emergency department (14.6% vs. 11.4%) (20).

Diabetes Complications

Complications of diabetes include neurological disease, peripheral vascular disease, cardiovascular disease, renal disease, endocrine/metabolic complications, ophthalmic disease, and other chronic complications (3). As children with diabetes grow older, the number and severity of disease-associated complications are likely to increase, as has been shown in adults with type 2 diabetes. Health care costs and utilization are higher among persons with a greater number of diabetes-related complications.

INTERNATIONAL PERSPECTIVE

Overall, diabetes-related costs and utilization vary by country and region. For example, blood glucose meters cost, on average, US $105 per glucose meter in the Western Pacific and US $61 in South and Central America (27). Similarly, a box of 50 blood glucose strips costs US $50 in North America and US $20 in Southeast Asia, and a box of 100 urine glucose strips costs US $20 in North America and US $5 in Southeast Asia. In some countries these supplies are subsidized or supplied free of charge to specific groups of people with diabetes. Insulin is crucial for survival to people with type 1 diabetes. The average cost of 100 insulin syringes is highest in North America, followed by South and Central America and Africa and is cheapest in Southeast Asia and Western Pacific (27). Insulin is available worldwide, but access differs by country due to taxes on insulin and other supplies needed for diabetes care (28).

Developed Countries

The World Health Organization estimates that more than 80% of expenditures for diabetes-related medical care are generated in the world's economically richest countries (29). The United States spends more than 50% of all global expenditure for diabetes care, whereas Europe accounts for another 25%; the remaining industrialized countries, such as Australia and Japan, account for most of the rest of diabetes care spending (29). These estimates account for none of the indirect costs of pain and suffering that people with diabetes, as well as their families and friends, incur.

European children with diabetes have higher hospitalization rates than comparable US children. In Germany, diabetes-related hospitalization costs were estimated to be US $506 per person-year, totaling US $12.4 million for German children aged 1 to 19 years. This constitutes a majority of total hospitalization costs associated with diabetes in Germany (8). Another German study showed that children and adolescents with diabetes onset between 1 and less than 15 years of age had significantly more hospital admissions (4.7 times) and hospital days (7.7 times) than nondiabetic control subjects. Another German study showed that 61.1% of the diabetic children and adolescents used diabetes-related medical ambulatory services at least once quarterly (30). Older children (ages 5 to <10 and 10 to <15 compared with ages 1 to <5) and females experienced a significantly increased number of hospital days; higher socioeconomic status was significantly related to a lower hospitalization risk and a decreased number of hospital days (9).

Developing Countries

Type 1 diabetes is particularly costly in terms of mortality in poor countries, because insulin is often not available (29). For example, in Zambia, a person diagnosed as needing insulin will live an average of 11 years, a person in Mali has a life expectancy of 30 months, and a person in Mozambique has only 12 months (29). Data on the direct medical costs of diabetes are not easily available for most developing countries. An extrapolation from developed countries suggests that in 2003, the direct costs of diabetes worldwide for people aged 20 to 79 years totaled at least US $129 billion and may have been as high as US $241 billion. Much of these costs were out-of-pocket because of these countries' lack of adequate health care infrastructures (29).

Among developing countries, medical costs are highest in Latin America and the Caribbean, where families pay 40–60% of diabetes care out-of-pocket. Similarly, in India, the poorest people with diabetes spend an average of 25% of their income on care (29). In Sudan, the mean annual income of the households was estimated at US $1222 and the median annual expenditure of diabetes care was US $283/ diabetic child, of which 36% was spent on insulin. Among families with a child with diabetes, 65% of total family expenditures on health were used for the diabetic child. Among all developing countries, the direct health care costs of diabetes range from 2.5% to 15.0% of annual health care budgets, depending on local prevalence and sophistication of the treatments available (1).

In developing countries, indirect costs of diabetes are at least as high, or even higher, than direct medical costs (31). Because the largest predicted rise in the number of people with diabetes in the next three decades will be among those in the economically productive ages of 20 to 64 years (32), the future indirect costs of diabetes are likely to be even larger than they are now (1).

GAPS IN THE LITERATURE

Type 2 Diabetes in Children

Until recently, type 2 diabetes was so rare among children and adolescents that very little data/literature was available on this population. Even today, there are not enough cases of type 2 diabetes in children and adolescents to adequately study health care cost and utilization in this population. What is known is that a majority of the patients diagnosed with type 2 diabetes in the pediatric population are obese (33), leading to initial treatment regimens for weight loss such as medical nutrition therapy. However, pharmacological therapy may also be initiated to enhance the effects of proper diet and exercise. Because progression of β-cell failure is anticipated with increased duration of disease, the number of treatments for glycemic control is likely to increase with age (32), which will inevitably increase medical care costs. In addition, due to increased frequency of the disease and earlier onset of complications, the financial burden to the population as a whole will rise (33). The long-term economic burden of type 2 diabetes in youth is currently unknown, because the likelihood of long-term complications and associated health care costs are unknown. Future studies are planned to collect information needed to examine this issue (34).

Data Limitations

No single data source exists on health care cost and utilization representative of children and adolescents with type 1 diabetes (3). Multiple data sources (Table 1) must be used; even then, meaningful interpretation of the data is limited by small sample sizes (3). In addition, the parents/guardians of children with diabetes are often our only source of information concerning indirect costs of disease and health care use. This may not capture the full impact the disease has on the child's quality of life.

Some examples of questions that remain unanswered because of limitations in the data are as follows:

- How much of total health care costs among youth is dedicated to diabetes?
- What are the estimated direct and indirect costs of diabetes in children with type 1 diabetes?
- What are the health care costs and utilization patterns by diabetes type?
- What are the health care costs by diabetes complication in children with type 1 and type 2 diabetes?
- How much will interventions cost and what will be their benefits?
- What would it cost to implement a program to prevent/control diabetes in children and adolescents?

The answers to most of these questions exist for adults with diabetes, but are lacking in children and adolescents with diabetes.

CONCLUSION

Diabetes is one of the most common chronic illnesses among children and adolescents (35); nonetheless, limited information is available concerning diabetes-related health care cost and utilization for this population. Diabetes is clearly an expensive disease to manage, both in costs for medical care and in quality of life. In general, research indicates an increasing trend in costs associated with diabetes due to advancing technologies. A complete picture of the health care costs and utilization in children with diabetes (both type 1 and type 2) is yet to be determined.

The contents of this chapter are solely the responsibility of the authors and do not necessarily represent the official views of the CDC.

REFERENCES

1. Narayan KMV, Zhang P, Kanaya AM, et al. Diabetes: the pandemic and potential solutions. In: Jamison DT, Breman JG, Measham AR, et al., eds. Disease Control Priorities in Developing Countries, 2nd ed. New York: Oxford University Press and The World Bank, 2006:591–603.
2. Songer TJ. Economic costs. In: Ekoe JM, Zimmet P, Williams R, eds. The Epidemiology of Diabetes Mellitus: An International Perspective. England: John Wiley and Sons, 2001:381–397.

3. Hogan P, Dall T, Nicolov P. Economic costs of diabetes in the US in 2002. Diabetes Care 2003; 26(3):917–932.
4. Zhang P, Imai K. The relationship between age and healthcare expenditure among persons with diabetes mellitus. Expert Opin Pharmacother 2007; 8(1):49–57.
5. Ning L, Samuels ME. Increased health care utilization associated with child day care among health maintenance organization and Medicaid enrollees. Ambul Child Health 2001; 7:219–230.
6. Songer TJ. The economics of diabetes care: USA. In: Alberti KGGM, Zimmet P, DeFronzo RA, eds. International Textbook of Diabetes Mellitus, 2nd ed. New York: John Wiley and Sons, 1996:1643–1654.
7. Aro S, Kangas T, Reunanen A, et al. Hospital use among diabetic patients and the general population. Diabetes Care 1994; 17(11):1320–1329.
8. Icks A, Rosenbauer J, Holl RW, et al. Hospitalization among diabetic children and adolescents and the general population in Germany. German Working Group for Pediatric Diabetology. Diabetes Care 2001; 24(3):435–440.
9. Icks A, Rosenbauer J, Haastert B, et al. Hospitalization among diabetic children and adolescents and non-diabetic control subjects: a prospective population-based study. Diabetologia 2001, 44(suppl 3), B87–B92.
10. http://www.cdc.gov/diabetes/statistics/index.htm#hospitalization. Accessed May 2007.
11. Palta M, LeCaire T, Daniels K, et al. Risk factors for hospitalization in a cohort with type 1 diabetes. Wisconsin Diabetes Registry. Am J Epidemiol 1997; 146(8):627–636.
12. http://www.ahrq.gov/data/hcup/highlight1/high1.htm. Accessed May 2007.
13. Minshall ME, Roze S, Palmer AJ, et al. Treating diabetes to accepted standards of care: a 10-year projection of the estimated economic and health impact in patients with type 1 and type 2 diabetes mellitus in the United States. Clin Ther 2005; 27(6):940–950.
14. Milton B, Holland P, Whitehead M. The social and economic consequences of childhood-onset type 1 diabetes mellitus across the lifecourse: a systematic review. Diabet Med 2006; 23(8):821–829.
15. Elrayah H, Eltom M, Bedri A, et al. Economic burden on families of childhood type 1 diabetes in urban Sudan. Diabetes Res Clin Pract 2005; 70(2):159–165.
16. Delamater AM, Albrecht DR, Postellon DC, et al. Racial differences in metabolic control of children and adolescents with type I diabetes mellitus. Diabetes Care 1991; 14(1): 20–25.
17. Hanson CL, Henggeler SW, Burghen GA. Race and sex differences in metabolic control of adolescents with IDDM: a function of psychosocial variables? Diabetes Care 1987; 10(3):313–318.
18. Currie J, Gruber J. Health insurance eligibility, utilization of medical care, and child health. Q J Econ 1996; 111(2):431–466.
19. Edwards LN, Grossman M. Adolescent Health, Family Background, and Preventive Medical Care. NBER Working Paper No. W0398, 1979.
20. Simpson L, Owens PL, Zodet MW, et al. Health care for children and youth in the United States: annual report on patterns of coverage, utilization, quality, and expenditures by income. Ambul Pediatr 2005; 5(1):6–44.
21. Todd J, Armon C, Griggs A, et al. Increased rates of morbidity, mortality, and charges for hospitalized children with public or no health insurance as compared with children with private insurance in Colorado and the United States. Pediatrics 2006; 118(2): 577–585.
22. Songer TJ, LaPorte R, Lave JR, et al. Health insurance and the financial impact of IDDM in families with a child with IDDM. Diabetes Care 1997; 20(4):577–584.
23. Taylor AK. Medical expenditures and insurance coverage for people with diabetes: estimates from the National Medical Care Expenditure Survey. Diabetes Care 1987; 10(1):87–94.
24. Songer TJ, DeBerry K, LaPorte RE, et al. International comparisons of IDDM mortality. Clues to prevention and the role of diabetes care. Diabetes Care 1992, 15(suppl 1):15–21.
25. Lorenzi G. Post-study access to health care has influenced glycemic control in the DCCT cohort. Diabetes 1996; 45(suppl 2):7A(abstr).
26. Drash AL. Clinical care of the patient with diabetes. What is the role of the diabetes professional? Diabetes Care 1994, 17(suppl 1):40–44.

27. http://www.eatlas.idf.org/Insulin_and_diabetes_supplies/Cost_of_diabetes_supplies/. Accessed April 2007.
28. http://www.eatlas.idf.org/Insulin_and_diabetes_supplies/Cost_of_insulin/. Accessed April 2007.
29. http://www.idf.org/home/index.cfm?node=41. Accessed April 2007.
30. Icks A, Rosenbauer J, Haastert B, et al. Direct costs of pediatric diabetes care in Germany and their predictors. Exp Clin Endocrinol Diabetes 2004; 112(6):302–309.
31. Barcelo A, Aedo C, Rajpathak S, et al. The cost of diabetes in Latin America and the Carribean. Bull World Health Organ 2003; 81(1):19–27.
32. King H, Aubert RE, Herman WH. Global burden of diabetes, 1995–2025: prevalence, numerical estimates, and projections. Diabetes Care 1998; 21(9):1414–1431.
33. Dolan LM. Type 2 diabetes in children and adolescents. In: Menon RK, Sperling MA, eds. Pediatric Diabetes. Boston: Kluwer Academic Publishers, 2003:61–88.
34. Songer TJ, Glazner J, Coombs L, et al. Examining the economic costs related to lifestyle and pharmacological interventions in youth with type 2 diabetes. Expert Rev Pharmacoeconomics Outcomes Res 2006; 6(3):315–324.
35. Bloom B, Dey AN, Freeman G. Summary health statistics for US children: National Health Interview Survey, 2005. Vital Health Stat 2006; 10(231):1–84.
36. http://www.ahrq.gov/data/mepsweb.htm#faq. Accessed May 2007.
37. http://www.cdc.gov/nchs/about/major/hdasd/nhdsdes.htm. Accessed May 2007.
38. http://www.cdc.gov/nchs/about/major/ahcd/faq.htm. Accessed May 2007.
39. Liese AD, D'Agostino RB Jr., Hamman RF, et al. The burden of diabetes mellitus among US youth: prevalence estimates from the SEARCH for Diabetes in Youth Study. Pediatrics 2006; 118(4):1510–1518.

Treatment Patterns in Youth with Diabetes

Harvey K. Chiu and Catherine Pihoker
*Division of Endocrinology, Children's Hospital and Regional Medical Center,
University of Washington, Seattle, Washington, U.S.A.*

INTRODUCTION

While insulin has long been the foundation of treatment in diabetes mellitus, over the past decade exciting modalities have become available in the therapeutic armamentarium. Within the spectrum of insulin options, new insulin analogs offer means to more closely reproduce normal physiologic insulin secretion than ever. The development of insulin pumps with continuous glucose monitoring brings closer the reality of a closed-loop system of glucose homeostasis. Type 2 diabetes mellitus (T2DM) in children and insulin resistance overlying features of type 1 diabetes mellitus (T1DM) are becoming increasingly common (1–4). Thus, the intervention paradigms available to address the pathophysiology of T2DM and insulin resistance, such as insulin sensitizers, are becoming more important in the pediatric diabetes population. New classes of medications, such as the incretins, offer the potential promise of β-cell preservation. Overall, new treatments and technologies enhance the ability to safely and effectively implement intensive treatment regimens. Intensive treatment is crucial to avoid the complications of poorly controlled diabetes mellitus, as clearly demonstrated by findings from the Diabetes Control and Complications Trial (5). This is particularly important as the number of children with diabetes, particularly with onset at very young ages, continues to rise.

MONITORING OF CHILDREN WITH DIABETES

Blood Glucose Monitoring
Monitoring of glucose levels is at the core of optimal diabetes management. A dizzying array of glucose meters is available on the market, and numerous studies point to the accuracy and utility of glucose meters (6–8). Glucose meters typically require a blood sample from a fingerstick, where a rich capillary network offers optimal blood sampling. Devices requiring volumes as low as 0.3 µL are now available. Glucose meters are also available that are able to sample blood from alternate sites such as the forearm, where fewer nerve endings may allow for less painful sample acquisition. The drawback in using non-fingerstick blood samples is a delay in the true glucose value (9), a concern during times of rapidly dynamic glucose changes. When hypoglycemia is suspected or at significant risk, the fingerstick should be the site of blood glucose acquisition.

Tissue/Interstitial Glucose Monitoring
The GlucoWatch G2 Biographer alarm (Cygnus Inc., Redwood City, California, U.S.) offers a noninvasive system designed to measures glucose values in near-real time. The GlucoWatch functions by "reverse iontophoresis," a process by which glucose is assayed through intact skin by applying an electroosmotic flow via a

low-level electrical current (10–11). The device alarms to hypoglycemic events by sensing both absolute glucose levels as well as downward trends in glucose. Limitations to the GlucoWatch system have resulted in its having lower than expected use in clinical practice. These limitations include an inability to sense absolute hypoglycemia, lack of precision or data when skin is warm and moist, as with exercise, and a relatively high rate of false alarms (12). However, noninvasive monitoring remains a desirable option for the pediatric population.

A promising adjunct has been the development of continuous glucose monitoring sensors (CGMS) by Minimed (Guardian®), Dexcom (STS®), and Abbott (Navigator®). Utilizing a subcutaneous probe, CGMS enables glucose sampling every few minutes. Benefits of CGMS include the detection of asymptomatic or nocturnal hypoglycemic episodes that would otherwise be underappreciated or unrecognized, postprandial hyperglycemia, as well as tracking trends in glucose levels (13,14). As CGMS has been used only in clinical research studies until very recently (15–17), the role of CGMS in clinical practice for children with diabetes is emerging.

Long-term Assessment of Glycemic Control: Hemoglobin A_{1c} and Fructosamine

Serum proteins are nonenzymatically covalently bound to glucose at a rate proportional to blood glucose concentrations. This principle allows for the measurement of average glycemic levels over a period of time correlating with the serum viability of a particular protein. The glycosylation of hemoglobin (Hb) enables an assessment of glycemic levels over two to three months, the duration of red blood cell viability. Glycated Hb comprises three species—HbA_{1a}, HbA_{1b}, and HbA_{1c}. HbA_{1c}, which represents the Amadori glycosylation of the terminal valine of each β chain of Hb, comprises about 80% of glycated HbA_1 and is the part that best represents the mean blood glucose values.

Fructosamine represents the glycosylation of albumin, a protein with a much shorter half-life than HbA_{1c}, and thus is able to represent glycemic control over the previous two to three weeks—a much shorter window of reference than HbA_{1c}. Fructosamine is susceptible to factors that affect its production and degradation—specifically nutritional status, hepatic disease, and renal disease.

For the past three decades, HbA_{1c} or glycated Hb have been the best measures of glycemic control in diabetes populations, useful for both individuals and population studies. Fructosamine is an alternative when HbA_{1c} may be inaccurate in any of the aforementioned scenarios, or perhaps when a short-term assessment of glycemic control may be desired, as in a very recent treatment change.

Blood and Urine Ketones

The appearance of ketones in blood or urine denotes insulin inadequacy, either through an absolute lack (such as insulin pump failure) or through exacerbation of insulin resistance, as in illness and the accompanying milieu of counterregulatory hormones and cytokines. With illness or hyperglycemia, ketone monitoring is advised for early detection and hopefully avoidance of diabetic ketoacidosis. Urine ketones are limited by the fact that they represent only acetoacetate and not β-hydroxybutyrate, the most prevalent ketone body in diabetic ketoacidosis. Capillary blood β-hydroxybutyrate meters are now available and may offer a more sensitive and earlier indication of insulinopenia (18). A capillary blood sample can be obtained rapidly, as opposed to the common challenge of obtaining a urine sample quickly in an infant or young child, and/or when severely dehydrated. Thus, though not universally used, assessment of blood ketones may be a superior to urine ketones as a measure of insulin deficiency, including in the emergency room setting (19).

TREATMENT GOALS

Goals of treatment for children as well as adults are published annually by the American Diabetes Association in the first supplement to *Diabetes Care* (20). Hypoglycemia is a particular concern in the pediatric population because detection of hypoglycemia may be more difficult, as it is often dependent on parent/caregiver to recognize symptoms when children are too young to express them. Also, severe hypoglycemia, especially if recurrent in young children or associated with seizure activity or coma, may predispose these patients to neurocognitive deficits (21–25).

While diet and physical activity are important components in the approach of the patient with diabetes mellitus, pharmacotherapy is essential for patients with T1DM, and is often necessary for those with T2DM. The treatment of T1DM requires the initiation of insulin at diagnosis. For the management of T2DM, the very different pathophysiology offers much more varied means of treatment. Figure 1 describes an overview of pharmacologic therapy for diabetes mellitus.

TYPE 1 DIABETES MELLITUS

T1DM represents a physiologic state of absolute or near-absolute insulinopenia, for which administration of exogenous insulin is the crux of treatment. Since the first administration of injectable insulin in a child in 1922 by Banting and Best (26–28), insulin pharmacology has evolved from bovine and pork sources to biosynthetic insulin to the numerous insulin analogs available today. Highly purified insulin preparations have largely eliminated the immunogenic complications associated with the early animal insulins, such as allergic reactions and immune-mediated insulin resistance. Table 1 summarizes available insulin types.

Regular Insulin

Regular insulin is solubilized by a complex with zinc. Multiple linkages, primarily hexamers, retard the availability of a subcutaneous injection such that action onset is usually at 30 minutes, with a peak after two to three hours and a typical duration of activity of four to six hours. Intravenously, the onset of effect is practically immediate, as the half-life lasts only a few minutes. The products Humulin R® and Novolin R® are unbuffered. The buffering provided by disodium phosphate in Velosulin® stabilizes the insulin in infusion pumps.

Neutral Protamine Hagedorn

Neutral Protamine Hagedorn (NPH) is an insulin of intermediate duration. Its solubility has been delayed by the neutralization of the acidic insulin with protamine, a basic protein. Slow absorption of insulin ensues with enzymatic breakdown of the protamine. Denaturization of the NPH may occur if the product is exposed to heat or if a vial is used for more than one month, and manifests as

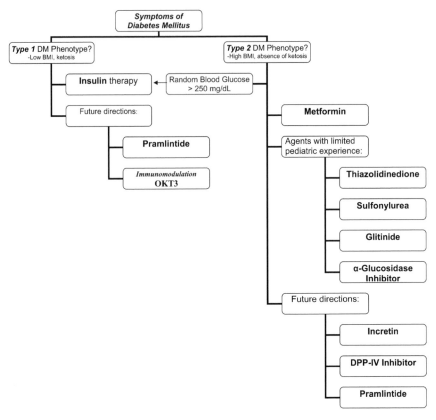

FIGURE 1 Overview of the pharmacologic treatment algorithm.

TABLE 1 Insulins and Duration of Actions at Typically Prescribed Doses

Insulin	Species source	Onset	Peak	Duration
Rapid-acting analog-insulin				
Lispro (Humalog®, Lilly)	Recombinant	15–30 min	30–90 min	3–5 hr
Aspart (Novolog®, Novo Nordisk)	Recombinant	15–30 min	1–3 hr	3–5 hr
Glulisine (Apidra®, Sanofi-Aventis)	Recombinant	20 min	30–90 min	1.5–3.5 hr
Inhaled Insulin (Exubera®, Pfizer)	Recombinant	10–20 min	30–90 min	3–5 hr
Short-acting insulin				
Regular (Humulin R®, Lilly; Novolin R®, Novo Nordisk; Velosulin®, Novo Nordisk)	Human	30–60 min	2–3 hr	4–6 hr
Intermediate-acting insulin				
NPH (Humulin N®, Lilly; Novolin N®, Novo Nordisk)	Human	1–4 hr	5–10 hr	10–16 hr
Long-acting insulin				
Glargine (Lantus®, Sanofi-Aventis)	Recombinant	1–2 hr	6–16 hr	20–24 hr
Detemir (Levemir®, Novo Nordisk)	Recombinant	1–2 hr	8–10 hr	5.7–23 hr

Source: From Refs. 41–50.

"clumping" in solution or "frosting" along the sides of the vial—an indication to use a new vial.

Insulin Analogs

Insulin lispro, aspart, and glulisine are modified, rapid-acting insulin analogs with comparable pharmacokinetics that remain as monomers and upon subcutaneous injection are absorbed rapidly (29–34). The structural differences of rapid-acting analogs relative to regular insulin have enabled their use in the rare cases of patients who have developed antibodies to regular insulin and subsequent allergy or severe insulin resistance. The rapid-acting insulins are delivered either by injection or through insulin pump to provide "bolus" insulin doses. This is the main feature of the "basal/bolus" insulin regimen described below.

Glargine and detemir are modified, long-acting, relatively peakless insulin analogs that are able to provide a basal insulin dose (35–38). Glargine is soluble at an acidic pH, but at the relatively neutral pH of a subcutaneous injection site, becomes relatively insoluble and forms an essentially 24-hour depot for insulin release. Insulin glargine has been suggested to not be mixed with short-acting insulin prior to injection because it may perturb the expected pharmacokinetics of these other insulins. However, a few studies (39,40) support the use of glargine mixed with rapid-acting analog insulin, in an effort to decrease the number of daily injections, albeit with perhaps a need for a higher dose of the rapid-acting analog insulin. Detemir is a more recent addition to the basal insulin class. Detemir insulin generally has a shorter duration of action, requiring twice daily dosing of detemir. This potential disadvantage is balanced by a possible more peakless profile than glargine (41) that may offer benefits of lower risk of severe hypoglycemia (42) and perhaps lower weight gain (43) than glargine insulin.

Some basic caveats to follow include the fact that onset and duration are affected by the absolute insulin dose. Studies demonstrate a fairly wide range in duration of detemir, a described "basal" insulin—from 5.7 to 23.2 hours—depending on the administered dose (37). Within the typical doses that these respective "rapid-acting" and "basal" analog insulins are being used, these insulins behave as typically described, but at the extremes of dosing, atypical pharmacokinetics may be observed.

Typical insulin injection sites include the abdomen, extremities, and buttocks. Absorption is most rapid from abdominal injection sites, followed by the extremities, and is slowest from the buttocks. Subcutaneous injection sites should be rotated on a regular basis to avoid lipohypertrophy, which may delay absorption and result in unpredictable insulin pharmacokinetics.

Inhaled insulin (44,45) was approved by the FDA for use in adults in 2006 for both T1DM and T2DM. The product available is Exubera®, marked in 1 mg and 3 mg blisters (comparable to approximately 3 U and 8 U of insulin, respectively) that are inhaled through a chamber device. However, current limitations make use of inhaled insulin impractical for treatment of pediatric patients. Doses of inhaled insulin are relatively large and can not be titrated with precision. Additional concerns are that insulin itself is a weak growth factor when bound to the insulin-like growth factor receptor, and cell proliferative effects are a theoretical question. Asthma, a common pediatric affliction, is also a contraindication. Inhaled insulin is yet to be approved in the pediatric or adolescent populations, but the promise for needle-phobic pediatric patients is interesting. In adult T2DM research studies, participants preferred the inhaled insulin over subcutaneous insulin (46–48). Because of its rapid onset and short duration of action, current inhaled insulin is only useful as prandial insulin, and hence a basal insulin still needs to be provided subcutaneously.

The choice of an insulin regimen is dependent on numerous factors, often balancing the attempts to mimic natural physiology with an individual patient's activities and social situation. In general, the insulin regimens may be dichotomized into two strategies: split/mixed and basal/bolus.

Split/Mixed Insulin Regimen

This traditional insulin regimen is based on the tenet of set doses of insulin at set times of the day, predicated on a fairly rigid carbohydrate consumption plan. The usual strategy is to provide a mixture of intermediate-acting insulin, such as NPH, with rapid- or short-acting insulin in two divided doses, given before breakfast and before dinner. Insulin peaks may occur between meals, necessitating the need for snacks. This regimen offers injections as few as twice a day (or three times, if the evening intermediate-acting insulin is administered at bedtime), and is attractive for families in whom circumstances preclude injections during the daytime, such as in the school-age child with no means of receiving an insulin injection at school. A significant downside is the relatively inflexibility of this regimen regarding caloric intake amounts and times. Food is consumed to match the insulin, rather than insulin being taken to match food intake. For this reason, the basal/bolus regimen is often preferred.

Basal/Bolus Regimen

This newer regimen has become popular with the advent of long-acting, relatively peakless insulin analogs. A basal amount of insulin is prescribed to inhibit hepatic gluconeogenesis and lipolysis. Bolus doses of rapid-acting insulin are then superimposed to control for glycemic surges associated with prandial carbohydrate intake.

Basal Insulin

Basal insulin typically represents 50% of the total daily insulin (TDI) dose, calculated at diagnosis of diabetes mellitus from an estimated initial TDI requirement of 0.5 to 1 U/kg body weight per day. When transitioning patients from a split/mix insulin regimen to a basal/bolus insulin regimen, the TDI requirement should be estimated to be 75–80% of the total split/mix insulin regimen, as often the insulin requirement is less with the basal/bolus regimen and such an insulin reduction will lower the risk of hypoglycemia in the transition.

Insulin glargine and insulin detemir are long-acting insulin analogs that are slowly and steadily absorbed from a depot subcutaneous injection site to provide a relatively peakless insulin release (35–38). The basal insulin is usually administered in the evening, as should these insulins not endure for an entire 24-hour period, prandial insulin given during the day will provide interval coverage. Though touted as "peakless," in some patients a small peak may be observed in the early hours after administration. In patients younger than six years of age, morning administration of basal insulin is a reasonable consideration. When the duration of basal insulin is less than 24 hours, the basal insulin is divided into twice-daily administration.

Bolus Insulin
As half of the TDI is provided as basal insulin, the remaining half essentially is provided as bolus insulin to cover prandial intake. Ideally, a specific amount of insulin is matched for a specific amount of carbohydrate intake (49). An initial estimation of this ratio can be made using a "500-rule." Using this rule, the quotient of 500 divided by the total insulin dose provides the amount of carbohydrates that a single unit of rapid-acting analog insulin will be expected to cover.

Correction Factor
A correction factor to normalize blood glucose values outside of the optimal range can also be calculated. With rapid-acting analog insulin, an "1800-rule" (50) can be utilized. The quotient of 1800 divided by the TDI dose will represent the glucose fall (in mg/dL) that 1 U of insulin will induce. This quotient can be used to estimate the additional insulin necessary for elevated blood glucose values, or conversely the amount of insulin that should be subtracted from an insulin dose if a glucose value below the target range is present.

The basal/bolus regimen, offers greater flexibility in the timing and amount of food intake relative to the split/mixed insulin regimen and results in fewer hypoglycemic events. Should social circumstances preclude administration of a midday injection, creative hybrid regimens have been used. For example, morning NPH may be added to the regimen to provide prandial coverage at midday. As oppose to a strict basal/bolus regimen, this would require a fixed carbohydrate content of the midday meal.

Continuous Subcutaneous Insulin Infusion
Continuous subcutaneous insulin infusion via insulin pumps in the pediatric population (51–53) offers flexibility in the appropriate motivated and committed patient and family. Insulin pumps can offer the advantage of decreasing the incidence of hypoglycemia relative to multiple-day insulin injections (54,55) and have proven a very viable option even in the preschool age group (56). Offering the most physiologic means of mimicking pancreatic physiology available, continuous subcutaneous insulin infusion affords great flexibility in the timing and amount of food consumed. Additionally, fluctuating basal insulin needs, such as increased needs during the dawn phenomenon or decreased needs during physical activity, can be titrated accordingly with the insulin pump. The flexibility offered by the insulin pump even allows for a regimen that allows the use of the pump overnight (57), a discontinuous "continuous" insulin infusion to take advantage of variable basal needs overnight, in combination with a multiple daily insulin injection regimen during the day to free the patient of the pump during daytime activities. Rapid-acting insulin (58–60) should be used with insulin pumps to offer this physiology.

The disadvantages of continuous subcutaneous insulin infusion are that there is no long-acting insulin, so that with interruption of insulin infusion, insulinopenia and potentially diabetic ketoacidosis can develop rapidly. Because of this possibility, families should be provided with an emergency prescription or supply of injectable basal and rapid-acting insulin on hand should a pump failure occur.

Starting Insulin Treatment

In a patient with long-standing diabetes mellitus completely devoid of endogenous insulin secretion and in the absence of significant insulin resistance, the TDI needs are, by definition of the "unit of insulin, 1 U/kg of body weight". Generally, the severity of presentation, including degree of hyperglycemia and ketosis as well as age, influence initial dose. During the pubertal growth spurt, as insulin resistance increases by 30%, daily insulin needs may approximate 1.5 U/kg of body weight. For a newly diagnosed diabetic patient, a prudent starting dose of insulin is typically 0.5 to 1 U/kg per day. Infants are usually more insulin sensitive and may require an initial total daily dose of <0.5 U/kg per day. Following the acute onset of T1DM, following resolution of the acute toxic hyperglycemic milieu (61,62), patients often enter a "honeymoon" phase in which the insulin requirements fall dramatically. The partial remission is defined as an insulin requirement <0.5 U/kg per day while maintaining very good glycemic control, e.g., HbA_{1c} <8%. The duration of this phase may last from weeks to months, but typically after one to two years, relapse eventuates into a requirement for increasing insulin needs that may reach 1 U/kg per day, or greater if there is an underlying level of insulin resistance. Insulin dose adjustments are made on the basis of the blood glucose values, and typically adjustments are no greater than 10% of the TDI dose.

Patients initiated on a split/mix regimen may be reasonably initiated on a regimen that divides the insulin into two administrations—two-third of the TDI dose before breakfast and one-third of the TDI dose before dinner. Of the morning dose, two-third should be provided as intermediate-acting NPH insulin and the remaining one-third should be provided as rapid-acting analog insulin. Of the evening dose, one-half should be provided as intermediate-acting NPH insulin and the remaining should be provided as rapid-acting analog insulin.

Surgery

Surgical, dental, or medical procedures often require a period of attenuated enteric intake. For patients on a split/mix regimen, the short or rapid-acting analog insulin should be withheld, and the NPH insulin should be administered at 50% of the usual dose (63). For patients on a basal/bolus regimen, the usual basal insulin dose should be administered, with usual correction doses provided as indicated. Prolonged cases may require a continuous intravenous insulin infusion with a dextrose-containing electrolyte solution. Different protocols have been published, but a reasonable regimen would be to provide insulin 0.025 to 0.03 U/kg per hour with an electrolyte solution containing 5–10% of dextrose, and with adjustments based on hourly glucose assessments targeting a glucose value 100 to 200 mg/dL.

Sick Day Management

From a diabetic standpoint, illness may be accompanied by a state of marked insulin resistance secondary to release of counterregulatory stress hormones as well as inflammatory cytokines. The primary challenges include (1) avoidance or correction of ketosis, avoiding diabetic ketoacidosis; (2) control of hyperglycemia; and (3) prevention of hypoglycemia that may ensue with efforts to confront the first two issues or due to poor oral intake. Vomiting may be due to the primary illness or more ominously to a secondary evolving diabetic ketoacidosis. Glucose assessments every two to three hours should be performed, together with ketone monitoring.

For patients with hyperglycemia and ketosis, a clinical scenario of diabetic ketoacidosis is likely developing. The initial goal is to suppress ketosis with the use of rapid-acting analog insulin boluses every three hours, provided the glucose values are at least 150 to 200 mg/dL to ensure that hypoglycemia does not ensue. For patients on a split/mix regimen of NPH/rapid-acting analog insulin regimen, this insulin bolus should be 0.1 times the TDI dose for moderate ketonuria, and 0.2 times the TDI for large ketonuria. For patients on a basal/bolus regimen or on an insulin pump, this insulin bolus should be 1.5 times the usual correction dose for moderate ketonuria, and 2 times the usual correction dose for large ketonuria. These insulin boluses are in addition to the usual doses of insulin Blood glucose values and ketones should be assessed one to three hours after each insulin bolus. Blood glucose levels of at least 200 mg/dL should be targeted, if necessary by consumption of clear sugar fluids, and hydration maintained. This protocol should be followed until ketonuria has remitted to at least the small level. The development of lethargy, confusion, or rapid, slow (Kussmaul's) respirations warrants immediate triage to a medical center.

TYPE 2 DIABETES MELLITUS

T2DM is a growing problem in pediatric diabetes, with a disproportionate affliction of non-Caucasian ethnicities as borne out by studies of Hispanic, Native American, Pacific Islander, Indian, and Australian aboriginal groups (64–66). T2DM represents a state of insulin resistance combined with relative insulin deficiency (67–68). Over the last decade, treatment of T2DM in the United States has markedly evolved as many new treatment regimens have been released. Insulin therapy, as described in the section on T2DM, can be used, but the relatively large armamentarium available to clinicians today allows for a varied approach to the treatment of the type 2 diabetic patient to target the true pathophysiology, rather than simply overcoming the individual physiologic deficiencies with an overwhelming insulin dosing. The newer medications have unique mechanisms of action. These include sensitizers at the hepatic or peripheral tissue level and incretins that restore the first-phase insulin response. Insulin secretagogues enhance deficient pancreatic β-cell activity. Other agents retard carbohydrate absorption. Table 2 provides an overview of the pharmacologic regimens available for T2DM.

Insulin Sensitizers with Predominant Hepatic Effects: Biguanides

Metformin is a biguanide with a primary effect of reducing hepatic glucose resistance, resulting in a subsequent decrease in gluconeogenesis and lower fasting glucose levels (69–72). Metformin also appears to enhance peripheral insulin-mediated glucose uptake (73,74) through the GLUT4 glucose transporter (75). The slight anorexic effect (76) results in a modest weight loss. Additional effects may include a decrease in gastrointestinal glucose uptake (77). Additionally, triglyceride reductions of as great as 50% have been noted in patients with hyper-triglyceridemia (78,79).

Side effects include transient nausea, abdominal discomfort, and diarrhea that are dose dependent. More significant is the rare risk of lactic acidosis, which occurs almost exclusively in the setting of renal insufficiency, where drug clearance becomes an issue. Hence metformin should be avoided in cases of renal insufficiency or acutely during potential renal compromise, such as acute dehydration or

TABLE 2 Summary of Treatment Options for Type 2 Diabetes Mellitus

Agent	Effect	Dose	Frequency	Glycemic control	Weight	Hypoglycemic risk	Randomized studies in youth	Comments
Biguanide								
Metformin	↑ Hepatic insulin sensitivity	1000–2550 mg	2–3 (1 with R form)	+++	↓	0	Yes	Gastrointestinal discomfort, rare risk of lactic acidosis
Thiazolidinedione								
Rosiglitazone	↑ Muscle/fat insulin sensitivity	4–8 mg	1	++	↑	0	Yes	Mild peripheral edema, ↑ LDL, ↑HDL
Pioglitazone	↑ Muscle/fat insulin sensitivity	15–45 mg	1	++	↑	0		Mild peripheral edema, ↑ HDL
Sulfonylurea								
First Generation								
Acetohexamide	↑ Insulin secretion	250–750 mg	1–2	+++	↑↑	↑↑		
Chlorpropamide	↑ Insulin secretion	250–500 mg	1	+++	↑↑	↑↑		Long duration, SIADH risk
Tolazamide	↑ Insulin secretion	100–1000 mg	1–2	+++	↑↑	↑↑		
Second Generation								
Glipizide	↑ Insulin secretion	2.5–40 mg	1	+++	↑↑	↑↑		Good with mild renal insufficiency
Glyburide	↑ Insulin secretion	2.5–20 mg	1	+++	↑↑	↑↑		
Glimepiride	↑ Insulin secretion	1–8 mg	1	+++	↑↑	↑↑		Good with renal insufficiency
Glitinide								
Repaglinide	↑ Insulin secretion	1–16 mg	3 (with meals)	+++	0/↑	↑		
Nateglinide	↑ Insulin secretion	180–360 mg	3 (with meals)	+++	0/↑	↑		
α-Glucosidase inhibitor								
Acarbose	Retards hydrolysis and uptake of	75–300 mg	3 (with meals)	+	0/↓	0		Gastrointestinal discomfort

Drug	Mechanism of action	Dose	Doses/day				Comments
Miglitol	Retards hydrolysis and uptake of complex carbohydrates	75–300 mg	3 (with meals)	+	0/↓	0	Gastrointestinal discomfort
Incretin pathway							
Exenatide	GLP-1 agonist ↑ insulin secretion ↓ gastric transit ↓ glucagon	10–20 µg	2	+++	↓	0	Possible pancreatic β-cell preservation
Sitagliptin	DPP-IV inhibitor ↑ insulin secretion ↓ gastric transit ↓ glucagon	25–50 mg	1	+	0	0	
Vildagliptin	DPP-IV inhibitor ↑ insulin secretion ↓ gastric transit ↓ glucagon	50 mg	1	+	0	0	
Amylin analog							
Pramlintide	↓ gastric transit ↓ glucagon	45–360 µg	3 (with meals)	++	0/↓	0	May also be used in T1DM
Insulin	↓ Hepatic gluconeogenesis	Unlimited	2–4	++++	↑↑	↑↑	Typically relatively large doses

Abbreviations: DPP IV, dipeptidyl peptidase IV; GLP-1, glucagon-like peptide; HDL, high-density lipoprotein; LDL, low-density lipoprotein; SIADH, syndrome of inappropriate antidiuretic hormone; T1DM, type 1 diabetes mellitus.

+++, represents on the spectrum of the relative effectiveness of glycemic change a particular agent may produce, based on a relative of "+" (least) to "++++" (greatest).

during the use of radiographic contrast materials. Other relative contraindications to metformin use include cardiopulmonary or hepatic insufficiency.

Metformin is currently the only oral hypoglycemic medication approved by the Food and Drug Administration in the pediatric population. A 16-week trial (80) at doses between 500 mg twice a day to 2000 mg total per day in patients between 10 and 16 years of age demonstrated an improvement in subjects treated with metformin relative to placebo when assessed for HbA_{1c} (7.5% vs. 8.6%, respectively; $p < 0.001$) as well as total serum cholesterol (−9.7 mg/dL vs. +0.7 mg/dL, respectively; $p = 0.043$). Side effects included diarrhea or abdominal pain in 25% of the subjects on metformin—an effect that significantly diminished with duration of treatment. Additionally, to enhance compliance, an extended-release, once-daily formulation is now available.

Insulin Sensitizers with Predominant Peripheral Tissue Effects: Thiazolidinediones

The thiazolidinedione class of drugs promotes insulin sensitization primarily through peripheral tissues muscle and fat. By binding and modulating a family of nuclear transcription factors—the peroxisome proliferator-activated receptors (PPAR-γs), which have a predominance in adipose tissue and a smaller presence in muscle and hepatic tissue (81)—the thiazolidinediones effect a gradual reduction in hyperglycemia over weeks to months correlated with decreasing insulin resistance and decreasing serum free fatty acid levels.

Thiazolidinediones are quite well tolerated. The predominant side effect is weight gain secondary to fluid retention, typically manifesting as mild to moderate edema. Lacking a side chain found in troglitazone, the first marketed thiazolidinedione, to which the hepatotoxic effects of troglitazone were attributed, two newer thiazolidinedione products are now available—rosiglitazone and pioglitazone. Hepatic transaminases should be assessed before initiating therapy and periodically thereafter to ensure that these levels do not exceed threefold the upper limit of normal.

In fact, recent literature suggests that the thiazolidinediones may prove efficacious in the treatment of nonalcoholic hepatic steatosis, a frequent comorbidity of T2DM (82–84). Though changes induced in the lipid profile with use of rosiglitazone may not be favorable, beneficial changes in the lipid profile have been observed with pioglitazone (neutral effect on total cholesterol and LDL, decrease in triglycerides, and increase in HDL) (85). This lipid effect may in part explain some cardiovascular concerns with rosiglitazone (86). Other conditions associated with increased insulin resistance, such as lipodystrophy (87) and polycystic ovarian syndrome (88,89), have demonstrated improvement with the use of thiazolidinediones. Additionally, thiazolidinediones may offer unique anti-inflammatory effects (90).

Studies have demonstrated the safety and efficacy of rosiglitazone in the pediatric population. In one 24-week study (91) of 195 pediatric patients aged 8 to 17 years comparing rosiglitazone and metformin, rosiglitazone was initiated at 2 mg twice a day and titrated up to maximal doses of 4 mg twice daily, with a decrease in HbA_{1c} of 0.25% (compared to 0.55% with metformin). Side effects were minimal, as one patient developed mild peripheral edema, and the average weight gain was 3 kg in the rosiglitazone cohort, compared with no weight gain in the metformin cohort.

The thiazolidinediones appear to have a somewhat lower effect on glycemic control than metformin, but may complement metformin or other modalities through a separate mechanism of action. Additional nonglycemic benefits of a thiazolidinedione may make this class an attractive adjunct.

Secretagogues of Insulin

All secretagogues of insulin on the market act through binding of the sulfonylurea receptor (SUR1) subunit of the adenosine triphosphate (ATP)-sensitive K+ channel on the plasma membrane of pancreatic β cells, resulting in closure of the channel and membrane depolarization (92). A voltage-dependent L-type Ca^{2+} channel subsequently opens, resulting in an intracellular calcium influx and a subsequent insulin release. The presence of viable pancreatic β cells is a prerequisite for this class, and hence these drugs are only relevant in T2DM but not T1DM.

Sulfonylureas

Sulfonylureas have been available since 1955. First-generation drugs include chlorpropamide, tolbutamide (no longer commercially available), tolazamide, and acetohexamide. Much more potent (93,94) and much more commonly used are the second-generation drugs, which include glyburide, glipizide, and glimepiride. Because of a predominantly hepatic metabolism, glipizide and glimepiride are preferred in the setting of renal insufficiency. Titrations of this class of drugs to a desired glycemic effect may be made as rapidly as every two to three days.

A retrospective analysis (95) of pediatric diabetic patients as young as 9.7 years assessed nine patients on sulfonylurea therapy. After a wide range of follow-up (3.2–52.9 months), sulfonylurea therapy did not appear to be associated with significant side effects. As would be expected from this class of drugs, a weight gain (31.2 kg/m^2 to 33.0 kg/m^2) was noted, and a decrease in the HbA_{1c} (10.2–9.0% after a mean of 16.5 months of follow-up) was described. Inherent to any insulin secretagogue is the risk of hypoglycemia. Sulfonylureas have been used very effective in monogenic diabetes, particularly MODY3 and neonatal diabetes due to mutations in KJCN11 (96,97).

Glitinides

Glitinides are represented by repaglinide (available in 0.5-, 1-, and 2-mg tablets) and nateglinide (available in 60 and 120 mg tablets). Both are biochemically unique from sulfonylureas and have a much more rapid effects, essentially offering prandial glycemic control, thus requiring use prior to each meal. Pediatric data are lacking, but adult studies suggest somewhat less potent effect than metformin (98,99).

Inhibitors of Carbohydrate Absorption: α-Glucosidase Inhibitors

α-Glucosidase inhibitors are represented by acarbose and miglitol. By inhibiting α-glucosidase at the brush border of the small intestine, carbohydrate metabolism and absorption is delayed, enabling the delayed insulin dynamics of diabetes mellitus to effect better glycemic control. Studies have demonstrated better post-prandial glycemic control in both T1DM and T2DM (100–104). Gastrointestinal side effects—including abdominal discomfort, borborygmi, flatulence, and diarrhea—may be limiting, and the decrease in HbA_{1c} has been modest at 0.5–1% (105). Pediatric studies (106,107) have demonstrated efficacy and safety in doses of acarbose up to 100 mg three times daily.

The Incretin Pathway

Incretins represent a class of gut hormones, glucagon-like peptide-1 (GLP-1) and gastric inhibitory polypeptide (GIP), which, upon enteric glucose stimulation, enhance insulin secretion (in effect restoring the first-phase insulin response lost in T2DM), attenuate glucagon secretion, and delay gastric emptying (108). Additional benefits include an anorexic effect and an anti-apoptotic effect on pancreatic β cells in animal models (109,110). The necessity of enteric glucose to effect the actions of glycemic control results in the absence of hypoglycemia, in the absence of other hypoglycemic-potentiating agents. Additionally, the anorectic effect results in weight loss, a useful adjunct in the typically overweight T2DM.

Two available classes of drugs act on this pathway—GLP-1 agonists and dipeptidyl peptidase IV (DPP-IV) inhibitors. A paucity of data in pediatric patients exists at present, but a study of normal subjects aged 15 to 28 years demonstrated effects similar to that observed in older diabetic cohorts (111). Exenatide is a GLP-1 agonist, whereas sitagliptin and vildagliptin are inhibitors of the enzyme—dipeptidylpeptidase IV—that degrades GLP-1. Exenatide appears to be somewhat more potent, with decreases in HbA_{1c} of 1–2%, although often accompanied by nausea. Minimal adverse effects have been noted with DPP-IV inhibitors, with decreases of HbA_{1c} of 0.5–1% observed (112).

Synthetic Analog of Amylin: Pramlintide

Amylin is a hormone co-secreted by the pancreatic β cell with insulin. Effects of amylin include a delay in gastric emptying, satiety, and an inhibition of post-prandial glucagon release, resulting in a significant control in postprandial glycemic control (113). Pramlintide is a synthetic analog of amylin (114), and has been used successfully in both T1DM and T2DM (115). Mild nausea may be seen, but hypoglycemia does not develop in the absence of another hypoglycemic-potentiating agent. A study in adolescent patients aged 12 to 18 years (116) demonstrated the efficacy and tolerability of pramlintide in pediatric patients.

COMBINATION THERAPY

Therapeutic regimens may offer synergistic effects when combined. Numerous combination tablets of pharmacologic agents used for diabetes mellitus have been actively marketed for the adult diabetic population, including combinations of metformin and glyburide (Glucovance®) (117) and combinations of metformin and rosiglitazone (Avandamet®) (118), Insulin itself has been marketed in combinations, such as BiAsp Insulin 70/30 (119), consisting of 70% NPH Insulin and 30% Aspart designed to offer a biphasic effect with the use of a single injection. Such combination preparations are designed to offer the convenience of fewer dosing requirements, with perhaps a synergistic effect.

A few studies have been performed in the pediatric diabetic population using combination therapy. Metformin has been studied (120) in obese type 1 pediatric patients on high doses of insulin, suggestive of a significant component of insulin resistance in addition to the absolute insulinopenia, and has been proven safe and effective in lowering insulin requirements in such patients. The combination of metformin and sulfonylureas appears to be efficacious in the pediatric type 2 diabetic population as well (117).

THERAPIES TO CHANGE THE NATURAL DISEASE COURSE

Currently, numerous agents are under investigation to potentially alter the natural disease course of diabetes mellitus. The immunomodulatory anti-CD3 monoclonal antibody HOKT3γ1 (Ala-Ala), also known as OKT3, interacts with CD-3 antigen, but blocks normal binding of the Fc receptor, thereby interfering with the normal immune response (121). Preliminary studies have suggested that OKT3 improves the course of T1DM mellitus in the first year of disease (122), and further studies are currently underway. Exenatide, as described previously, offers the potential for pancreatic β-cell preservation (109–111), and may hold promise for altering the disease course of both T1DM and T2DM; current studies to investigate this effect are in progress.

CONCLUSION

Treatment options for youth with diabetes mellitus have markedly evolved especially over recent years. A wide array of monitoring devices for glycemic control exists, and the advent of CGMS brings us closer to a closed-loop system that mimics natural physiology. Numerous advances have provided "designer" insulins, or in the case of T2DM, alternative therapies. Exciting efforts to modulate the natural disease course are underway. Intrinsic to any pharmacologic interventions is embracing a healthy lifestyle. Optimal treatment of diabetes mellitus requires an integrated approach that involves a commitment from the physician, registered dieticians, social workers, pharmacy, the family, and most importantly the patient.

REFERENCES

1. Gungor N, Hannon T, Libman I, et al. Type 2 diabetes mellitus in youth: the complete picture to date. Pediatr Clin North Am 2005; 52(6):1579–1609.
2. Waldhor T, Schober E, Rami B. Regional distribution of risk for childhood diabetes in Austria and possible association with body mass index. Eur J Pediatr 2003; 162:380–384.
3. Wilkin TJ. The accelerator hypothesis: weight gain as the missing link between type 1 and type 2 diabetes. Diabetologia 2001; 44:914–922.
4. Laron Z. Type 2 diabetes mellitus in childhood—a global perspective. J Pediatr Endocrinol Metab 2002; 15(suppl 1):459–469.
5. The Diabetes Control and Complications Trial Research Group. The effect of intensive treatment of diabetes on the development and progression of long-term complications in insulin-dependent diabetes mellitus. N Engl J Med 1993; 329:977–986.
6. The Diabetes Research in Children Network (Directnet) Study Group. A multicenter study of the accuracy of the One Touch Ultra home glucose meter in children with type 1 diabetes. Diabetes Technol Ther 2003; 5(6):933–941.
7. Arabadjief D, Nichols JH. Assessing glucose meter accuracy. Curr Med Res Opin 2006; 22(11):2167–2174.
8. Rivers SM, Kane MP, Bakst G, et al. Precision and accuracy of two blood glucose meters: FreeStyle Flash versus One Touch Ultra. Am J Health Syst Pharm 2006; 61(15):1411–1416.
9. Jungheim K, Koschinsky T. Glucose monitoring at the arm: risky delays of hypoglycemia and hyperglycemia detection. Diabetes Care 2002; 25:956–960.
10. Potts RO, Tamada JA, Tierney MJ. Glucose monitoring by reverse iontophoresis. Diabetes Metab Res Rev 2002; 18(suppl 1):S49–S53.
11. Tierney MD, Tamada JA, Potts RO, et al. Clinical evaluation of the GlucoWatch biographer: a continual, non-invasive glucose monitor for patients with diabetes. Biosens Bioelectron 2001; 16(9–12):621–619.

12. Tsalikian E, Kollman C, Mauras N, et al. GlucoWatch G2 Biographer alarm reliability during hypoglycemia in children. Diabetes Technol Ther 2004; 6(5):559–566.

13. Wiltshire EJ, Newton K, McTavish L. Unrecognized hypoglycaemia in children and adolescents with type 1 diabetes using the continuous glucose monitoring system: prevalence and contributors. J Paediatr Child Health 2006; 42(12):758–763.

14. Maia FF, Araujo LR. Efficacy of continuous glucose monitoring system (CGMS) to detect postprandial hyperglycemia and unrecognized hypoglycemia in type 1 diabetic patients. Diabetes Res Clin Pract 2007; 75(1):30–34.

15. Yates K, Hasnat Milton A, Dear K, et al. Continuous glucose monitoring-guided insulin adjustment in children and adolescents on near-physiological insulin regimens: a randomized controlled trial. Diabetes Care 2006; 29(7): 1512–1517.

16. Lagarde WH, Barrows FP, Davenport ML, et al. Continuous subcutaneous glucose monitoring in children with type 1 diabetes mellitus: a single-blind, randomized, controlled trial. Pediatr Diabetes 2006; 7(3):159–164.

17. Melki V, Ayon F, Fernandez M, et al. Value and limitations of the Continuous Glucose Monitoring System in the management of type 1 diabetes. Diabetes Metab 2006; 32(2): 123–129.

18. Federici MO, Benedetti MM. Diabetes Res Clin Pract 2006; 74(suppl 2):S77–S81.

19. Taboulet P, Deconinck N, Thurel A, et al. Correlation between urine ketones (acetoacetate) and capillary blood ketones (3-beta-hydroxybutyrate) in hyperglycaemic patients. Diabetes Metab 2007 Feb 20 (Epub).

20. American Diabetes Association. Standards of medical care in diabetes—2007. Diabetes Care 2007; 30(suppl 1):S4–S41.

21. Rovet JF, Ehrlich RM, Hoppe M. Intellectual deficits associated with early onset of insulin-dependent diabetes mellitus in children. Diabetes Care 1987; 10:510–515.

22. Seidl R, Birnbacher R, Hauser E, et al. Brainstem auditory evoked potentials and visually evoked potentials in young patients with IDDM. Diabetes Care 1996; 19: 1220–1224.

23. Soltesz G, Acsadi G. Association between diabetes, severe hypoglycaemia, and electroencephalographic abnormalities. Arch Dis Child 1989; 64:992–996.

24. Rovet JF, Ehrlich RM. The effect of hypoglycemic seizures on cognitive function in children with diabetes: a 7-year prospective study. J Pediatr 1999; 134:503–506.

25. Bjorgaas M, Gimse R, Vik T, et al. Cognitive function in type 1 diabetic children with and without episodes of severe hypoglycaemia. Acta Paediatr 1997; 86:148–153.

26. Banting FG, Best CH. The internal secretions of the pancreas. J Lab Clin Med 1922; 7:251–266.

27. Banting FG, Best CH. Pancreatic extracts. J Lab Clin Med 1922; 7:464–472.

28. Banting FG, Best CH, Collip JB, et al. Pancreatic extracts in the treatment of diabetes mellitus. Can Med Assoc J 1922; 12:141–146.

29. Kaku K, Matsuda M, Urae A, et al. Pharmacokinetics and pharmacodynamics of insulin aspart, a rapid-acting analog of human insulin, in healthy Japanese volunteers. Diabetes Res Clin Pract 2000; 49:119–126.

30. Mudaliar SR, Lindberg FA, Joyce M, et al. Insulin aspart (B28 asp-insulin): a fast acting analog of human insulin: absorption kinetics and action profile compared with regular human insulin in healthy nondiabetic subjects. Diabetes Care 1999; 22:1501–1506.

31. Plank J, Wutte A, Bunner G, et al. A direct comparison of insulin aspart and insulin lispro in patients with type 1 diabetes. Diabetes Care 2002; 25:2053–2057.

32. Skyler JS. Insulin treatment. In: Lebovitz HE, ed. Therapy for Diabetes Mellitus and Related Disorders. Alexandria, VA: American Diabetes Association, 1998:186–203.

33. Becker RHA, Frick AD, Wessels DH, et al. Pharmacodynamics and pharmacokinetics of a new, rapid-acting insulin analog, insulin glulisine. Diabetes 2003; 52(6):A110(1) (abstr 471-P).

34. Frick A, Becker R, Wessels D, et al. Pharmacokinetic and glucodynamic profiles of insulin glulisine following subcutaneous administration at various injection sites. Diabetes 2003a; 52(6):A199(1) (abstr).

35. Lepore M, Pampanelli S, Fanelli C, et al. Pharmacokinetics and pharmacodynamics of subcutaneous injection of long-acting human insulin analog glargine, NPH insulin, and

ultralente human insulin and continuous subcutaneous infusion of insulin lispro. Diabetes 2000; 49:2142–2148.

36. Luzio S, Dunseath G, Peter R, et al. Comparison of the pharmacokinetics and pharmacodynamics of biphasic insulin aspart and insulin glargine in people with type 2 diabetes. Diabetologia 2006; 49(6):1163–1168.
37. Plank J, Bodenlenz M, Sinner F, et al. A double-blind, randomized, dose-response study investigating the pharmacodynamic and pharmacokinetic properties of the long-acting insulin analog detemir. Diabetes Care 2005; 28(5):1107–1112.
38. Russel-Jones D, Simpson R, Hylleberg B, et al. Effects of QD insulin detemir or neutral protamine hagedorn on blood glucose control in patients with type 1 diabetes mellitus using a basal-bolus regimen. Clin Ther 2004; 26(3):724–736.
39. Fiallo-Scharer R, Horner B, McFann K, et al. Mixing rapid-acting insulin analogues with insulin glargine in children with type 1 diabetes mellitus. J Pediatr 2006; 148:481–484.
40. Kaplan W, Rodriguez LM, Smith OE. Effects of mixing glargine and short-acting insulin analogs on glucose control. Diabetes Care 2004; 27(11):2739–2740.
41. Klein O, Lynge J, Endahl L, et al. Albumin-bound basal insulin analogues (insulin detemir and NN344): comparable time action profiles but less variability than insulin glargine in type 2 diabetes. Diabetes Obes Metab 2007; 9(3):290–299.
42. Pieber TR, Treichel HC, Hompesch B, et al. Comparison of insulin detemir and insulin glargine in subjects with type 1 diabetes using intensive insulin therapy. Diabet Med 2007; 24(6):635–642 (Epub).
43. Peterson GE. Intermediate and long-acting insulins: a review of NPH insulin, insulin glargine and insulin detemir. Curr Med Res Opin 2006; 22(12):2613–2619.
44. McMahon GT, Arky RA. Inhaled insulin for diabetes mellitus. N Engl J Med 2007; 356:497–502.
45. Patton JS, Bukar JG, Eldon MA. Clinical pharmacokinetics and pharmacodynamics of inhaled insulin. Clin Pharmacokinet 2004; 43:781–801.
46. Cappelleri JC, Cefalu WT, Rosenstock J, et al. Treatment satisfaction in type 2 diabetes: a comparison between an inhaled insulin regimen and a subcutaneous insulin regimen. Clin Ther 2002; 24:552–564.
47. Rosenstock J, Cappelleri JC, Bolinder B, et al. Patient satisfaction and glycemic control after 1 year with inhaled insulin (Exubera) in patients with type 1 or type 2 diabetes. Diabetes Care 2004; 27:1318–1323.
48. Sadri H, MacKeigan LD, Leiter LA, et al. Willingness to pay for inhaled insulin: a contingent valuation approach. Pharmacoeconomics 2005; 23:1215–1227.
49. Halfon P, Belkhadir J, Slama G. Correlation between amount of carbohydrate in mixed meals and insulin delivery by artificial pancreas in seven IDDM subjects. Diabetes Care 1989; 12:427–429.
50. Stoller WA. Individualizing insulin management. Three practical cases, rules for regimen adjustment. Postgrad Med 2002; 111(5):51–66.
51. Litton J, Rice A, Friedman N, et al. Insulin pump therapy in toddlers and preschool children with type 1 diabetes. J Pediatr 2002; 141:490–495.
52. Maniatis AK, Klingensmith GJ, Slover RH, et al. Continuous subcutaneous insulin infusion therapy for children and adolescents: An option for routine diabetes care. Pediatrics 2001; 107:331–356.
53. Plotnick LP, Clark LM, Brancati FL, et al. Safety and effectiveness of insulin pump therapy in children and adolescents with type 1 diabetes. Diabetes Care 2002; 25: 2053–2057.
54. Boland EA, Grey M, Oesterle A, et al. Continuous subcutaneous insulin infusion. A new way to lower risk of severe hypoglycemia, improve metabolic control, and enhance coping in adolescents with type 1 diabetes. Diabetes Care 1999; 22:1779–1784.
55. Bode BW, Steed RD, Davidson PC. Reduction in severe hypoglycemia with long-term continuous subcutaneous insulin infusion in type 1 diabetes. Diabetes Care 1996:19: 324–327.
56. Bougberes PF, Landier F, Lemmel C, et al. Insulin pump therapy in young children with type 1 diabetes. J Pediatr 1984; 105:212–217.

57. Kaufman FR, Halvorson M, Kim C, et al. Use of insulin pump therapy at nighttime only for children 7–10 years of age with type 1 diabetes. Diabetes Care 2000; 23:579–582.
58. Bode BW, Strange P. Efficacy, safety, and pump compatibility of insulin aspart used in continuous subcutaneous insulin infusion therapy in patients with type 1 diabetes. Diabetes Care 2001; 24:69–72.
59. Melki V, Renard E, Lassmann-Vague V, et al. Improvement of HbA$_{1c}$ and blood glucose stability in IDDM patients treated with lispro insulin analog in external pumps. Diabetes Care 1998; 21:977–982.
60. Renner R, Pfutzner A, Trautmann M, et al. Use of insulin lispro in continuous subcutaneous insulin infusion treatment. Results of a multicenter trial. German Humalog-CSII Study Group. Diabetes Care 1999; 22:784–788.
61. Unger RH, Grunder S. Hyperglycemia as an inducer as well as a consequence of impaired islet cell function and insulin resistance: implications for the management of diabetes. Diabetologia 1985; 28:119–121.
62. Rossetti, Giaccari A, DeFronzo RA. Glucose toxicity. Diabetes Care 1990; 13:610–630.
63. Rhodes ET, Rerrari LR, Wolfsdorf JI. Perioperative management of pediatric surgical patients with diabetes mellitus. Anesth Analg 2005; 101:986–999.
64. Boyko EJ, de Cowten M, Zimmer PZ, et al. Features of the metabolic syndrome predict higher risk of diabetes and impaired glucose tolerance: a prospective study in Mauritius. Diabetes Care 2000; 23:1242–1248.
65. Ramachandran A, Snehalatha C, Latha E, et al. Rising prevalence of NIDDM in an urban population in India. Diabetologia 1997; 40:232–237.
66. O'Dea K. Westernization, insulin resistance and diabetes in Australian aborigines. Med J Aust 1991; 155:258–264.
67. DeFronzo RA. The triumvirate β-cell, muscle, liver: a collusion responsible for NIDDM. Diabetes 1988; 37:667–687.
68. Savage PJ, Dippe SE, Bennett PH, et al. Hyperinsulinemia and hypoinsulinemia: insulin responses to oral carbohydrate over a wide spectrum of glucose tolerance. Diabetes 1975; 24:362–368.
69. Silverstein JH, Rosenbloom AL. Treatment of type 2 diabetes mellitus in children and adolescents. J Pediatr Endocrinol Metab 2000; 13(suppl 6):1403–1409.
70. De Fronzo RA, Goodman AM. Efficacy of metformin in patients with non-insulin-dependent diabetes mellitus. The Multicenter Metformin Study Group. N Engl J Med 1995; 333:541–549.
71. Bailey CJ. Biguanides and NIDDM. Diabetes Care 1992; 15:755–772.
72. Inzucchi SE, Maggs DG, Spollett GR, et al. Efficacy and metabolic effects of metformin and troglitazone in type II diabetes mellitus. N Engl J Med 1998; 338:867–872.
73. Rossetti L, DeFronzo RA, Gherzi R, et al. Effect of metformin treatment on insulin action in diabetic rats: in vivo and in vitro correlations. Metabolism 1990; 39:425.
74. Schernthaner G. Improvement in insulin action is an important part of the antidiabetic effect of metformin. Horm Metab Res Suppl 1985; 15:116–120.
75. Klip A, Leiter LA. Cellular mechanisms of action of metformin. Diabetes Care 1990; 13:696–704.
76. Clarke BF, Duncan LJP. Comparison of chlorpropamide and metformin treatment on weight and blood glucose response of uncontrolled obese diabetics. Lancet 1968; 1:123–126.
77. Caspary WF, Creutzfeldt W. Analysis of the inhibitory effect of biguanides on glucose absorption: inhibition of sugar transport. Diabetologia 1971; 7:379–385.
78. Wu MS, Johnston P, Sheu WH, et al. Effect of metformin on carbohydrate and lipoprotein metabolism in NIDDM patients. Diabetes Care 1990; 13:1–8.
79. Schneider J, Erren T, Zofel P, et al. Metformin induced changes in serum lipids lipoproteins and apoproteins in non-insulin-dependent diabetes mellitus. Atherosclerosis 1990; 82:97–103.
80. Jones KL, Arslanian S, Peterokova VA, et al. Effect of metformin in pediatric patients with type 2 diabetes mellitus: a randomized controlled trial. Diabetes Care 2002; 25:89–94.

81. Vidal-Puig A, Considine R, Jimenez-Linan M, et al. Peroxisome-proliferator activated receptor gene expression in human tissues: effects of obesity, weight loss, and regulation by insulin and glucocorticoids. J Clin Invest 1997; 99:2416–2422.
82. Harrison SA. New treatments for nonalcoholic fatty liver disease. Curr Gastroenterol Rep 2006; 8(1):21–29.
83. Roden M. Mechanisms of Disease: hepatic steatosis in type 2 diabetes—pathogenesis and clinical relevance. Nat Clin Pract Endocrinol Metab 2006; 2(6):335–348.
84. Wang CH, Leung CH, Liu SC, et al. Safety and effectiveness in type 2 diabetes patients with nonalcoholic fatty liver disease. J Formos Med Assoc 2006; 105(9):743–752.
85. Yamasaki Y, Kawamori R, Wasada T, et al. Pioglitazone (AD-4833) ameliorates insulin resistance in patients with NIDDM. AD-4833 glucose clamp study group, Japan. Tohoku J Exp Med 1997; 183:173–183.
86. Nissen SE, Wolski K. Effect of rosiglitazone on the risk of myocardial infarction and death. N Engl J Med 2007; 356(24):2457–2471.
87. Ludtke A, Heck K, Genschel J, et al. Long term treatment experience in a subject with Dunnigan-type familial partial lipodystrophy: efficacy of rosiglitazone. Diabet Med 2005; 22(11):1611–1613.
88. Azziz R, Ehrmann D, Legro RS, et al. Troglitazone improves ovulation and hirsutism in the polycystic ovary syndrome: a multicenter, double blind, placebo-controlled trial. J Clin Endocrinol Metab 2001; 86:1626–1632.
89. Ghazeeri G, Kutteh WH, Bryer-Ash M, et al. Effect of rosiglitazone on spontaneous and clomiphene citrate-induced ovulation in women with polycystic ovary syndrome. Fertil Steril 2003; 73:562–566.
90. Esposity K, Ciotola M, Carleo D, et al. Effect of rosiglitazone on endothelial function and inflammatory markers in patients with the metabolic syndrome. Diabetes Care 2006; 29(5):1071–1076.
91. Saenger P, Kenneth J, Guissou D, et al. Benefits of rosiglitazone in children with type 2 diabetes mellitus. Paper presented at The European Society for Paediatric Endocrinology/Lawson Wilkins Pediatric Endocrine Society 7th Joint Meeting, September 21–24, 2005, Lyon, France.
92. Boyd AE III. Sulfonylurea receptors, ion channels and fruit flies. Diabetes 1988; 37: 847–850.
93. Melander A, Bitzen P-O, Faber O, et al. Sulphonylurea antidiabetic drugs: an update of their clinical pharmacology and rational therapeutic use. Drugs 1989; 37:58–72.
94. Skillman TG, Feldman JM. The pharmacology of sulfonylureas. Am J Med 1981; 70: 361–372.
95. Benavides S, Striet J, Germak J, et al. Efficacy and safety of hypoglycemic drugs in children with type 2 diabetes mellitus. Pharmacotherapy 2005; 25(6):803–809.
96. Pearson ER, Liddell WG, Shepherd M, et al. Sensitivity to sulphonylureas in patients with hepatocyte nuclear factor-1 alpha gene mutations: evidence for pharmacogenetics in diabetes. Diabet Med 2000; 17(7):543–545.
97. Sagen JV, Raeder H, Hathout E, et al. Permanent neonatal diabetes due to mutations in KCNJ11 encoding Kir6.2: patient characteristics and initial response to sulfonylurea therapy. Diabetes 2004; 53(10):2713–2718.
98. Horton E, Clinkingbeard C, Gatlin M, et al. Nateglinide alone and in combination with metformin improves glycemic control by reducing mealtime glucose in type 2 diabetes. Diabetes Care 2000; 23(11):1660–1665.
99. Riddle M. Glycemic management of type 2 diabetes: an emerging strategy with oral agents, insulin, and combinations. Endocrinol Metab Clin N Am 2005; 34:77–98.
100. Vierhapper H, Bratusch-Marrain A, Waldhause W. α-Glucosidase hydrolase inhibition in diabetes. Lancet 1978; 2:1386.
101. Hanefeld M, Fischer S, Schulze J. Therapeutic potentials of acarbose as first-line drug in NIDDM insufficiently with diet alone. Diabetes Care 1991; 14:732–737.
102. Walton RJ, Sherif IT, Noy GA, et al. Improved metabolic profiles in insulin-treated diabetic patients given an α-glucoside hydrolase inhibitor. BMJ 1979; 1:220–221.
103. Dimitriadis G, Hatziagelaki E, Ladas S, et al. Effects of prolonged administration of two new α-glucosidase inhibitors on blood glucose control, insulin requirements and breath

hydrogen excretion in patients with insulin-dependent diabetes mellitus. Eur J Clin Invest 1988; 18:33–38.

104. Arends J, Willms BH. Smoothening effect of a new α-glucosidase inhibitor, BAY m 1099, on blood glucose profiles of sulfonylurea-treated type II diabetic patients. Horm Metab Res 1986; 18:761–764.

105. Chiasson J, Josse R, Hunt JA, et al. The efficacy of acarbose in the treatment of patients with non-insulin-dependent diabetes mellitus: a multicenter controlled clinical trial. Ann Intern Med 1994; 121(12):928–935.

106. Mangiagli A, Campisi S, De Sanctis V, et al. Effects of acarbose in patients with beta-thalassaemia major and abnormal glucose homeostasis. Pediatr Endocrinol Rev 2004; 2(suppl 2): 276–278.

107. Zung A, Zadik Z. Acarbose treatment of infant dumping syndrome: extensive study of glucose dynamics and long-term follow-up. J Pediatr Endocrinol Metab 2003; 16(6): 907–915.

108. Drucker DJ. Enhancing incretin action for the treatment of type 2 diabetes. Diabetes Care 2003; 26:2929–2940.

109. Farilla L, Hui H, Bertolotto C, et al. Glucagon-like peptide-1 promotes islet cell growth and inhibits apoptosis in Zucker diabetic rats. Endocrinology 2002; 143:4397–4408.

110. Li Y, Hansotia T, Yusta B, et al. Glucagon-like peptide-1 receptor signaling modulates beta cell apoptosis. J Biol Chem 2003; 278:471–478.

111. Limb C, Tamborlane WV, Sherwin RS, et al. Acute incretin response to oral glucose is associated with stimulation of gastric inhibitory polypeptide, not glucagon-like peptide in young subjects. Pediatr Res 1997; 41:364–367.

112. Drucker DJ, Nauck MA. The incretin system: glucagon-like peptide 1 receptor agonists and dipeptidyl peptidase-4 inhibitors in type 2 diabetes. Lancet 2006; 368(9548): 1696–1705.

113. Young AA. Amylin's physiology and its role in diabetes. Curr Opin Endocrinol Diabetes 1997; 4:282–290.

114. Kruger DF, Gloster MA. Pramlintide for the treatment of insulin-requiring diabetes mellitus: rationale and review of clinical data. Drugs 2004; 64:1419–1432.

115. Ryan GJ, Jobe LJ, Martin R. Pramlintide in the treatment of type 1 and type 2 diabetes mellitus. Clin Ther 2005; 27(10):1500–1512.

116. Heptulla RA, Rodrigues LM, Bomgaars L, et al. The role of amylin and glucagon in the dampening of glycemic excursions in children with type 1 diabetes. Diabetes 2005; 54 (4):1100–1107.

117. Glyburide/metformin (Glucovance) for type 2 diabetes. Med Lett Drugs Ther 2000; 42(1092):105–106.

118. Del Prato S, Volpe L. Rosiglitazone plus metformin: combination therapy for Type 2 diabetes. Expert Opin Pharmacother 2004; 5(6):1411–1422.

119. Urakami T, Morimoto S, Owada M, et al. Usefulness of the addition of metformin to insulin in pediatric patients with type 1 diabetes mellitus. Pediatr Int 2005; 47(4): 430–433.

120. Ray JA, Vantine WJ, Rose S. Insulin therapy in type 2 diabetes failing oral agents: cost-effectiveness of biphasic insulin aspart 70/30 vs. insulin glargine in the US. Diabetes Obes Metab 2007; 9(1):103–113.

121. Chatenoud L, Ferran C, Legendre C, et al. In vivo cell activation following OKT3 administration: systemic cytokine release and modulation by corticosteroids. Transplantation 1990; 49:697–702.

122. Herold KC, Hagopian W, Auger JA, et al. Anti-CD3 monoclonal antibody in new-onset type 1 diabetes mellitus. N Engl J Med 2002; 346(22):1692–1697.

20 Psychosocial Issues in Childhood Diabetes

Barbara J. Anderson
Department of Pediatrics, Baylor College of Medicine, Houston, Texas, U.S.A.

INTRODUCTION

The scope of this chapter is on the psychosocial tasks of the developing child and adolescent with type 1 diabetes (T1DM) and related behavioral research. To date, there has been very little behavioral research focused on youth with type 2 diabetes (T2DM) as this cohort of youth has only begun to appear in larger numbers in the past decade (1). The focus here is on psychosocial issues across the different stages of child and adolescent development, with an emphasis on the family system as one of the most critical—and potentially modifiable—psychological and social influence on the developing child with T1DM. Throughout the development of the child and adolescent with T1DM, we focus on identifying psychosocial factors that put the child with T1DM at increased risk for adverse health outcomes.

Psychosocial Issues

The concept of "psychosocial" first came into widespread use in the mid 1900s by Erik Erikson, who theorized that the lifespan is divided into eight stages of "psychosocial development" (in contrast to the stages of "psychosexual development" as discussed by Freud) (2–3). At each stage Erikson was interested in how social and cultural factors influence the manner in which an individual resolves the conflicts brought about by biological maturation. The focus of Erikson's theory is on how children interact with their social environment and how these social interactions affect the child's developing sense of self. In each stage the child confronts a new challenge, with the possibility of successful mastery which results in a healthy personality and successful interactions with others, and prepares the child for the challenges of the next stage. Failure to successfully master the challenges of a stage can result in a reduced ability to complete further stages and in a more unhealthy personality and sense of self.

It is well documented that the daily demands of the complex diabetes regimen affect the developing child as well as family life throughout the pediatric age range (4–6). In this chapter, the focus is on identifying and understanding how growing up with diabetes affects the psychosocial tasks that the child confronts at each developmental stage. To be consistent with the psychosocial research literature in pediatric diabetes, we divide child and adolescent development into three major stages: early childhood (0–5 years); the school-age period (6–10 years); and early to mid adolescence (11–16 years). For each stage of development we identify the central psychosocial tasks as defined by Erikson, and other developmental theorists, followed by a review of what research has demonstrated about the major psychosocial challenges facing the child with diabetes at each of these life stages. Emphasis will be given to research which has linked specific aspects of the child's family/social environment to healthy psychological functioning as well as optimal glycemic control. In addition, for each stage, psychosocial risk factors will be identified that are associated with adverse health outcomes in children with diabetes.

Psychosocial Tasks in Early Childhood (0–5 years)

During the first year of life, the central psychosocial task is for the infant to establish a strong and trusting emotional attachment with the primary caregiver(s). In the next developmental period, children between two and four years have two central developmental tasks: 1) to separate from the primary caregiver in order to establish him/herself as a separate person and develop a sense of autonomy, and 2) to develop a sense of mastery over the environment as well as the confidence that he/she can act upon and affect the physical and social environment. Following the toddler years, preschoolers in the fourth to fifth years of life build upon this newly established autonomy to explore and begin to master the world outside the home (2).

Psychosocial Research on the Very Young Child with Diabetes

There have been no large, well-controlled studies of diabetes in infancy and only one longitudinal study is available, which followed very young children with diabetes between one and four years of age and their parents prospectively (7). There are, however, several small, qualitative studies that illustrate the potential impact of diabetes on the infant-parent relationship. In one qualitative study, mothers of infants with diabetes reported a diminished bond with their children and a loss of the ideal mother-child relationship (8). In another small, descriptive study, mothers reported feeling 'constant vigilance' because their infants were so dependent on them to manage the disease and to recognize dangerous glycemic fluctuations (9). These authors also report that chronic stress and lack of social support put mothers of infants with diabetes at risk for physical and emotional problems. Because of the demands of daily management, many parents are unable to leave their infants in the care of others (8–9). Moreover, finding "relief" caregivers who are competent and comfortable caring for a young child with diabetes is often extremely difficult (10).

Wysocki et al. (11) investigated maternal reports of the psychological adjustment of a sample of 20 children with diabetes between two and six years of age using the Child Behavior Checklist (CBCL) (12). Compared to a normative sample, children with type 1 diabetes showed significantly more "internalizing" behavior problems such as depression, anxiety, sleep problems, somatic complaints, or withdrawal. Wysocki et al. also noted that the mothers of very young children with diabetes reported more parenting stress when contrasted with a nondiabetic standardization sample. In contrast, Northam et al. (7) found no significant deviations from normative scores on any scale of the CBCL at diagnosis or 1 year later in a sample of 18 children less than 4 years of age. However, neither study assessed children's behavior independent of maternal report. Similar to the findings of Wysocki et al. (11), recently Powers et al. (13) also found higher stress levels in parents of very young children with diabetes compared to parents of very young nondiabetic children.

Anderson et al. (14) reported that in a sample of 106 very young children with diabetes (with an average age of 4.6 years and average disease duration of 1.2 years), children received two or more injections per day from their parents, and on average, parents monitored their child's blood glucose level four times daily, with a range of one to seven blood glucose checks per day. Thus, it is clear that the daily demands of caring for diabetes create a heavy burden for parents of very young children with diabetes. In a larger sample of parents of very young children,

Anderson et al. (14) reported that among the most significant concerns these parents identified were the added stress on the family system and the problem of differentiating changes in the child's behavior due to blood glucose fluctuations from normal behavioral changes in young children.

Several authors (11,15) have reported that mothers of very young child with diabetes report more concerns about identifying hypoglycemia when compared with parents of older children and adolescents with diabetes. Early studies by Ryan et al. (16–18) and Rovet et al. (19) documented mild, cognitive deficits that were associated with severe recurrent hypoglycemia in very young children with diabetes. However recent research, some based on advances in brain imaging techniques (20), has recently led Ryan to hypothesize that while early onset of diabetes is a potent predictor of neurocognitive dysfunction, it may be that "chronic hyperglycemia" in very young children with diabetes is as damaging to the developing brain as severe, "recurrent hypoglycemia" (21).

Recently continuous subcutaneous insulin infusion therapy (CSII), or "pump" therapy has increasingly been used in very young children with diabetes. Several studies have shown that insulin pump therapy is a safe alternative to multiple daily insulin injections and may improve quality of life for families of very young children with diabetes (22–26). CSII may reduce the rate of severe hypoglycemic reactions among young children (24–26). In these studies, the reported satisfaction with pump therapy and improved quality of life were likely due to a reduction in marked fluctuating blood glucose levels and a reduction in severe hypoglycemic events and resultant reduced parental anxiety. CSII also allows greater convenience and lifestyle flexibility, with respect to basic family routines such as timing of meals.

Three small randomized studies comparing pump therapy to multiple daily injections concluded that pump therapy did not result in significantly better glycemic control (27–29). In two of these studies more mild-moderate hypoglycemia was observed in the pump-treated children (28,29). Both of these studies also documented trends for improvements in parent-reported diabetes-related quality of life (28,29). Similarly, Jeha et al. reported that pump therapy is very acceptable to motivated and well-educated parents and does not result in any additional parenting stress (30).

Based on these studies, it appears that CSII therapy is an effective and safe alternative for very young children. As with all pediatric diabetes management issues, the decision to start pump therapy in a very young child must be individualized to each family's lifestyle and to parental abilities.

In this first decade of the twenty-first century, it seems that the most appropriate approach to the care of very young children with diabetes—both from a psychosocial as well as physical health perspective—is to strive for optimal glycemic control, while avoiding severe hypoglycemia, through an individualized plan of intensive insulin therapy that is sensitive to minimizing stress on the parents and on the family system (21,31).

Psychosocial Tasks in the School-Age Period (6–10 years)

The primary developmental tasks of the school-age child are: making a smooth adjustment from the home to the school setting; forming close friendships with children of the same sex; developing new intellectual, athletic, and artistic skills; and forming a positive sense of self (2).

Psychosocial Research on School-Age Children with Diabetes

Studies of school-age children with diabetes have linked low self-esteem and poor social-emotional adjustment to poorly-controlled diabetes (31,32). Herskowitz-Dumont et al. (33) found that recurrent diabetic ketoacidosis (DKA) over eight years post-diagnosis was associated with significantly higher ratings of behavior problems and lower levels of social competence. Liss et al. (34) found that children who had been hospitalized with DKA in the preceding year reported lower levels of self-esteem and social competence than children who had no DKA in that period. Significantly more youths in the DKA group met the diagnostic criteria for at least one psychiatric disorder (88% vs. 28%).

Participation or attendance in school is disrupted if the child has chronically poor glycemic control (35). Frequent school absences may result in educational setbacks and interfere with peer relationships and self-esteem (36). In addition, minimizing the occurrence of hypoglycemia at school is crucial in light of studies indicating that memory and concentration may continue to be impaired even after the physical symptoms of hypoglycemia have subsided (37).

A recent study using the well-validated Child Health Questionnaire (CHQ) reported that psychosocial indices of well-being were better for children aged 5 to 11 years with type 1 diabetes in good glycemic control (with HbAlc less than 8.8%) (38). Data from Sweden and the United States document that severe hypoglycemia was associated with the lowest health-related quality of life in children and their parents (39–41). It seems to be critical for school-age children with diabetes to have treatment regimens that are minimally interruptive to the child's school day and which balance the benefits of optimal control against the child's developmental needs and the risks of hypoglycemia.

The family has frequently been studied as the primary psychosocial influence on school-age children with diabetes. Waller et al. conducted one of the first empirical studies of families with children with diabetes under the age of 12 years (42). Among school-age patients, more diabetes-related family guidance and control were linked to better metabolic outcomes, and diabetes-related parental warmth and caring were important for optimal outcomes. Liss et al. also found that children hospitalized with DKA reported less diabetes-related parental warmth and caring (34). Family variables that are not diabetes-specific, such as conflict, stress, and family cohesion, have also been linked to glycemic control and adherence behavior in school-age children with T1DM (43–49). Family environments that are more structured and rule-governed have been shown to be associated with better glycemic control in school-age children with type 1 diabetes (50). Frequently, high levels of family stress have been shown to correlate with poorer glycemic control in children under 12 years of age (49). In contrast, Kovacs et al. have not found relationships between general family factors and metabolic control or treatment adherence in a longitudinal study of school-age children (51). However, a second longitudinal study of school-age children with newly-diagnosed diabetes by Jacobson et al. (44,52) revealed that the child's perception of family conflict measured at diagnosis was the strongest predictor of poor adherence to insulin administration, meal planning, exercise, and blood glucose monitoring tasks over a four-year follow-up period.

The connection between family conflict, the child's adherence to the treatment regimen, and glycemic control was also examined by Miller-Johnson et al. (46). Parent-child conflict was a significant correlate of both adherence and glycemic control. The authors suggested that conflict may interfere with glycemic control by disrupting treatment adherence.

In a recent study of parenting styles, regimen adherence, and glycemic control in 4- to 10-year-olds with type 1 diabetes and their parents, "authoritative parenting" characterized by parental support and affection was related to better regimen adherence and glycemic control (53). Authoritative parenting, in which conflict is minimized as parents set consistent, realistic limits on children's behavior while displaying warmth and sensitivity to their child's needs and feelings, has been linked to improved behavioral outcomes in general child development as well as in diabetes-specific adjustment of school-age children (54). There is mounting empirical evidence that parental involvement in diabetes management is required throughout the school-age developmental period for the child's physical and psychosocial well-being (55–58).

Grey et al. studied 8- to 14-year-old children newly diagnosed with diabetes and a nondiabetic, peer comparison group (59). Children's adjustment problems at diagnosis disappeared at one year post-diagnosis, but reappeared at two years post-diagnosis, a pattern similar to that found by Kovacs et al. (60–64). Grey et al. argued that, while adjustment immediately after diagnosis is crucial, their data suggest that a second "critical period" of adjustment occurs in the second year after diagnosis, and that intervention is important during the critical second year of life with diabetes for prevention of psychosocial and metabolic deterioration (59).

Psychosocial Tasks in Early to Middle Adolescence (11--16 years)

The psychosocial tasks of early adolescence include adapting to the sudden physical changes that come with puberty; establishing a new role in the family, gaining positive acceptance by peers; and developing more abstract reasoning and critical thinking skills (64). Beginning with Erikson (3), the earliest theories of psychosocial aspects of adolescent development emphasized discontinuity, turmoil, and independence from parental influence (65). However during the last decade, theorists have argued that issues of attachment and interpersonal relationships during adolescence have been overlooked. There is a new theoretical focus on "interdependence" and the development of healthy interpersonal relationships during early adolescence. New theories of early adolescent development are emerging based on models of self-regulation as opposed to freedom from parents (66,67). A consensus appears to be developing among investigators concerned with early adolescent development that engagement with, rather than separation from, parents during early adolescence enhances academic performance and ego development, and reduces vulnerability to negative peer influences (68). In summary, current developmental theories identify the major psychosocial task of the early adolescent period as movement away from dependence on the family, not toward independence, but rather, toward interdependence. Furthermore, this interdependence does not require that adolescents distance themselves emotionally from parents, but rather requires a reorganization in which family members renegotiate roles and redistribute responsibilities within the family system.

Psychosocial Research on Early to Mid Adolescents with Diabetes

Optimal glycemic control is more difficult to establish and maintain during the early and middle adolescent period because of the normal 'insulin resistance' that occurs during puberty (69). In addition to this basic biological phenomenon, the normal developmental tasks involving transitions in family roles and peer relationships that occur during early and middle adolescence often interfere with adherence to the diabetes treatment regimen. Young adolescents frequently seek a new level of separation from their parents, while simultaneously attachments to peers intensify. In recent family studies, it has been documented that there is an erosion of parental involvement and support for diabetes management tasks over the early- and middle-adolescent years (56–58). Empirical research has documented a steady decrease in adherence to diabetes treatment over the early adolescent period (70–72). However, empirical studies have shown that young adolescents who have more parental involvement, monitoring, and teamwork in diabetes management tend to achieve and maintain better diabetes outcomes (73–76). Social support from peers and siblings can also contribute to adolescents' treatment adherence and adaptation to diabetes (77–80).

Supportive parental behavior must be individualized depending on the adolescent's developmental level, temperament, and the unique circumstances of each family. Parental involvement, can, at times, undermine healthy adolescent self-care behavior, as in the behavioral interaction cycle of "miscarried helping" that occurs when parental help that is given shames, blames, or humiliates the adolescent with diabetes (81). In the context of a chronic illness such as diabetes, "miscarried helping" can escalate parent-adolescent conflict, which undermines adolescent adherence and positive medical outcomes.

While metabolic deterioration occurs predictably during this period of adolescence, there is convincing evidence that improved metabolic control during this period of adolescence has the potential to reverse early complications of diabetes, such as neuropathic and gastrointestinal complications, and may aid in the prevention of diabetic nephropathy and diabetic retinopathy (82).

Interventions with Early to Middle Adolescents with Diabetes

Two themes emerge from the recent research on early to middle adolescents with diabetes and their families; first, sustaining appropriate levels of parental involvement in diabetes management; and second, minimizing parent-adolescent conflict, are important for positive health outcomes over this developmental period. Given the importance of the family system for optimal psychological and glycemic outcomes in adolescents during this stage of development, it is not surprising that a number of family-centered interventions have been implemented with youngsters aged 11 to 16 years and their families.

Behavioral family systems therapy. Behavioral family systems therapy (BFST) is a family-focused intervention that employs multidimensional methods of treatment to improve family communication and problem-solving skills (83). The BFST model has been adapted to the treatment of youths with T1DM to promote family-based skills in an effort to improve diabetes management and glycemic control (84). Wysocki et al. conducted a randomized, controlled trial of BFST that included 10 family sessions over a three-month period and found subsequent improvement in certain family processes (e.g., improved communication, reduced conflict). These effects were observed for up to one year post-treatment (85). However, it was not until they adapted the original intervention model to be diabetes-specific (BFST-Diabetes, BFST-D) that improvements in adherence and diabetes control occurred (86).

Adolescents were randomized to one of three conditions: BFST-D, a multi-family support group, or standard care. In BFST-D, individual families received 12 sessions across 6 months from a psychologist trained in the BFST model. Sessions focused on problem-solving, communication, cognitive restructuring, and functional-structural family therapy (86). Additional components of BFST-D include behavioral contracting around diabetes management tasks, goal setting, diabetes education, psychoeducation, parental participation in simulated diabetes tasks (e.g., monitoring and treating simulated hypoglycemia), and possible extension to the social networks of the youth. Immediate post-treatment results indicated that for adolescents who were in the poorest control at baseline (HbAlc > 9.0%), families in the BFST-D condition had lower levels of diabetes-specific conflict and significantly greater improvement in HbA1c than did adolescents in the other two groups. Most important, adolescents in the BFST-D condition showed significant improvements in self-management behaviors when compared to adolescents in the other two conditions.

In an exploratory pilot study, Harris et al. adapted the original BFST model to a home-based intervention focused on a very high-risk population—adolescents with T1DM in chronic poor metabolic control with a pattern of missing diabetes clinic appointments (87). Ten 90-minute sessions of BFST therapy were delivered in the home setting to the adolescent and parent over a period of five to eight weeks. Assessments of psychological, family, adherence, and glycemic control variables were made immediately following the intervention and again after six months. Immediate post-treatment results indicated improvement in general parent-teen conflict and diabetes-specific family conflict; however, these gains were not sustained at the six-month follow-up. Moreover glycemic control remained unchanged from baseline to initial post-treatment assessment as well as at the six-month follow-up point (88). The importance of this intervention is its focus on a high-risk group of pediatric patients for whom traditional medical and psycho-educational services had consistently failed.

Multisystemic therapy. Another intervention focused on the high risk group of adolescents with T1DM in very poor control and their families was carried out by Ellis et al. who looked at the effectiveness of multisystemic therapy (MST) in improving health outcomes in poorly controlled adolescents with T1DM (89). MST is an intensive, home-, school- and community-based form of psychotherapy, originally developed for youth with severe antisocial behavior problems (90). Adolescents with HbAlc > 8% were randomized to two conditions: the MST condition for six months of intensive home-based family psychotherapy and standard diabetes medical care, or the control condition of standard diabetes medical care only. Immediate post-treatment results at six months indicated that youth in the MST condition monitored their blood glucose levels significantly more often, had fewer inpatient hospitalizations and showed a significant improvement in metabolic control when compared with control subjects receiving standard medical care. In addition, participation in MST therapy significantly reduced diabetes-related stress in adolescents (91).

Coping skills training. Only one published intervention has been carried out in the context of pediatric patients receiving intensive diabetes therapy (92). In an intervention to strengthen the coping skills of youth with diabetes who were beginning a program of intensive management, Grey et al. randomly assigned adolescents tone of two groups: intensive insulin therapy along with a small group program of structured social problem-solving skills training (or Coping skills training, CST) or to a program of intensive diabetes management alone (92). While parents were not directly involved in the intervention process, the CST program was designed to increase the adolescent's sense of competence and mastery by learning and practicing more effective diabetes-related social behaviors related to parents as well as peers. For example, the sessions focused on "skills that help adolescents to negotiate with family members over treatment responsibilities" (p. 112). Four weekly meetings were followed by monthly visits for a total of 10 social skills training sessions delivered by a trained mental health professional. Follow-up assessments of glycemic control and quality of life made at 3 months and 12 months indicated that adolescents in the social problem-solving skills training intervention had improved HbAlc and reported higher quality of life than adolescents undergoing intensive diabetes treatment without this behavioral intervention (93). At one year, adolescents in the CST condition had significant improvements in diabetes self-efficacy. The control condition received the CST intervention after the one-year study; thus no longer term outcome data are available. The research by Grey et al. is important in that it demonstrated that CST helped adolescents to optimize the initiation and maintenance of a program of intensive therapy over one year.

Care ambassador intervention. Studies have documented that adverse short-term (poor metabolic control) and long-term (retinopathy and nephropathy) outcomes occur when patients with diabetes become lost-to-follow-up or have infrequent encounters with their medical team (94–97). Thus, effective, inexpensive approaches aimed at increasing ambulatory medical visits for youth with T1DM are needed. To address this need, in 1998, Laffel et al. published the results of a two-year longitudinal study utilizing a Care Ambassador intervention compared with standard care (98). Study participants were youth, aged 10 to 15 years, with T1DM who were randomly assigned to either a Care Ambassador Intervention group or to standard multi-disciplinary care. Subjects in the two groups were followed prospectively for 24 months or until they dropped-out of care. The Care Ambassador intervention was specifically designed to help patients and their families receive ambulatory diabetes care as prescribed by the patient's usual diabetes health care team. A Care Ambassador assisted the families with their appointment scheduling and confirmation and helped them with questions concerning billing or insurance by directing the families to the appropriate personnel. The primary task of the Care Ambassadors was to monitor the clinic attendance of intervention patients and provide telephone or written outreach to families after missed or canceled appointments. The Care Ambassadors had no formal medical education and provided no prescriptive medical advice. During the study, the intervention group had significantly more diabetes visits compared to the standard care group. The increased clinic visit frequency was associated with improved outcomes, as evidenced by a shift in the distribution of glycemic control towards lower HbAlc values and a 50% reduction in the risk of severe hypoglycemia and hospital/ER use in the intervention group compared with standard care.

In 2003, Svoren et al. sought to further evaluate the Care Ambassador Intervention model and to determine whether this intervention supplemented by psychoeducational modules could further improve outcomes (99). This study again found that the Care Ambassador intervention increased clinic visit frequency.

However, only youth assigned to receive the psychoeducational modules experienced significantly reduced rates of short-term adverse outcomes and demonstrated improved control.

Family-focused teamwork intervention. Studies have also shown the importance of developmentally appropriate family involvement around diabetes management for optimizing glycemic control and preventing acute and chronic complications in youth with diabetes (57,58). In 1999, Anderson et al. demonstrated that parent involvement in diabetes management tasks could be strengthened through a low-intensity Family Teamwork intervention integrated into routine follow-up diabetes care (100). Moreover, the study found that, despite increased engagement between parent and teen focused around diabetes tasks, diabetes-related family conflict simultaneously decreased while glycemic control improved compared with the comparison group.

In 2003, Laffel et al. reported the results of a randomized, controlled trial that further evaluated this family-focused intervention aimed at optimizing glycemic control, minimizing diabetes-related family conflict, and maintaining quality of life in youth with T1DM (101). Children and adolescents, 8 to 17 years of age, with T1DM for ≤6 years were randomly assigned to either a family-focused teamwork intervention or to standard multidisciplinary diabetes care. Both study groups were seen at three- to four-month intervals and were followed prospectively for one year. The intervention for the families in the teamwork condition focused on the importance of parent-child responsibility-sharing for diabetes tasks and ways to avoid conflict that undermines such teamwork. The intervention specifically targeted increased parent involvement with blood glucose monitoring and insulin dosing. After one year, the HbA1c in the teamwork intervention group did not deteriorate and was significantly lower than the HbA1c in the group receiving standard care. Furthermore, although parent involvement was maintained or increased in the families receiving the teamwork intervention, no increase in diabetes-related family conflict or any negative impact on quality of life was found. After two years, the Teamwork group demonstrated better glycemic control and quality of life compared with the standard care group (102).

Psychopathology in Adolescents with Diabetes

Evidence as to the prevalence of psychopathology (depression, eating disorders, anxiety disorders, and behavior disorders) in adolescents with diabetes is contradictory with some studies documenting increased prevalence (103–106) while other studies find no higher prevalence of psychopathology in adolescents with diabetes than in the general population of adolescents (107,108). For example, evidence as to the prevalence of major depressive illness in adolescents with T1DM is contradictory, with some studies reporting a prevalence rate of two to three times the rate of depression as in the general population of adolescents (109) while the more recent SEARCH for Diabetes in Youth multicenter study (110) reported that the incidence of depressed mood in adolescence with diabetes is no higher than in the general population of healthy adolescents (111). This variation among reports of the prevalence of depression in adolescents with diabetes may be due to differences in study design, the diagnostic or screening instrument used, and the diagnostic or cutoff criteria employed (112). However, recent reports consistently document that the presence of psychopathology in adolescents with diabetes is associated with poorer glycemic control (113,114) and increased incidence of hospitalizations (115,116) which put the adolescent in poor glycemic control at increased risk for diabetes-related complications (117).

Female adolescents with diabetes are at increased risk of developing an eating disorder or subclinical eating disorder than aged-matched adolescents without diabetes (118,119). Eating disorders, especially insulin under-dosing or insulin omission is linked to poor glycemic control and the development of diabetes-related complications (120). Disruptive behavior disorders have also been reported in adolescents with diabetes (121,122). Moreover, adolescents with disruptive behavior problems were found to be twice as likely to have a glycosylated hemoglobin level above 9% (122). In summary, it is clear that adolescents with type 1 diabetes who also have a psychiatric diagnosis are at increased risk for poor glycemic control and the development of diabetes-related complications. Moreover, there is evidence that a negative developmental trajectory around diabetes management during adolescence may persist into early adulthood, accelerating the risk of long-term medical and psychological complications of diabetes (123,124). Given the number of innovative interventions which target adolescents with T1DM, it is notable that there have been no published intervention trials with this very high-risk group of adolescents. Clearly there is a great need for screening and intervention programs for adolescents with T1DM and psychiatric comorbidities, such as depression and eating disorders.

CONCLUSIONS

In a recent and elegant review of the literature on emotional well-being and quality of life in childhood diabetes, Cameron and Northam (125) trace the childhood precursors of adolescent outcomes in T1DM and make a strong case for earlier screening and interventions with this patient population. The research literature reviewed in this chapter also documents the all-encompassing impact of T1DM and its complex daily treatment regimen on the psychosocial tasks of the developing child as well as on the family system. This clearly provides a strong base of evidence for the allocation of psychosocial resources, such as social workers, psychologists, psychiatrists, and child life specialists for our youngest patients with diabetes and their families as well as at diagnosis and early in the disease course for patients and families at high-risk for adverse health outcomes.

REFERENCES

1. Anderson BJ, Cullen K, McKay S. Quality of life, family behavior, and health outcomes in children with type 2 diabetes. Pediatr Ann 2005; 34:722–729.
2. Erikson EH. Childhood and Society. 2nd ed. New York: Norton, 1963.
3. Erikson EH. Identity, Youth and Crisis. New York: Norton, 1968.
4. Wolfsdorf JI, Anderson BA, Pasquarello C. Treatment of the child with diabetes. In: Kahn CR, Weir G, eds. Joslin's Diabetes Mellitus. 13th ed. Philadelphia: Lea Febiger, 1994:430–451.
5. Silverstein JH, Johnson S. Psychosocial challenge of diabetes and the development of a continuum of care. Pediatr Ann 1994; 23:300–305.
6. Anderson BJ, Auslander WF. Research on diabetes management and the family: a critique. Diabetes Care 1980; 3:696–702.
7. Northam E, Anderson P, Adler R, et al. Psychosocial and family functioning in children with insulin-dependent diabetes at diagnosis and one year later. J Pediatr Psychol 1996; 21:699–717.

8. Hatton DL, Canam C, Thorne S, et al. Parents' perceptions of caring for an infant or toddler with diabetes. J Adv Nurs 1995; 22:569–577.

9. Sullivan-Bolyai S, Deatrick J, Gruppuso P, et al. Constant vigilance: mothers' work parenting young children with type 1 diabetes. J Pediatr Nurs 2003; 18:21–29.

10. Kushion W, Salisbury PJ, Seitz KW, et al. Issues in the care of infants and toddlers with insulin dependent diabetes mellitus. Diabetes Educ 1991; 17:107–110.

11. Wysocki T, Huxtable K, Linscheid TR, et al. Adjustment to diabetes mellitus in preschoolers and their mothers. Diabetes Care 1989; 12:524–529.

12. Achenbach TM, Edelbrock CS. Manual for the Child Behavior Checklist and Revised Child Behavior Profile. Burlington, VT: University of Vermont Press, 1983.

13. Powers SW, Byars KC, Mitchell MJ, et al. Parent report of mealtime behavior and parenting stress in young children with type 1 diabetes and in healthy control subjects. Diabetes Care 2002; 25:313–318.

14. Anderson BJ, Loughlin C, Goldberg E, et al. Comprehensive, family-focused outpatient care for very young children living with chronic disease: lessons from a program in pediatric diabetes. Child Serv Social Policy Res Prac 2001; 4:235–250.

15. Banion CR, Miles MS, Carter MC. Problems of mothers in management of children with diabetes. Diabetes Care 1983; 6:548–551.

16. Ryan C, Vega A, Longstreet C, et al. Neuropsychological changes in adolescents with insulin-independent diabetes. J Consult Clin Psychol 1984; 52:335–342.

17. Ryan C, Longstreet C, Morrow L. The effects of diabetes mellitus on the school attendance and school achievement of adolescents. Child Care Health Dev 1985; 11: 229–240.

18. Ryan C, Vega A, Drash A. Cognitive deficits in adolescents who developed diabetes early in life. Pediatrics 1985; 75:921–927.

19. Rovet JF, Ehrlich RM, Hoppe M. Intellectual deficits associated with early onset of insulin-dependent diabetes mellitus in children. Diabetes Care 1987; 10:510–515.

20. Ferguson SC, Blane A, Wardlaw JM, et al. Influences of an early-onset age of type 1 diabetes on cerebral structure and cognitive function. Diabetes Care 2005; 28:1431–1437.

21. Ryan CM. Why is cognitive dysfunction associated with the development of diabetes early in life? The diathesis hypothesis. Pediatr Diabetes 2006; 7:289–297.

22. Shehadeh N, Battelino T, Galatzer A, et al. Insulin pump therapy for 1-6 year old children with type 1 diabetes. Isr Med Assoc J 2004; 6:284–286.

23. DiMeglio LA, Pottorff TM, Boyd SR, et al. A randomized, controlled study of insulin pump therapy in diabetic preschoolers. J Pediatr 2004:145; 380–384.

24. Litton J, Rice A, Friedman N, et al. Insulin pump therapy in toddlers and preschool children with type 1 diabetes mellitus. J Pediatr 2002; 141:490–495.

25. Saha ME, Huuppone T, Mikael K, et al. Continuous subcutaneous insulin infusion in the treatment of children and adolescents with type 1 diabetes mellitus. J Pediatr Endocrinol Metab 2002; 15:1005–1010.

26. Tubiana-Rufi N, de Lonlay P, Bloch J, et al. Remission of severe hypoglycemic incidents in young diabetic children treated with subcutaneous infusion. Arch Pediatr 1996; 3:969–976.

27. Fox LA, Buckloh LM, Smith SD, et al. A randomized controlled trial of insulin pump therapy in young children with type 1 diabetes. Diabetes Care 2005; 28:1277–1281.

28. Wilson DM, Buckingham BA, Kunselman EL, et al. A two-center randomized controlled feasibility trial of insulin pump therapy in young children with diabetes. Diabetes Care 2005; 28:15–19.

29. Weinzimer SA, Swan KL, Sikes KA, et al. Emerging evidence for the use of insulin pump therapy in infants, toddlers, and preschool-aged children with type 1 diabetes. Pediatr Diabetes 2006; 7:15–19.

30. Jeha GS, Karaviti LP, Anderson BJ, et al. Insulin pump therapy in preschool children with Type 1 diabetes mellitus improves glycemic control and decreases glucose excursions and the risk of hypoglycemia. Diabetes Technol Ther 2005; 7:876–884.

31. Johnson SB. Psychological factors in juvenile diabetes: a review. J Behav Med 1980; 3:95–116.

32. Ryden O, Nevander L, Johnsson P, et al. Family therapy in poorly controlled juvenile IDDM: effects on diabetes control, self-evaluation, and behavioral symptoms. Acta Paediatr 1994; 83:285–291.
33. Herskowitz-Dumont R, Jacobson AM, et al. Psychosocial predictors of acute complications of diabetes in youth. Diabet Med 1995; 12:612–618.
34. Liss DS, Waller DA, Kennard BD, et al. Psychiatric illness and family support in children and adolescents with diabetic ketoacidosis: a controlled study. J Am Acad Child Adolesc Psychiatry 1998; 37:536–544.
35. Balik B, Haig B, Moynihan PM. Diabetes and the school-aged child. Am J Matern Child Nurs 1986; 11:324–330.
36. Pond JS, Peters ML, Pannell DL, et al. Psychosocial challenges for children with insulin-dependent diabetes mellitus. Diabetes Educ 1995; 21:297–299.
37. Puczynski MS, Puczynski SS, Reich J, et al. Mental efficiency and hypoglycemia. J Dev Behav Pediatr 1990; 11:170–174.
38. Wake M, Hesketh K, Cameron FM. The Child Health Questionnaire in children with diabetes: cross sectional survey of parent and adolescent reported functional health status. Diabet Med 2000; 17:700–707.
39. Cameron FJ. The impact of diabetes on health-related quality of life in children and adolescents. Pediatr Diabetes 2003; 4:132–136.
40. Nordfeldt S, Jonsson D. Short-term effects of severe hypoglycemia in children and adolescents with type 1 diabetes. A cost-of-illness study. Acta Paediatr 2001; 90:137–142.
41. Marrero DG, Guare JC, Vandagriff JL, et al. Fear of hypoglycemia in the parents of children and adolescents with diabetes: maladaptive or healthy response? Diabetes Educ 1997; 23:281–286.
42. Waller D, Chipman JJ, Hardy BW, et al. Measuring diabetes-specific family support and its relation to metabolic control: a preliminary report. J Am Acad Child Psychol 1986; 25:415–418.
43. Marteau TM, Bloch S, Baum JD. Family life and diabetic control. J Child Psychol Psychiatry 1987; 28:823–833.
44. Hauser ST, Jacobson AM, Lavori P, et al. Adherence among children and adolescents with insulin-dependent diabetes mellitus over four-year longitudinal follow-up: II. Immediate and long-term linkages with the family milieu J Pediatr Psychol 1990; 15:527–542.
45. Auslander WF, Bubb J, Rogge M, et al. Family stress and resources: potential areas of intervention in children recently diagnosed with diabetes. Health Soc Work 1993; 18:101–113.
46. Miller-Johnson S, Emery RE, Marvin RS, et al. Parent-child relationships and the management of diabetes mellitus. J Consult Clin Psychol 1994; 62:603–610.
47. Jacobson AM, Hauser ST, Lavori P, et al. Family environment and glycemic control: a four-year prospective study of children and adolescents with insulin-dependent diabetes mellitus. Psychosom Med 1994; 56:401–409.
48. Goldston DB, Kovacs M, Obrosky S, et al. A longitudinal study of life events and metabolic control among youths with insulin-dependent diabetes mellitus. Health Psychol 1995; 14:409–414.
49. Viner R, McGrath M, Trudinger P. Family stress and metabolic control in diabetes. Arch Dis Child 1996; 74:418–421.
50. Cohen DM, Lumley MA, Naar-King S, et al. Child behavior problems and family functioning as predictors of adherence and glycemic control in economically disadvantaged children with type 1 diabetes: a prospective study. J Pediatr Psychol 2004; 29:171–184.
51. Kovacs M, Kass RE, Schnell TM, et al. Family functioning and metabolic control of school-aged children with IDDM. Diabetes Care 1989; 12:409–414.
52. Jacobson AM, Hauser ST, Lavori P, et al. Adherence among children and adolescents with insulin-dependent diabetes mellitus over four-year longitudinal follow-up: I. The influence of patient coping and adjustment. J Pediatr Psychol 1990; 15:511–526.
53. Davis CL, Delamater AM, Shaw KH, et al. Parenting styles, regimen adherence, and glycemic control in 4- to 10-year-old children with diabetes. J Pediatr Psychol 2001; 26:123–129.

54. Anderson BJ. Family conflict and diabetes management in youth: clinical lessons from child development and diabetes research. Diabetes Spectr 2004; 17:22–26.

55. Weissberg-Benchell J, Glasgow AM, Tynan WD, et al. Adolescent diabetes management and mismanagement. Diabetes Care 1995; 18:77–82

56. Anderson BJ, Auslander WF, Jung KC, et al. Assessing family sharing of diabetes responsibilities. J Pediatr Psychol 1990; 15:477–492.

57. Wysocki T, Taylor A, Hough BS, et al. Deviation for developmentally appropriate self-care autonomy. Association with diabetes outcomes. Diabetes Care 1996; 19:119–125.

58. Anderson B, Ho J, Brackett J, et al. Parental involvement in diabetes management tasks: relationships to blood glucose monitoring adherence and metabolic control in young adolescents with insulin-dependent diabetes mellitus. J Pediatr 1997; 130:257–265.

59. Grey M, Cameron ME, Lipman TH, et al. Psychosocial status of children with diabetes in the first 2 years after diagnosis. Diabetes Care 1995; 18:1330–1336.

60. Kovacs M, Iyengar S, Goldston D, et al. Psychological functioning of children with insulin-dependent diabetes mellitus: a longitudinal study. J Pediatr Psychol 1990; 15:619–632.

61. Kovacs M, Iyengar S, Goldston D, et al. Psychological functioning among mothers of children with insulin-dependent diabetes mellitus: a longitudinal study. J Consult Clin Psychol 1990; 58:189–195.

62. Kovacs M, Feinberg TL, Paulauskas S, et al. Initial coping responses and psychosocial characteristics of children with insulin-dependent diabetes mellitus. J Pediatr 1985; 106:827–834.

63. Kovacs M, Finkelstein R, Feinberg TL, et al. Initial psychological responses of parents to the diagnosis of insulin-dependent diabetes mellitus in their children. Diabetes Care 1985; 8:568–575.

64. Newman BM, Newman PR. Development through life: a psychosocial approach. Homewood, Ill: Dorsey Press, 1975.

65. Blos P. The adolescent passage. New York, NY: International Universities Press, 1979.

66. Hill JP. Research on adolescents and their families: past and prospect. In: Irwin CE, ed. Adolescent Social Behavior and Health. San Francisco, CA: Jossey-Bass, 1987:13–32.

67. Gilligan C. Adolescent development reconsidered. In: Irwin CE, ed. Adolescent Social Behavior and Health. San Francisco, CA: Jossey-Bass, 1987:63–92.

68. Resnick MD, Bearman PS, Blum RW, et al. Protecting adolescent from harm: findings from the National Longitudinal Study on Adolescent health. JAMA 1997; 278:823–832.

69. Amiel SA, Sherwin RS, Simonson DC, et al. Impaired insulin action in puberty: a contributing factor to poor glycemic control in adolescents with diabetes. N Engl J Med 1986; 315:215–219.

70. Johnson SB, Silverstein J, Rosenbloom A, et al. Assessing daily management of childhood diabetes. Health Psychol 1986; 5:545–564.

71. Harris, MA, Wysocki T, Sadler M, et al. Validation of a structured interview for the assessment of diabeges self-management. Diabetes Care 2000; 23:1301–1304.

72. Thomas AM, Peterson J, Goldstein D. Problem solving and diabetes regimen adherence by children and adolescents with IDDM in social pressure situations: a reflection of normal development. J Pediatr Psychol 1997; 22:541–561.

73. Allen DA, Tennen H, McGrade BJ, et al. Parent and child perceptions of the management of juvenile diabetes. J Pediatr Psychol 1983; 8(2):129–141.

74. Ingersoll G, Orr DP, Herrold AJ, et al. Cognitive maturity and self-management among adolescent with insulin-dependent diabetes mellitus. J Pediatr 1986; 108:620–623.

75. Palmer D, Berg CA, Wiebe DJ, et al. The role of autonomy and pubertal status in understanding age difference in maternal involvement in diabetes responsibility across adolescence. J Pediatr Psychol 2004; 29:35–46.

76. Weibe DJ, Berg CA, Korbel C, et al. Children's appraisals of maternal involvement in coping with diabetes: enhancing our understanding of adherence, metabolic control, and quality of life across adolescence. J Pediatr Psychol 2005; 30:167–178.

77. Shroff-Pendley J, Kasmen LJ, Miller DL, et al. Peer and family support in children and adolescents with type 1 diabetes. J Pediatr Psychol 2002; 27:429–438.

78. La Greca AM, Auslander WF, Greco P, et al. I get by with a little help from my family and friends: adolescents' support for diabetes care. J Pediatr Psychol 1995; 26:279–282.

79. Greco P, Shroff-Pendley J, McDonnell K, et al. A peer group intervention for adolescents with type 1 diabetes and their best friends. J Pediatr Psychol 2001; 26:485–490.

80. Bearman KJ, La Greca AM. Assessing friend support of adolescents' diabetes care: the diabetes social support questionnaire-friends version. J Pediatr Psychol 2002; 27: 417–428.

81. Anderson BJ. Coyne JC. "Miscarried helping" in the interactions between chronically ill children and their parents. In: Johnson JH, Johnson SB, eds. Advances in Child Health Psychology. Gainesville, FL: University of Florida, 1991:167–177.

82. White NH, Waltman SR, Krupin E, et al. Reversal of neuropathic and gastrointestinal complications related to diabetes mellitus in adolescent with improved metabolic control. Pediatrics 1981; 99:41–45.

83. Robin AL, Foster SL. Negotiating parent-adolescent conflict: a behavioral family systems approach. New York: Guilford, 1989.

84. Wysocki T, Harris MA, Greco P, et al. Randomized, controlled trial of behavior therapy for families of adolescents with insulin-dependent diabetes mellitus. J Pediatr Psychol 2000; 25:23–33.

85. Wysocki T, Greco P, Harris MA, et al. Behavior therapy for families of adolescents with diabetes: maintenance of treatment effects. Diabetes Care 2001; 24:441–446.

86. Wysocki T, Harris MA, Buckloh LM, et al. Effects of behavioral family systems therapy for diabetes on adolescents' family relationships, treatment adherence, and metabolic control. J Pediatr Psychol 2006; 31:928–938.

87. Harris MA, Mertlich D. Piloting home-based behavioral family systems therapy for adolescent with poorly controlled diabetes. Children's Health Care 2003; 32:65–79.

88. Harris MA, Harris BS, Mertlich D. Brief Report: In-home family therapy for adolescents with poorly controlled diabetes: failure to maintain benefits at 6-month follow-up. J Pediatr Psychol 2005; 30:683–688.

89. Ellis DA, Frey M, Narr-King S, et al. Use of multisystemic therapy to improve regimen adherence among adolescent with type 1 diabetes in chronic poor metabolic control: a randomized controlled trial. Diabetes Care 2005; 28:1604–1610.

90. Henggeler SW, Schoenwalk DS, Borduin CM, et al. Multisystemic Treatment of Antisocial Behavior in Children and Adolescents. New York: Guilford Press, 1998.

91. Ellis DA, Frey M, Narr-King S, et al. The effects of multisystemic therapy on diabetes stress among adolescents with chronically poorly controlled type 1 diabetes: findings from a randomized, controlled trial. Pediatrics 2005; 116:826–832.

92. Grey M, Boland E, Davidson M, et al. Short-term effects of coping skills training as adjunct to intensive therapy in adolescents. Diabetes Care 1998; 21:902–914.

93. Grey M, Boland E, Davidson M, et al. Coping skills training for youth with diabetes mellitus has long-lasting effects on metabolic control and quality of life. J Pediatr 2000; 137:107–113.

94. Krolewski AS, Warram JH, Christlieb AR, et al. The changing natural history of nephropathy in type I diabetes. Am J Med 1985; 78:785–794.

95. Jacobson AM, Adler AG, Derby L, et al. Clinic attendance and glycemic control. Study of contrasting groups of patients with IDDM. Diabetes Care 1991; 14:599–601.

96. Graber AS, Davidson P, Brown AW, et al. Dropout and relapse during diabetes care. Diabetes Care 1992; 15:1477–1483.

97. Jacobson AM, Hauser ST, Willett J, et al. Consequences of irregular versus continuous medical follow-up in children and adolescents with insulin-dependent diabetes mellitus. J Pediatr 1997; 131:727–733.

98. Laffel L, Brackett J, Ho J, et al. Changing the process of diabetes care improves metabolic outcomes and reduces hospitalizations. Qual Manag Health Care 1998; 6:53–62.

99. Svoren B, Butler D, Levine B, et al. Reducing acute adverse outcomes in youths with type 1 diabetes: a randomized, controlled trial. Pediatrics 2003; 112:914–922.

100. Anderson BJ, Brackett j, Ho J, et al. An office based intervention to maintain parent-adolescent teamwork in diabetes management: impact on parent involvement, family conflict, and subsequent glycemic control. Diabetes Care 1999; 22:713–721.

101. Laffel LM, Vangsness L, Connell A, et al. Impact of ambulatory, family-focused teamwork intervention on glycemic control in youth with type 1 diabetes. J Pediatr 2003; 142:409–416.
102. Butler DA, Volkening LK, Milaszewski K, et al. Family-focused teamwork intervention for youth with Type 1 diabetes (T1DM) positively impacts A1c and quality of life (QoL): results of a 2-year randomized controlled trial. Diabetes 2006; 55:A421.
103. Kovacs M, Goldston D, Obrosky DS, et al. Psychiatric disorders in youths with IDDM: Rates and risk factors. Diabetes Care 1997; 20:36–44.
104. Kovacs M, Obrosky DS, Goldston D, et al. Major depressive disorder in youths with IDDM: a controlled prospective study of course and outcome Diabetes Care 1997; 20:45–51.
105. Northam EA, Matthews LK, Anderson PJ, et al. Psychiatric morbidity and health outcomes in type 1 diabetes—perspectives from a prospective longitudinal study. Diabet Med 2005; 22:152–157.
106. Blanz B, Rensch-Riemann B, Frotz-Sigmunc D, et al. IDDM is a risk factor for adolescent psychiatric disorders. Diabetes Care 1993; 16:1579–1587.
107. Jacobson AM, Hauser ST, Willett JB, et al. Psychological adjustment to IDDM: 10-year follow-up of an onset cohort of child and adolescent patients. Diabetes Care 1997; 20; 811–818.
108. Bryden KS, Peveler RC, Stein A, et al. Clinical and psychological course of diabetes from adolescence to young adulthood: a longitudinal cohort study. Diabetes Care 2001; 24:1536–1540.
109. Gray M, Whittemore R, Tamborlane W. Depression in type 1 diabetes in children: natural history and correlates. J Psychosom Res 2002, 53:907–911.
110. The SEARCH for Diabetes in Youth Study Group. SEARCH for diabetes in youth: a multi-center study of the prevalence, incidence and classification of diabetes mellitus in youth. Control Clin Trials 2004; 25:458–471.
111. Lawrence JM, Standiford DA, Loots B, et al. Prevalence and correlates of depressed mood among youth with diabetes: the SEARCH for Diabetes in Youth Study. Pediatrics 2006; 117:1348–1358.
112. Dantzer C, Swendsen J, Maruice-Tison S, et al. Anxiety and depression in juvenile diabetes: a critical review. Clin Psychol Rev 2003; 23:787–800.
113. Hassan K, Loar R, Anderson BJ, et al. The role of socioeconomic status, depression, quality of life, and glycemic control in type 1 diabetes mellitus. J Pediatr 2006; 149: 526–531.
114. Lernmark B, Persson B, Fisher L, et al. Symptoms of depression are important to psychological adaptation and metabolic control in children with diabetes mellitus. Diabet Med 1999; 16:14–22.
115. Rewers A, Chase HP, Mackenzie T, et al. Predictors of acute complications in children with type 1 diabetes. JAMA 2002; 287:2511–2518.
116. Stewart SM, Emslie GJ, Klein D, et al. Depressive symptoms predict hospitalization for adolescents with type 1 diabetes mellitus. Pediatrics 2005; 115:1315–1319.
117. Diabetes Control and Complications Trial Research Group. The effect of intensive diabetes treatment on the development and progression of long-term complications in insulin-dependent diabetes mellitus. N Engl J Med 1993; 329:977–998.
118. Jones JM, Lawson ML, Daneman D, et al. Eating disorders in adolescent females with and without type 1 diabetes: cross sectional study. BMJ 2000; 320:1563–1566.
119. Steel JM, Young RJ, Lloyd GC, et al. Abnormal eating attitude in young insulin-dependent diabetics. Br J Psychiatry 1989; 155:515–521.
120. Rydall AC, Rodin GM, Osmsted MP, et al. Disordered eating behavior and micro-vascular complications in young women with insulin-dependent diabetes mellitus. N Engl J Med 1997; 336:1849–1854.
121. Goldston DB, Kelley AE, Reboussin DM, et al. Suicidal ideation and behavior and noncompliance with the medical regimen among diabetic adolescents. J Am Acad Child Adolesc Psychiatry 1997; 36:1528–1536.
122. Leonard BJ, Jang YP, Savik K, et al. Psychosocial factors associated with levels of metabolic control in youth with Type 1 diabetes. J Pediatr Nurs 2002; 7:28–37.

123. Wysocki T, Hough BS, Ward KM, et al. Diabetes mellitus in the transition to adulthood: adjustment, self-care, and health status. J Dev Behav Pediatr 1992; 13:194–201.
124. Bryden KS, Peveler RC, Stein A, et al. Clinical and psychological course of diabetes from adolescence to young adulthood. Diabetes Care 2001; 24:1536–1540.
125. Cameron FJ, Northam EA. Childhood precursors of adolescent outcomes in type 1 diabetes mellitus. J Pediatr Endocrinol Metab 2005; 18:223–234.

Index